Frederick Guttmann R.

While every precaution has been taken in the preparation of this book, the publisher assumes no responsibility for errors or omissions, or for damages resulting from the use of the information contained herein.

C-O-V-I-D, THE BIGGEST CONSPIRACY IN HISTORY

First edition. April 8, 2024.

Copyright © 2024 Frederick Guttmann.

ISBN: 979-8231346516

Written by Frederick Guttmann.

COVID

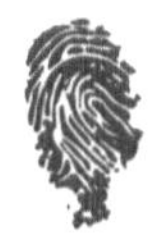

THE BIGGEST CONSPIRACY OF THE HISTORY

Frederick Guttmann Ramirez
COVID, The Biggest Conspiracy in History
Contact: frederickguttmann@gmail.com
Web: www.frederickguttmann.com[1]
487 pages

Cover: Frederick Guttmann and Cristian Aldana
First edition: Cali, Colombia – February/March 2021
Second edition: Tenerife, Spain – August 2021

---

1.   *http://www.frederickguttmann.com*

INDEX

THANKS

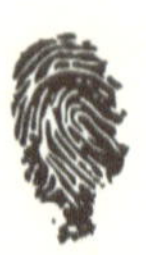

A year and a half ago I began this investigation after connecting the dots of deeply suspicious aspects regarding this epidemic that was said to have attacked a large part of humanity, leading to a prolonged confinement in almost all countries. I cannot even remotely take credit for this arduous work of study, analysis and data collection. It is the first time in my more than 12 years as a writer that I have had the collaboration of a thesis and agglomeration of documentation with the help of many people, especially friends and students.

I owe much of this compilation and discovery to the tireless work of a Colombian friend, José Omar Osorio. He has lived in England for many years, and I know him personally because we met several times on the island of Tenerife, where we were both also living. José has always had a great hunger for knowledge and has dedicated himself to seeking the truth and sharing it despite the ridicule he received and seeing himself alone in his understanding of the Truth. Courage, friend, your work has not been in vain and you will soon see the fruit of your sacrifice and effort!

My sister Kersten, who works in the world of the health system, and is a strong opponent of vaccination, has provided me with many data and reports, as well as her own comments on the plot that is developing from the elite, especially from the US. .USA, where she resides. In fact, I had been aware for a long time of what was said about the dangers of vaccines, but it was not until the wave of global "covid" propaganda that I saw why Kersten was so passionate about the issue. I also want to thank my friend and partner in the Neo Eden project, Jean Paul Luna, with whom I share in the city of Cali (Colombia), who has provided me with very valuable information regarding the Deep State. And of course, to Razedick Bertrand, from Honduras, who has bravely resisted for at least 7 years, enduring ridicule, criticism and disapproval since we began developing interviews for the Stereo Amor radio station in Tegucigalpa. It is thanks to him that much of my work has been able to be distributed throughout the world, especially Spanish-speaking, and through whom a revival has been fostered in many people of the Honduran people regarding the Truth.

Likewise, I want to dedicate a few letters to a great friend, who, although I did not have the pleasure of meeting in person, was a faithful student and companion from a distance from Argentina. Victim of the great plot against humanity and the framework of deception by the elites that we are experiencing, Víctor Manuel, followed my work for many years. He promoted the Truth with his acquaintances and created a beautiful group that is now the source of great work done to promote the Truth. His students and former partner remember him not only for the great person he was in this incarnation but for the mission he carried out and the seed he left on the ground that has borne great fruit. From here we all thank you and wish you a transition to your next place of work where the Holy Spirit takes you with you.

Since the beginning of 2020, ProjectMagen members have been sharing information that, thanks to social networks, has been aired and reached a large number of groups and individuals. And collecting the necessary information, collecting from everywhere, I have put together this work. Given the extensive volume of material, I have asked for help in compiling data and transcribing many contents that were in audio and video. However, I have had to remove much of the material and simply leave links to the content, due to the extensive content. In that order of things I want to thank the participation of Daniel Martínez, a great friend, financial support and partner of the Neo Eden kibbutz project (eco villages that we are promoting in Colombia), a Colombian resident in Valencia (Spain), as well as Jessica Valladares from Honduras, Ruth López from Venezuela, Andri García from Mexico - a student who has been with me for more than 8 years -, Laady Pedraza from the USA, Karime Rojas from Australia, and also Carl Ulises from the USA. These Students collaborated with me with many transcriptions. I also thank my great English friend Graham Hodgkinson, thanks to whose support I was able to focus for almost half a year on my work without distractions to begin my research and bombardment of information.

Before embarking on this last stage of my life, I went through a tribulation where I could count on the support – in most cases from a distance – of my mother (Meeky), Razedick, Javier Asuar, Laura Gómez, Ruth López , from Graham, from Daniel Martínez and from my great friend of 20 years of acquaintance, Abiam Francisco Palomares, another great researcher and colleague from the Canary Islands, with whom I founded the EnergyAngels youth urban dance association. Thanks to David - yoga and reiki teacher - neighbor of the town where I lived for a while in Candelaria (beautiful place in Tenerife on the beach) , a deeply spiritual man with a great inner light, a true teacher, who was placed by the angels in the place and time it should be. His words and intervention at the right time loosened the moorings for my new life to take off. And thank you to the most fabulous and positive angel I have ever known in this incarnation at this time, Judit Besay, my daughter in this life, who has given me encouragement, hope, light, love and strength, especially when I have needed it most.

I also wish to send a lot of light to those who have received me since I left Tenerife, Spain. Thank you to those who have not had a "muzzle" while I have "threshed" (1st Cor. 9,9; 1st Tim. 5,18) and prepared the ground for the subsistence of those of us who have to resist what is coming to the world in these years , like Daniel Martínez and his cousin and former officer of mine at the 'Almirante Cristóbal Colón' Naval Academy, Hamber Martínez, Marcela and Captain Juan Carlos Torres, as well as the collaboration of his cousin Diego, who received me in Valencia for 3 weeks and where we begin the following preparations for the Neo Eden project. To Javier Asuar, an Argentine colleague of mine in Energy Angels, when we were professionally dedicated to BreakDance, who with Sandra - his partner - invited me to Santiago de Compostela. To Laura Gómez, a friend of almost 15 years who also welcomed me in Barcelona, and whom I appreciate and admire very much, and to her mother, Ino Lorente, and her sister, Elena. I had the pleasure of meeting his father, who made his transition a year ago. May the Light guide you. Likewise, to my sister Kersten and her fabulous chicks who welcomed me in Florida, USA, and to my aunt Valby. There are also Judit Fagerlund and my disciplined student Joel García, who welcomed me in Santo Domingo, Dominican Republic, a country of beautiful beaches.

Thanks also to Ricardo Martínez and Manuel Ignacio and their family, who received me in Neiva, Colombia, to begin the study of the implementation of the Neo Eden project, as well as to Paola – Daniel's mother – and his sister Marta. Thanks to my parents (Félix and Meeky) and my brother Erwin and his wife Sandra, who have received me in Cali, and the support of Jean Paul, Juanito, David "Oso" Albarracín and Gissele, Jefferson and Jhonny Casañas in Cali, as well as well as Rodrigo León and his sister Carolina, and Mauro, thanks to whom we studied a wing of the project not far from Bogotá. And of course, infinite thanks to all the Hondurans who welcomed me there. The words fall short. To the whole family - and Stereo Amor team - from Razedick Bertrand, to Klarissa, Ericka, Pamela Ypsilanti, Deymi, Jefrey Ortiz, Leticia Valladares, Daysi, Lorena Valladares, Mildred, Enrique Hernández, Nestor and Gabriela Vega, Heydi Vega, Heydi Tosta, Edgardo, Edinson Bonilla, Héctor Barnica, Tony Pineda, Alan, Claude Cardona, Claudia Fiallos, Michelle Bertrand, Mirian Olivera, Daniel Funes, Christian Alexander, Astrid O'Connor and Adolfo. It was a unique and beautiful welcome, and a human warmth and trust that I had never received. A huge hug.

Lastly, and not least, I want to thank the financial support that has been a pillar so that I can dedicate myself to this titanic work, those who have bought my books, have tithed me, have offered me or collaborated financially in other areas, such as trips, PCR tests required at airports, transportation, accommodation, diets, etc., on these last trips. It is the work of Truth, which in this time brings strong struggles of all kinds and which have forged my character, they have given me an experience that I would not have received otherwise and the maturity and awareness necessary to prepare myself and many for the which could be considered the most terrible decade that humanity on this globe will ever know. My family, as well as those who supported from Valencia and Honduras were a cornerstone in paying for the tickets from one country to another. May they be as prosperous and blessed as they have enriched my life, supports like Daniel Martínez, Jordi - honest conspiracy theorist who, although he is a crazy Dutchman who will not even know that he is being used by the Holy Spirit, "will have a prophet's reward" (Matthew 10,41) - Celina Quiriarte from Mexico, who for years supported the cause despite her own family difficulties, and to my students who were in 2020 trusting in my personal virtual advice: Ricardo Sabogal from New Jersey, Angelina Rodríguez from Texas, and Esther from Tegucigalpa, Honduras. Thank you for your financial support because in addition to the fact that "the worker is worthy of his salary" (Luke 10:7), he is also worthy of being honored for his service and dedication.

Thank you for having the courage to read this and share it with others. Thank you for contributing to this cause, since part of the proceeds from the sale of this manuscript will finance our 'Neo Eden' eco-village project. And without further ado, let's get started...

INTRODUCTION

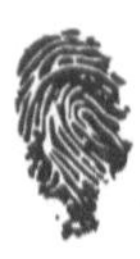

In December 2019, the world's news broadcasts reported alarming news: a new disease seemed to have appeared in Asia, killing several people. In a few weeks the supposed virus was said to have spread and begun to infect people on the European continent. In less than two months the spread across the planet was a fact. But hey, some things didn't add up.

Information had begun to spread about 5G antenna installations around which dead birds were seen - and recently horses were affected in Europe - where cases of this new virus that was said to have come from China began to occur. Two Chinese reporters and a scientist reportedly brought to light in October 2019 that the city of Wuhan had been the first to install 5G antennas and posed a health hazard, causing nausea, headaches, fevers, diarrhea and vomiting. . The three people were arrested by the government and imprisoned for three weeks, after which time they were released and a few days later they died of the "bug." What was happening? The tycoon George Soros had invested 16 billion dollars to pay the world's governments and news media to take control of the planet by an organization called the 'Deep State'.

The truly "powerful" do not have a Facebook profile, nor have you heard that about their names. Or you would have even imagined where they came from and what philosophy they have. I warn you that if you do not have an open mind and are not willing to throw away your previous beliefs to know the Truth, as it is, then this book is not for you. On the contrary, if you want to know what is happening, what is behind it and where it is going to end, this content that you will read will break your mold and it will be impossible for you not to want to be part of the "prophets of our time", who are announcing this new Deep State "gospel" of Truth and its agenda for a draconian New World Order. This manuscript can be the gateway to a unique opportunity, for you and your close ones and contacts, to be part of the Light that is spreading in this time when the Darkness wants to destroy our race and our planet.

I. THE UNDERLYING POWER

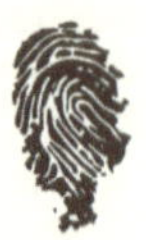

<< Put on the whole armor of God, so that you can stand firm against the wiles of the devil. For we do not fight against flesh and blood,
*but **against the archons, against the authorities, against the masters of the world of darkness of this age, against spirits of iniquity in the heights of heaven**. Therefore take up the whole armor of God,*
<u>that you may be able to withstand in the evil day, and having finished all, to stand</u>. >>
(Apostle Paul to the Ephesians, chapter 6:11-13, New Testament, Bible)

To understand a plot you must have information about the context of the events. When a neophyte in serious research comes across something incoherent according to the belief system in which they have been educated, they assume that said information is not "logical." Who or what standard determines that something is, or is not, logical? What is "denialism", or "respirationism"? What is a "conspiracy theory"? Denying a fact like those surrounding contemporary history comes first from cognitive dissonance, and second from fear and helplessness. You don't want to accept that something like this is possible and find yourself unable to change it. But what is a conspiracy theory? An assumption that assumes there is a large scale plot. In effect, however, the use of this appreciation has been deliberately distorted at a social level to give it a mocking or discrediting tone. In truth, all known history has been developed with conspiracies, but the mind wants to deny the seriousness of current events and the magnitude of what it would imply for these conspiracy "theories" to be true.

I have observed how in less than 2 years a large part of the people who were skeptical of what I warned them about have changed their attitude towards me. Those who laughed are no longer seen. The amount of information collected gives a certain security to say uncomfortable things, because you know that one day critics will thank you for the courage you had in saying things even at the risk of being labeled and belittled. Accustomed to ridicule and criticism, I will not beat around the bush to openly explain to you what is happening - if you do not know it, or if you do know it, if you do not know the whole story -, and it will be the reader's judgment on himself to ridicule my words or give rise to your intuition and objective reasoning. Since I can remember I have been passionate about literature and I have read so many books of all types of genres that I have lost count. Various subjects caught my attention powerfully. Such is the case of ancient history and the mysteries of the universe. I found since I was a teenager in my readings that there was what Carl G. Jung would call "archetypes", in ancient people – and even in current iconography – a fixation with certain elements of nature, which, of a symbolic nature, were mostly present in its cultural aspects. Among this iconography were animals, and among the animals, reptiles always stood out, in order of seniority. These were symbols of wisdom, mostly the archetype of the serpent and the dragon (which in cases are exactly the same). Do you know about the Mayan or Aztec culture? Then you will have heard of its main deity: Quetzalcoatl (Kulkulkan), the feathered serpent.

The Bible - which is nothing more than a brief library of Jewish literature - describes the first zoomorphic being as a

Nachash, or copper serpent. Greek mythology speaks of the first supernatural beings called Giants, who were half anthropomorphic and half reptiles. The Egyptians described the first creator gods as reptiles and amphibians. The Amerindians also had creator gods with a reptilian appearance. In distant Asia the main gods had a pantheon of supernatural dragons, capable of creating, speaking and thinking – and even flying. These dragons were a form of intelligent deity, and they were not the only ones: Nu-Güa, one of the creator goddesses of humanity, according to Chinese tradition, was half anthropomorphic and half dragon. In Australia, the aborigines relate that in the time of Los Sueños, before there were settlers in that region, there were gods who came from heaven who represented two reptilian races that fought over the expanses of Australia with their flying chariots, attacking each other with weapons so powerful that they turned the green island in a gigantic desert. These types of descriptions appear extensively in the mythology of North America, Mongolia, Africa, Turkey... everywhere. In fact, the oldest Sumerian tablets ever found say that before the Earth was populated by gods or men, "reptiles had descended from heaven."

If it weren't disconcerting enough, emerald tablets found in the Yucatan describe thousands of years ago how the leaders of the islands of Atlantis were subverted by anthropomorphic reptiles from the underworld that were not exactly the same physical material as human bodies. The description seems to denote numinous or incorporeal creatures that only masters could discover using mystical powers. This seems far-fetched if it is not compared with engravings, figures, descriptions, materials and other strange evidence that have become known to the world and of which I speak at length in my saga, 'The Sakla Rebellion' (4 books on comparative mythology and censored archeology and paleontology). The Hopi Indians of Arizona tell a fascinating story that coincides with that of other remote cultures, where they describe that zoomorphic, snake-like beings came to our planet thousands of years ago and settled in caves under the surface, and that at one time they arrived the precursor races of the human being, beings "from the stars", and there was a bloody thermonuclear combat between both races, which devastated Mongolia, the Sahara and other regions that were forested, turning them into deserts until the present. There are accounts of this in the mythical Hindu Mahabharatha, and physical evidence of radiation in the destroyed cities that were found in Pakistan, mentioned in the "myth."

Yes, this type of story would seem like a tribal legend if it weren't for the fact that it coincides with the same thing that Hindus say. In the remote Vedanta culture, the race of the Nagas is described, the anthropomorphic reptiles that live underground on our planet. It is enough to see the linguistic relationship of the Sanskrit Nagas with the Hebrew Najash (serpent), which is the way in which the Hebrew myth refers to the "demon" who tempted the couple in the garden of Eden. In ufology the presence of reptilians is patent, and comes to life outside of science fiction when compared with testimonies of military officers, testimonies of secret service agents and classified documents regarding government investigations called Black Ops. Why would they all agree to invent something like that? If they are telling the truth, the real existence of reptilians became public knowledge thanks to the courage of these people in important positions in places like the US. It was known that there have been secret government agreements with various races from other worlds since 1954, since when Russia and England have also had them. It is even argued that the Israeli government would also have been in contact with alien races at the present time. The Germans had already had these contacts before and during WWII. I do not expect you to believe me because I say it, I intend to say things as I have recorded them, because a wise man said, <<you will know the truth and the truth will set you free>>.

It is extremely important that things are understood without reservations or fears, because time proves right to those who have it. I do not say this from arrogance, ego or pride but with all good intentions. One day all this will be public knowledge and it will stop being a "paranoid fantasy." In my work 'Wandering Stars, the History of the UFO Phenomenon' (2010) I collect an overwhelming amount of reports, documents, testimonies and evidence in general of the presence of extraterrestrial entities and pan-dimensional beings on Earth. The cases of people who report having been abducted by non-human entities are so large that governments such as the US and the United Kingdom dedicated research groups between the 60s and 90s to concisely evaluate the phenomenon. Many of these "abductors" were reptilians. Testimonies from people who worked in Black Ops (covert operations) describe in detail these individuals and their unpleasant presence operating in underground facilities in the US, specifically in the main one of ambivalent use (terrestrial and draconian), 'Dulce', located on Archuleta Mesa on the border between Colorado and New Mexico. The US would have been working with at least 4 races out of 60 that they are aware of that would have been coming to our world, and one of them is the Lacerta. They are the ones the apostle Paul spoke of, calling them "the authorities" and the "archons."

According to ufology and whistleblowers who have worked in secret operations, the lacerta are part of a reptilian race originating from the Thuban system (Alpha type), in the constellation of the Dragon (Draco), also known as Alfasirians. .

In my research on this matter, and which I address in 'The Sakla Rebellion', I mostly explain the relationship of all these themes with the Bible and Gnostic texts, to make it clear once and for all that it is not a conspiratorial or conspiratorial assumption. boring people who want to create ridiculous novels or new trends. That's what the Deep State wants you to believe. The fact of removing this from ridicule is crucial to understanding what we are talking about and how all this leads us to the Truth of what is happening in the world, and as I have said, it is irrelevant whether from the reader's angle I am ridiculed or vilified. for exposing these facts without taboos or shame. The Truth will prevail and come to light because <<there is nothing hidden that remains unrevealed, nor anything secret that will not be made known>> (Ihoshua, aka 'Jesus'). But you can delve deeper into this subject by reading RA Boulay's research work, 'Flying Snakes and Dragons, The History of the Human Reptilian Past' (2003), which addresses many complementary areas to the summary that I gave you in the introduction of this book. You will begin to understand what the apostle Paul meant when he said that our fight is against beings of darkness that come from the "high heavens", from regions light years from Earth.

A fight that is not against "flesh" or "blood"? This means that, on the one hand, our true potential enemies are not primarily on this planet, and on the other hand, that these entities do not belong, in essence, to the matter or corporeality that we know. In the film 'Monsters, Inc.' (Monsters SA, by Pixar & Disney, 2001), the energy of human beings is absorbed by entities that are "on the other side", in a parallel dimension or plane. These "monsters" prefer the energy of children, which is more powerful than that of adults, but the predilection is over fear (which produces the expensive adrenochrome). They show that laughter is much stronger in energy, but the hidden message must be fully understood. Fear, sadness, suffering, food offerings, murder, war, sexual pleasure and torture have been an elixir for these "entities", called jinn by the Arabs, tzitzimime by the Aztecs, shed or siir by the Hebrews, daimon by the Greeks, druj by the Celts, asura by the Vedanta or Hindus, gallu by the Sumerians, hatayw by the Egyptians or yaoguay by the Chinese.

There are many categories of these beings (see 'The Sakla Rebellion III, The Fallen'), but my point with this parenthesis is that it was not out of madness or boredom that so many cultures had - even in many parts of our present - a fixation obsessive and compulsive to carry out horrendous actions to receive favors from their "gods". It is necessary to be clear that these "gods" were not the ones who demanded these offerings, rituals, sacrifices and holocausts, but the Shedu (siirím, lilitu, rujim, ruchot ha-temaa), so mentioned in Semitic and Akkadian folklore that later became evoked in texts from the Old Testament, or Tanak. Sadly, these customs remain, and these psychopathic aberrations are carried out in satanic rites, in secret societies, in the high levels of Freemasonry, in the hermetic orders to which the richest and most powerful people on this globe belong.

If it says that the draconians have tried to control various races for thousands of years in this part of the Milky Way, and many of their lackeys and servants are entities from the planes of error, that is, thought-forms, disembodied souls and daemons (shedu, druj, jinn, demons), quite a few of which were created in the image and likeness of their masters. It is not trivial that the people of our past spoke of them and the Bible describes them as 'the ancient serpent', 'leviathan', 'the dragon', 'devil' or 'satan', who must return for the Final Battle, at Har-Megiddo (Armageddon). Logically, this will displease Christians, Catholics and many other religious groups who want to see things from a "gassy", "romantic", "legalistic" and "sensationalist" perspective. According to the biblical book of Revelation, the Ancient Serpent, called the Dragon (the Balaur of Romanian mythology), has "seven heads", as described in Gnostic texts (circa 2nd-3rd century AD). In the Sumerian Enuma-Elish, or account of the creation of our solar system, it speaks of the reptilians facing the gods in a pitched battle when our planet was still in full geological formation. These gods would have defeated the reptilians, and just as can be seen from Mayan stories, Gnostic texts or the Orphic stories of Ancient Greece, among others, the reptilians would then have been thrown to the bottom of the Earth.

A group of draconians would have been forced underground, but they would not remain idly by. The inhabitants of the neighborhood of Cairo (Egypt), called Mary's Tree, where work on the city's subway began, report that when these facilities were in the process of being drilled, the workers saw humans with tails walking at the end of the tunnels - where no one was supposed to be (apart from because they were the only ones in the place, and at that depth) -, and that the president of the country was aware of it. It was also known that it had been discovered that effectively 100 meters below Cairo there was a metropolis of anthropomorphic beings with tails and reptilian appearance. In California, an underground reptilian city was discovered on January 29, 1934 - as reported by the Los Angeles Time - just below Hollywood. The same with caves in Cappadocia, Turkey, whose legends attribute to humanoid reptiloids. The American Indians were also no strangers to these stories and the existence of these caves. If this is not enough to make you think, you should check your ability to keep an open mind: for the Hopi Indians of Arizona, reptilians exist and have been living in underground galleries under the USA for thousands of years.

What do the lacerta want? Domination. According to ufology, the draconians appeared millions of years ago in the Draco constellation (in the Alpha Draconis star system) and at that time they were the most technologically advanced in the entire galaxy. As the Gnostic texts relate, they believed that they were the only ones in existence and considered themselves animisms "God", sovereign and the pure royal race (note the correlation with the biblical passage of the prophet Ezekiel, chapter 28). When they learned of the existence of humans (in a system in the Lyra constellation), they went there and massacred them, destroying 3 planets populated by our most remote ancestors. The massacre was so unexpected, brutal, and unique in the peaceful history of the Milky Way that a Confederation of Worlds was created to discuss the problem and evaluate solutions. The Draconians wanted total domination of the galaxy and had the greatest technology possible to achieve it: time travel and hyperspace jumps. They became obsessed with genetic engineering and attacked Orion. The inhabitants there resisted them for 5,000 years. Finally, Orion would have fallen to the Draconians, even though they were the numerical majority, given that the Draconians would be using time travel to frustrate all the Orionite battles. Orion, however, would become a lackey of the draconians. The Draconians would use genetic engineering to modify the structure and bodies of the Orionites and all other victims who fell to their empire.

With these three weapons (time travel, jumps to hyperspace and genetic engineering) the reptilians became masters and lords of the Orion Arm. Powerless, the Confederacy asked for help from the Andromeda galaxy alliance, a call first attended to by the Zenetaen race. According to information received by channeling groups of extraterrestrial entities, the Milky Way received support from the future and from another universe, the Source Universe, from which this universe was produced. There, at that time, the fight between "good and evil" began, and is the origin of the appearance of biblical stories such as the arrival of the deity Jehovah and the archangels Gabriel or Michael. I know this sounds like science fiction, but I have corroborated this information throughout more than 10 years of research, and this has been consistent with classified information and the testimonies of people in high positions and ranks in the field of politics, military forces, intelligence and clandestine investigations. I myself was skeptical of all this and even made fun of those who spoke of reptilians. I had to eat my words when I started to investigate the matter and "connect the dots". The information was overwhelming and there was no room for doubt. The Satan of the monotheistic religion was a psychological appreciation relative to the ego of each conscious being, and in the phenomenal field he was personified by an alliance of anthropomorphic reptiles from another dimension located in the direction of the terrestrial polar north.

Or what do you think demons are? Not all, as I explain in 'The Sakla Rebellion III, The Fallen', but many of them are precisely the draconians. In ancient descriptions such as the Emerald Tablets of Thoth, The Gospel of Valentinus, the works of Nag Hammadi, the Ars Goetia or the Testament of Solomon, it is seen that the appearance of these main demons, or arch-demons, is reptilian, "spirits." " of ophidic and draconic appearance. The same can be seen by reviewing books on witchcraft, spells, astrology, demonology and Satanism. If you want to understand the legends of Romanian vampires and dragons, here it is. It is said that the supremacy of the draconians was mocked when there were casualties in their own ranks, among the highest positions. In this way, Confederate espionage gained ground and the confrontations began to become even. However, the war is not over. The Orionites became the area most faced with this problem. Conflicts in Orion persist. They came to Earth in the past and brought genetically altered soldiers, whose height was over 2.50 m tall. Their mission was to establish a monarchy on our planet and subdue humans, who would see these individuals as gods and obey them. This is the "blue blood". The ancient lacerta were already here, but there were other "fallen" ones when these giants came, who chose human women to be the wombs of their offspring.

Many famous characters from prehistory emerged from this hybrid race, such as the semi-god heroes of mythology or emperors. This persisted until today, being the origin of royal families, especially in Europe. That is the aristocracy that calls itself the Illuminati, many of whom are said to be Jews, but as the apostle Paul noted, "they came out from among us, but they are not of us," and they called them Jesus and John the Baptist, " serpents, generation of vipers," who "call themselves Jews, but they are not." This is the great secret that the royal castes hide, and that has also been discovered on numerous occasions through letters from themselves, where they confess it: they are a Nephilim lineage (since Illuminati is not 'enlightened' in Latin, but in fact It means in the Semitic language "the descendants of the Ilu", and Ilu was the name of the Anunnaki/Nephilim). It is stated that on several occasions these draconian beings were expelled from our world, as reported in texts such as the Bible, but there is one event that is consistent with the topic in question that concerns us: the Return of the Dragon. The apostle John says that <<the dragon was cast down to the Earth>>, addressing a future prophecy, not a past one.

By falling to our planet he would side with the Global Government, called in the Bible 'Thirion' (beast, creature, wild animal, monster) and Belial, whom the Arabs know as Dajjal, the Jews as Armilius and the Christians like the Antichrist. The return of the draconians is also described in texts from the Egyptian Library of Nag Hammadi and in the Scandinavian Völuspá. The Völuspá is the prosaic Viking Age that tells the story of the final battle between good and evil, or Ragnarök or Gottendamerung (the biblical Armageddon). There the ancient serpent (Jörmungandr), who since its creation has wanted to devour the Tree of Life (the Yggdrasil), confronts Thor, and both fall in battle.

The death of almost all the gods and demons (reptiloids from another dimension) would reflect the involvement of various non-human races, starting with the coalition of several feuding races of gods. These gods are largely extraterrestrials from other dimensions and planets, as described in detail in the work Oahspe, from 1882. Already in the mid-70s of the 20th century, great researchers such as the Swiss Erich von Däniken presented it in works such as as 'Chariots of the Gods', or Zecharia Sitchin later in works such as 'The Twelfth Planet'. Since then the literature on the aforementioned has been widely extensive and well documented, even in the Bible: <<the kingdom of heaven suffers violence and the violent shake it.>> (Gospel of Matthew, chapter 11,12) If not You've seen an episode of the series 'Ancient Aliens' (from the History Channel), think again. They may sound bigoted, but much of what they say is actually documented in military reports.

The proto-Hebrew prophet Enoch had already spoken of this reptilian empire, being the first to define its two parties: Leviathan and Behemoth. The various stories say that in the battle for the sovereignty of our solar system thousands of years ago, the Lacerta empire that wanted to dominate here faced a coalition of Light on the part of the Confederacy, and after a crushing defeat, a part of the draconians was forced to flee, known since then as 'Fugitive Serpent Leviathan' (the Dragon Leviathan), and the other fled to the depths of the Earth, to hide in dungeons, and was called 'Tortuous Serpent Leviathan' (the Behemoth Dragon). This story is described in detail in Vedanta (Indian) literature, when you read where Brahma (the Hindu Jehovah) defeats Vala (Satan) by dividing him into two: Rahu and Katu (Rahab/Behemoth and Leviathan). According to rabbinic eschatology, Leviathan must return at the end of time and attempt to procreate – figuratively speaking – with Behemoth, who is under the hills of the planet, and if they unite they will bring the world to destruction. According to this Jewish legend, Behemoth and Leviathan were separated by the Most High god in prehistory before they procreated, because if they had done so, it would have meant the destruction of the world. But now he will let them unite again, and at the height of his power the Almighty will fall with his arm upon them and destroy them in the battle of Gog Magog, and the bodies of these dragons will lie on the surface for years, as a testimony to all. nations for generations to come.

Meanwhile, the Behemoth - or 'the Beast' - operates from "below", and the Leviathan, from "above". They have not yet been allowed to unite, but Revelation speaks of that for 3 and a half years they will be working together on our globe, and at the end of this time the Lord (the Confederacy) will come upon them with all his power, and they will be destroyed. This is commented on in various prophecies, one of them revealing that "God" also has powers that serve him, and that they come from a world that is located at great distances in the galaxy: <<They come from a distant Earth, from the last of the heavens, Yahweh and the

instruments of his indignation...>> (Isaiah 13:5, RVA 60) We can also observe the description of these events in the Sibylline Oracles of ancient Greece, but I will now move on to the next point of this explanation without further detours, and I leave the rest of the research work on this matter to you.

I must add that according to military and contact sources, ET the Dragon (the Ancient Serpent) uses technology as its main, favorite and efficient weapon, and thus has been subduing hundreds of races for millions of years. It is argued that planet Earth was chosen long ago as a paradise of experimentation and experience for millions of souls developing in our galaxy. The anthropomorphic dragons have therefore wanted to subjugate us using their advances and scientific development. They would have implemented another technology that they learned over time: psychic. They understood that it is possible to use energy fields, waves and magnetism that propagate through space. It is the same effect that religion might attribute to the power of prayer and fasting, or in what is called faith, the Law of Attraction, or the various types of use of meditation or focusing. Ufology states that reptilians (alphadraconians) cannot create with their minds, humans can. They know it, and that makes them afraid of us, which is why, among other things, they prevent our race from knowing that mystery: that we **are creators, and our potential lies in our mind, in the power of our thoughts-ideas, emotions-feelings. and belief system-convictions** .

They, however, would know how to use psychic technology to intervene on the psyche from anywhere at a distance. This is more complex than the other technological systems they have, but they have been used especially for sabotage on human beings who pose a threat to their sovereignty. It should be noted that the use of this psychic technology is ineffective against the technology of the Plejaren, the Pleiadian race. Now I'll tell you about the good ones.

As I have learned from multiple military and contact reports, when the wars in the Lyra star system began, the so-called Galactic Confederation created a research group and other defense groups to protect the galaxy from the Dragon threat. In Gnostic culture this Dragon is personified as Sakla, Ialdabaot or Jaldabaoz (the Jah-Bul-On of Freemasonry), in Judaism it is called Samael, but on a general or collective level it is called the Devil or Satan. It must be clarified that Satan is a cultural and folkloric idea that was used to refer to what we, after the psychology works of Jung and Freud, call the 'Ich' (the ego), but since we speak in parameters of duality, the antagonistic of good is generalized as Satan, or Ahriman (as Zoroaster defined him). Although, this is not Lucifer (Luzbel), Baphomet, Beelzebub (Baal-Zebub), Iblis or Mastema. I speak at length about him in 'The Rebellion of Sakla II, The Serpent', whoever he is appears as an individual, a character, not a group, but he falls into the category of personification of the ego, that is, of what he is. collectively understood as a concept or idea of Satan or Devil.

That said, the issue must be taken to the opposite side of the scale. Just as the Dragon is said to have 7 hierarchs or gods of the lacerta, so 7 princes from another universe would have been chosen to serve the Light. Groups from Andromeda, Aldebaran, Arthur and the Pleiades were the main ones to participate in helping the victims of draconian tyranny. They represent the army of Light, and are also consciousnesses of other dimensions. Some of the Draconians and Pleiadians are beings of matter that we know and dwell on planets as we understand them. However, most are of higher dimensions, and usually live in motherships several kilometers in diameter not made of baryonic matter, some come from the future and others from a universe prior to and superior to this one. All this information includes former military personnel, former secret service officers, classified documents and people who claim to have had contact with this type of alien intelligence.

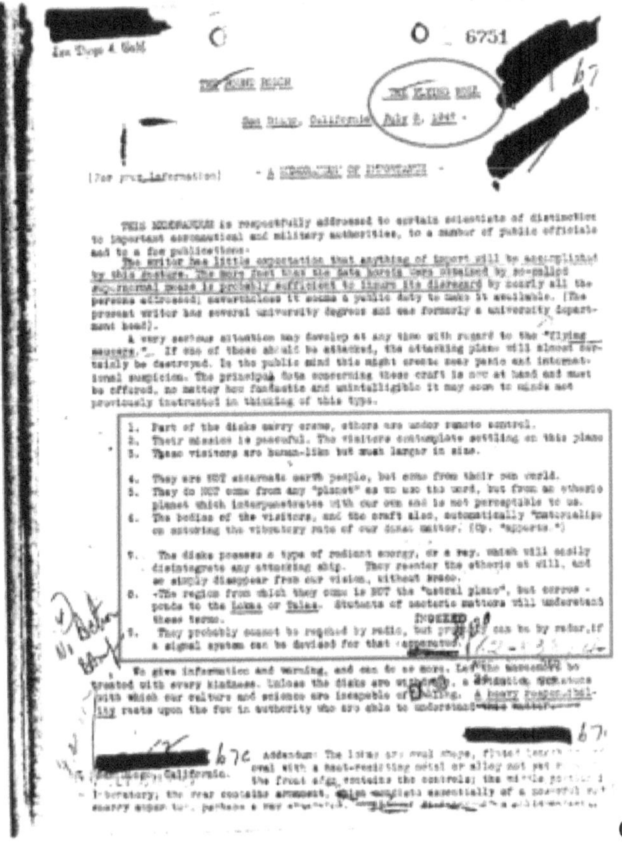

On the next page you can see an FBI document from July 8, 1947, where this intelligence agency already had knowledge of the existence of these pan-dimensional entities, their nature, their ships, their origin and their intentions. This is just a mere example of the large number of records that exist on this matter, and which, for obvious reasons of space and capacity, I cannot add to the volume of this work.

Unlike the draconians, the beings of light belong to much higher dimensional planes, some of them inhabiting etheric worlds whose diameter sometimes far exceeds the volume of several star systems combined. These worlds are not visible because they belong to Dark Matter and their potential is Dark Energy, as current science would call it. In terminology, they are not "dark" because of something bad but because they are not visible, and some of the places where they dwell are timeless vortices from which they do their work in consciousnesses/ civilizations like ours. Etheric worlds of this type have a hexagonal shape, as described in the work Oahspe (1882), but, as I say, not all beings of "light" are from etheric worlds (and by "light" I do not mean to be "lightbulb beings"... I speak figuratively). There are non-material substances between the baryon and etheric atomic structure, which I call "psychic matter", which is divided into 3 groups, one of which is visible, and is what nebulae and quasars are made of. However, many beings of light, which some call good extraterrestrials, are what religion called "angels", although not all of these << ministering spirits>> are angels, in the sense of the use of the term (Greek 'aggelou ': emissary, herald or messenger) nor in the transcendent sense of the term. Some of them are anthropomorphic, but others are not. However, Fourth Density beings, like them, and higher, have at least two appearances, which change at will. They are metamorphic creatures.

Coinciding with the information kept by the teachers of India, this universe would be composed of 7 dimensions and various planes for each dimension, which are intertwined with all the electromagnetic fields throughout it. This pattern is repeated in other universes, but with some varying cosmic rules. The mineral world belongs to the state of First Density, or first dimension; the plant and animal world constitute the Second;

We are now in the Third, just like the so-called "extraterrestrials" that inhabit physical worlds; The Fourth Density is what the Bible calls the state of "Resurrection" (the Nirvana of Buddhism), but it has nothing to do with Third Density matter, but with a higher wavelength vibration of consciousness, and from there Many of the so-called ascended masters come, angels, Orionites and Draconians, among many; The Fifth Density is that of the so-called "gods"; The Sixth is of the unified consciousnesses and those who have moved away from the duality of the ego projection; The Seventh is the path to the Infinite and the Superior Universe (our origin, since our souls come from those worlds there). The Dragon has servants of Second, Third and Fourth Density, and its "lords" are in Fifth Density. Among the planes of reality are the 'Loka', or kingdoms-heavens-worlds that constitute a hierarchy or multi-level structure where consciousness is experienced (you can see this in Vedanta literature shared by various schools of Hindu thought).

I am fully aware that possibly all this is new for you, and even hard to digest, but believe me when I tell you that without this introduction you will not understand the context of this book and, above all, who you are, what you do. here and where you are going. Have patience and a little faith (trust), because I know well why I am showing you this Star Trek novel that seems to have nothing to do with a supposed virus that attacks humanity.

Now, the structural basis of the planes through which souls travel are 7 essential Loka (heavens-worlds in Sanskrit) that seem to fold into 31 planes of existence. The soul transits through these states until it cuts Samsara (reincarnations) through the transition from Moksha (absence of ego, the gateway to the Fourth Density) to the Buddha state, or Nirvana, Complete Awakening (activation of the body of Fourth Density). Ergo, the

Ancient Serpent also has consciousnesses and thought-forms of parallel planes of Lower Dimensions (called Thalas in Vedanta culture), which are defined as Third Level Spirits in 4 categories, among which are the Impure (demons of high rank) . lower), Light (problematic, known as imps, gnomes, goblins), False Instruction (they do not know the truth, they give misinformation), Neutral and Hitters or Disruptors (they act on matter, like poltergeists). For its part, the state of Sixth Density is out of reach of draconians, as well as the Seventh. They have their adonim (lords) in Fifth Density only because they were created there by the Universal Matrix at the beginning of the Big Bang (but that is extensive to cover here, I recommend parts 2 and 4 of the saga 'The Sakla Rebellion' to understand all this dynamics).

These 7 dimensional states correspond to the 7 bodies that the Adamic consciousnesses possess: Atmic, Budhiko, Causal, Mental, Astral, Vital and Physical, or Buddhic, Etheric, Light, Ectoplasm, physical vehicle, Physical Body Complex, and Chemical . We have these 7, but only the third is activated at this moment (and will be until the moment of what biblical translations have called "Resurrection", or the Awakening/Enlightenment of Buddhism and Taoism), and it is the one we see . Just as the reptilians have lackeys from Planes of Error, the Light has servants from intermediate planes, which are First Level Spirits of 4 categories: Benevolent, Wise, Protectors and Superiors. In the same way there are transcended beings or ascended masters, who having reached the Buddha state of Nirvana operate as Second Level Spirits helping from Fourth Density towards the distortions of that dimension or in the affairs of lower dimensions like ours, in Third. In this sense, I recommend my work 'Transcendencia' (2016) for greater detail.

Several thousand years ago the Ancient Serpent used the children of the Nephilim (the fallen, giants) to oppress terrestrial humanity through submission to the authorities, as is now happening again since 2020: consented dictatorship (the people docilely accept be tyrannized). We can see this even in false democracy, because the Illuminati (the structure that develops from the power of human-draconian monarchies) are the ones who direct the affairs of our planet. You will wonder how it is possible that they are here and have not been expelled by the Confederacy. I recommend the work of Zecharia Sitchin, 'The Wars of Gods and Men' (2007) and that of William Bramley, 'Gods of Eden' (1993). Now you will know. The Draconians essentially use the Orionites for all their movements. While the Earth was in what some cultures call the Shemu-An (gestation) state it was used as a source of mineral resources, but when "sapiens sapiens" avatars were created and brought here from Mars, the Confederacy intervened. There were various political and moral discussions of the Confederation (Milky Way and Andromeda) about management with our planet, since it was determined that at that point there should no longer be intervention. The Sowers, in charge of life processes, had come from Alpha Centauri and Southern Cross (of the Swan constellation) to alkalize our oceans and introduce spores so that biological and multicellular life could begin to develop (see my work 'Creation vs. Evolution ', 2012). Then the Orian Geneticists (Orionites) arrived and created various biological races. The dinosaurs were a draconian experiment on Mars, using their own DNA.

By mentioning Mars I am telling you that until a couple of tens of thousands of years ago that planet was quite active (and NASA has known this for decades). Now, when there were "humans" on Earth, the Confederation prohibited intervention and influence over them. But before that arrival the Alphadraconians sent their emissaries from the Orian monarchy to review the behavior of the homo sapiens. The Orians discovered that humanity was too intelligent and became afraid (they thought we could surpass them and one day take away their dominion). They decided to exterminate entire groups of homo sapiens using climate technology. Thus they extinct the Cro-Magnons and Neanderthals, as well as the first genotypes created in the laboratory: homo erectus (homo ergaster, homo antecessor). They produced a new race at the expense of the previous ones, but this time, of the 12 strands of DNA they possessed, the Orian geneticists removed 10 strands from humanity, leaving them with only 2, thus preventing them from awakening their consciousness and surpassing their creators. For thousands of years man wandered in ignorance like a caveman, without direction or understanding. Regarding this, you can read these details in the 'Epic of Gilgamesh', from Babylonian literature, which coincides with the story of the origin of man from the Kolbrin canon (Celtic and Egyptian ancestral records). This is where the Aztec and Mayan legends about the first men come from. Jehovah then intervened so that the Paa-Tal (our soul race) - who were on their way to incarnate - had a proper bodily vehicle and a lucid mind. Jehovah's team made genetic improvements in Homo Sapiens, highlighting the introduction of the FOX-P2 gene, which allowed them to speak, in addition to other genetic patterns that made man capable of immortality.

I use the name 'Jehovah' because I understand that is the one you are familiar with, but that was not his name, and he was not a single individual. It was a group of several princes with a superior with them, who came from the confederation. They were identified first with the image of a leaf inside a circle, and then with the name El-Shadai and El-Alion. Later in the time of Mashah (Moses) his name was known, 'Adonai Tzabaot' (which translated into Spanish means 'Lord of Hosts'). This group was thereafter identified as IHVH (Yaheveh), although linguistic corruption gave rise to forms such as Jehovah or Yahweh. Its intention was to reflect the existence of a true god, different from the others (the Orionite factions), which identified a greater one: The ONE. It is from the ONE, or Perfect One, that the 22 universes that exist were produced. Seeing what Iaheveh achieved sparked a series of conflicts between the Iaheveh group and the Orionites (if you ever read or heard about the Anunnaki called Enki and Enlil, the myth came from these conflicts) . The Orionites known in the "alien conspiracy theory philosophy" as the En.Ki camp, dedicated themselves to a great work of disinformation and deception about the reputation of En.Lil (the mythology of the group of Iaheveh, or Jehovah). Thanks to this misinformation agenda, an idea of En.Lil - or Zeus, according to the Greek version - who had a bad character, was angry, avenging, punishing, dictatorial, infallible, etc. became popular. Come on... the bipolar god of Western religions.

The impotent Orians wanted to continue using humans as labor for their mining and pleasure work, but without risking revolts or seditions against the tyranny of their masters. However, the Draconians devised a master plan that is still directed by their Earth arm, the Illuminati/DeepState: control of humanity. The first thing was to plunge the human race into hardship, forced labor, worries, diseases, climatic disagreements, plagues, natural disasters and wars. They incited tribal groups against each other to exterminate each other. They introduced lethal laboratory-made viruses and thus decimated the population. With their climatic weapons they used the weather against men and ruined their crops. Through the Orian influence they seduced some and others into fornication, and encouraged them towards the pleasures of hallucinogenic smoke and mushrooms, alcoholic beverages and witchcraft. They perverted humanity to such a degree that their life was a daily apocalypse, and anarchy was common life. Humanity got fed up and lashed out at "their masters." Everywhere the people armed themselves against the giants. There was great mortality. The frightened gods did not want to be involved or destroy their creation and be left without labor and pleasure. In a change of power of the assembly of gods on Earth it was determined to cleanse the planet. Using geomagnetic technology the poles were reversed causing an immediate "Ice Age".

After the flood caused, few survived. Atlantis (Poseidonis) sank and every vestige of Lemuria (Mu) was swallowed by the sea. From the 5 continents of that time, 5 shipping companies with a total of 138 vessels representing the survival of what was left of the 7 original avatar-races disembarking in new places to begin again. The Pleiadians came to help many in planning their escape from the disaster. You must understand this to understand the analogy of our present that I will explain to you later, because history tends to repeat itself. The first United Nations Organization was then founded between the Indus Valley and Mesopotamia. Established by King Nimrod. The capital of the world in the Sumerian city of Babili (Babel) united the survivors in the same idea: a single feeling. The draconians who remained underground encouraged the political leaders of these cities to build a shuttle, supposedly to commemorate the world's victory over destruction and honor the planetary union. The true intention was to create a pan-dimensional energy system focused to infinity to be an exit route from Earth for the captured draconians. The Confederation changed its plans and dissolved, each one went to a different region of the Earth and over time their common language (pre-Sanskrit Tamil) was deformed to give shape to the languages of the world.

The great capitals had sunk in the flood, including Atlantis and Kumari-Kandam, but the priestly caste left for Hyperborea, while Dyehuty (known in Egyptian mythology by the Greek name 'Thoth') and Argot were helped by Ra to erect the Great Pyramid, the main one in a chain of hundreds of pyramids spread throughout the planet. Thousands of years later the Draconians altered the design and erected other structures with another alignment to coincide with Rigel in Orion and Thuban in Draco. On the recommendation of Totmes - his father -, Dyehuty had established a Kemite priesthood in Egypt to safeguard the mysteries of the Kingdom of Heaven protected in Atlantis. The draconians infiltrated spirits of error who posed as gods and deceived the priests.

The Orionites founded new dynasties in the emerging nations, one for each of the children of the royal line. The preeminent Orionite monarchy interbred with the Betasirian monarchy, creating the Nebaru (Niburian, or those of Nibiru) lineage, and they considered themselves the legitimate heirs of our planet. They brought their children to be lords of each of the great metropolises they built on each continent. They took this to mirror the institutional order operating in the galaxy. Thus they were divided into 5 sections of the Earth, being the adonim (adonai, lords) over the mortals. They once again subjected humanity to servitude, fear and veneration. Investigations conducted by the Confederacy revealed the abuse of Orian authority on humanity and the stratagems of subjugation and tyranny perpetuated once again against man. The Confederacy decided it was time to intervene. The application of universal Non-Intervention policies in the development of evolving Third Density races was once again violated. It was then sent to 5 groups 3,300 years ago, among which were again the groups Iaheveh (Jehovah) and Ra.

Iaheveh (Jehovah) went to the Paa-Tal incarnated in the descendants of the Hebrew patriarch Abraham, with whom he already had a follow-up with some Pleiadian spies, who were helping an ancestral priesthood, an image of a heavenly one, called the Melki-Tzedek priesthood. Ner (Noah's brother) had then been high priest of this order, but in the days of Abraham there was another pontiff, maximum of this order, who went to meet Abraham after the victory of the coalition that supported Abraham in the war against Kedar. -Laomer (see Gen. 14:7). Abraham therefore came from this priestly family ancestry. For his part, Ra, who had helped the Atlanteans before the flood, continued wanting to help the Kemites (later called Egyptians), having his base of operations on the planet we call Venus.

The attempts of Ra and Iaheveh (Jehovah) to help were thwarted by the strong Orian and Draconian influence, both from off-planet and from the surface and below it. The sabotage was too intense, to the point that it was not possible to clarify to the Israelite prophets from whom the "divine" messages really came. The Orians used the name of Iaheveh (Jehovah) to send their own confusing messages to the prophets, sowing airs of racial elitism, dualism, divine wrath, everlasting punishments and damnations, and vengeance on enemies. For their part, the Egyptians worshiped the Ra group as a god, which made them retreat, since that was not their intention. However, the Ra group since then only showed themselves from their ships "flying" over the cities, and they operated psychically, without showing themselves physically again so as not to encourage idolatry. The group of Iaheveh (Jehovah) and Ra appear to have joined forces when the Terra-Santorini volcano exploded, and attacked Egypt, where the draconians had made their refuge. A new battle on land against the Orians drove the reptiles back, but they had groups operating from Canaan that were waiting for the Israelite people to destroy them. Earth conflicts between extraterrestrial and terrestrial groups continued decade after decade and century after century for a long time.

Finally Ra and Iaheveh (Jehovah) left Earth and both groups moved on to the next octave of consciousness, leaving the work to new generations sent by the Confederacy with new ideas. Ra and Iaheveh no longer belong to this universe, as we understand it. The Confederacy was aware that the Dragon would not give in, neither on our planet nor on the many others on which they create oppression. It was then accepted that the invariant probability-possibility line was the paradigm known as 'Har-Magedon'. For thousands of years, Confederate allies who also use time travel have used it against the Dragon. The Dragon knows the Har-Magedon plan and makes constant interventions in the space-time continuum towards the past to alter events in his favor, which is in turn neutralized and/or altered by the Confederacy. Basically it is a war in time, or more correctly, in times. The draconians know that by mathematical equation their days are numbered, but they have played with the advantage of time travel to anticipate ambushes, operations to capture their leaders, military defeats, etc. This has meant that the end of the conflict has lasted for millions of years.

When in the mid-70s it was seen in the MJ-12 (Shadow Government) that the use of time travel was possible with the Montauk project, it was then terrestrial governments that began to use this technology, which later was used by the Illuminati to foresee all the variables of space-time continuity to achieve a successful New World Order. This was used both for research in time with chrononauts, and to take people to colonies established on the Moon (Adam Base) and Mars (Eve Base), according to the secret project 'Alternative 2', which the secret organization MJ-12 developed with the help of SIV (Vatican secret service) investigations for human survival in the face of Har-Magedon. However, the technology for the Montauk project was not achieved by the US alone, but was provided to them by the Beta-Sirians. This angered the Orians, who wished to gain the upper hand over humanity. Since 1954 it was evident to the main governments of Earth that we were at a disadvantage compared to extraterrestrial races, and the Orians used this for blackmail of various kinds. Thousands of years ago the Orians took the Zetae (or 'Zetareticulans') and Rigellians captive, and exterminated almost all of their males, leaving only females. They genetically manipulated them, leading their endemic race to near extermination. They put microchips in the back of their heads and used them as puppets for their purposes. In 1931 they were sent to our solar system to establish contact, but had to keep their distance due to Confederate control.

The contact attempts of the Thule and Vril organization of Nazi Germany established communication with them and received technological and logistical help (the Feuerball, or Foo-Fighters, were an example of the result of that assistance to hinder the coordination and air maneuvers of the Allies). This spurred Adolf Hitler to take over Europe, trusting in extraterrestrial help. The Allies found out about this, so both the US and the USSR also sought to establish contact (at that time spirits of darkness had already been intervening in the minds of the scientists of the secret Manhattan project to develop the atomic bomb in Los Alamos). Both nations received the same model agreement, which consisted of the exchange of farm animals for genetic experiments, in exchange for alien technology. In reality, few animals were mutilated and the experiments were carried out on Soviet and American soil with humans, who were kidnapped and taken to their ships to suffer horrible traumatic experiences. The commission in charge of extraterrestrial affairs in the US shadow government reported this to the "gray" emissaries, who recognized their lack of ethics and were not prejudiced in recognizing their deeds.

A list of abducted people was required and that they at least not remember the traumas of the experiments to which they were subjected. This was not obeyed either. According to galactic law, if you establish an agreement with a race, and give rise to intrusion under a legal document, it cannot be invalidated. Consequently, the Confederacy could not intervene to annul the treaty. The US was in trouble. As Naval Intelligence officer Milton William Cooper explains in his work 'Behold A Pale Horse', the agreements signed with the Rigellians since 1954, under the consent of then-President Dwight Eisenhower, were the death certificate. Since then, not only Grays but Orionites and Draconians operated from Earth's soil, and began to act with impunity. In bases like Area 51 there were various compartmentalized levels for different investigations. Reverse technology was used to analyze the use of flying saucers of extraterrestrial origin for military purposes. At other levels children were used for experiments in remote viewing, precognition and vivid dreaming (later carried out by British intelligence, MI6, with the Mannequin project). Also the use of paranormal abilities, such as telekinesis or telepathy. In another plant, genetic experiments were carried out, creating hybrids, clones and chimeras. They were provided with scientific knowledge 50 years ahead of where we were in 1960. Tests began on remote wave Tesla technology, weather weapons, psychic technology, mind control, use of lasers, night vision, invisibility materials, antigravity, development of micronuclear weapons, biological weapons and motion sensors.

The operational factions of the Dragon had been using the armed conflicts in our world to antagonize the people, thus managing to avoid civil revolutions against the hegemony of the Illuminati power. The Orionites, specifically, were responsible for the creation of radical sects and the manipulation of religions with the aim of indoctrinating devotees and brainwashing them, depriving them of essential knowledge and the ability to judge themselves. To improve this the Grays (Rigellians, Zetae) began to take trips to the Earth's past to alter momentous events. The Confederation personally warned several world leaders at a symposium, but their desire for power prevented them from giving in, largely due to the tensions of the Cold War. In 1953, members from the Confederacy presented evidence to demonstrate that they were the angels of the Bible and that they had been watching over our world since ancient times, and they showed the terrestrial commission as proof a three-dimensional holographic color recording of the crucifixion. of Ihoshua (Jesus). Given the fear of vulnerability, and that the help that the Pleiadians offered was subject to nuclear disarmament, there was no agreement with them. The offer from "the bad guys" was in the best interest of US policies. The draconians wanted to encourage the use of technology as they had already achieved on other peoples in the galaxy, thus getting humanity to exterminate itself and its leaders to first submit to them. Draconians are not interested in political leaders or leaders of social movements. They are not interested in anyone but themselves. At the right moment they make the leaders themselves, having finished their function in the script, also destroy each other.

The Draconians infiltrated the Vatican, as it was clear for millennia that a religious awakening threatened the Illuminati monopoly. Thus the Jesuits were born, and they entered every great nation to control the media, the entertainment industries (television series, movies, music industry, pornography) and the education and science systems (colleges, universities and research centers).). In this way they took control of all the media so that no one knew the truth, those who told it were ridiculed and what was there was altered. The draconians encouraged in their lackeys the system of loans, debt and interest, which created the banking systems, so that their lackeys were over every economic and financial structure. Progressively these banksters (banking gangsters) indebted all nations and linked themselves with corporate industries. The multinationals in turn preyed on the smaller ones, leaving a few above all the others. Now we saw some mega-rich masters of the banks and mega-rich masters of corporations (such as the pharmaceutical industry) with more power than the governments themselves. This is how they began to buy world leaders to sign agreements and establish laws based on Illuminati ideals, which are none other than draconian ideals. The world progressively became a huge corporation, a technocratic dictatorial system, protected by its own laws. And technology continued to increase, also being protected by bought politicians, so that techno-surveillance and law enforcement obeyed the same Illuminati interests. Well, thank you for having an open mind and getting to this point. Once the above has been explained, let's now get into the matter...

II. PROBLEMS AND SOLUTIONS

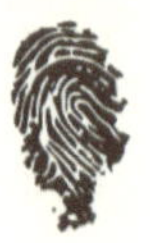

The terrestrial draconian structure (the so-called Illuminati) had to deal with various issues. For them, the problem of human beings is serious, and represents a huge headache. We are too intelligent, we have an unsurpassed reasoning capacity, we have spiritual moral principles, we are empathetic when we are not under pressure, we tend towards love, service , teamwork, unity, we do not accept injustice, we have an abundant creativity, we tend towards mercy, kindness, we have emotional systems that neutralize draconian technology (love, joy, laughter, happiness, affection, kindness, dance, music, art, sport, creativity, imagination, protection instinct, friendship). For centuries they have tried to reduce this, but it is not easy for them on a large scale, nor permanently, and they know that it is enough for one to wake up to encourage awakening in others like a virus. Our biomagnetic field is our main defense. These drawbacks are added to the fact that since there are more than 7,000 million human beings on Earth, the ability to control all of them becomes very complex, despite the growing technology and artificial intelligence itself that can be used. serve.

Anything that is not under digital network control is not easy to keep track of, much less manipulate. For this reason we must begin to talk about the famous 'New World Order', which is the opposite of human intuition, instinct or intuitive capacity, spiritual values or the analytical and critical criteria of Adamic reasoning. It is something like what the apostle John would have called "the Spirit of the Antichrist" (understanding by 'spirit' the collective idea, social conscience, or mentality; and 'antichrist' as the philosophy or idea itself contrary to the awakening of conscience or social unification, everything that is opposed to morality, love, the common good and goodness). The power of this "beast" of the Apocalypse lies in advanced technology. That is, everything is moving to data and numbers (the 'Internet of Things'), without feelings or emotions, the power of Artificial Intelligence, reaching artificial "consciousness", without humanity. Also hidden behind this curtain is the intention to create a transhuman race, as the Orionites are said to have done with the inhabitants of the planets of the Rigel and Zeta Reticuli systems.

In this sense, the 'Agenda 2030' operation comes into action, the cornerstone of which has been a large number of implementations to carry out human depopulation on a genocidal scale. We go point by point knowing the pieces of this chess game with which the so-called Illuminati intends to 'Checkmate' our race. The Draconians are said to lead the Orionites, the Orionites the Black Monks and Druids of the Satanic Draconian Priesthood on Earth, operating from secret military installations on the Moon. The Illuminati is the structure of the Orian monarchy on our planet, and under the Illuminati and the Black Monks are organizations such as the NSA (US National Security Agency) and groups such as MJ-12 (Majestic-12). Underneath these are the structures of the Deep State (the Deep State, or dark government agency of the Illuminati that operates over all these devices on Earth), such as The Round Table , the CFR (Council on Foreign Relations of the USA), the TC (or 'Trilateral Commission'), the Knights of Rhodes, the Jesuits and the Political Zionists (or 'Elders of Zion'), and under them the Bilderberg Club, the UN, the WHO (World Health Organization) and NATO, always in pyramid style. The hierarchical structure is broader and more branched but you can see it in my books 'Recognizing the Time of the End' and 'Armageddon, E-5', or by investigating the exhibitions of whitleblowers (snitches, divulgers, moles).

The Illuminati structures all these movements through various secret societies, which in turn use intelligence agencies, such as the CIA (which had originally been created under executive orders of the NSC in order to investigate the UFO phenomenon) and the banking leadership. Since the Illuminati constitutes the royal draconian lineage on Earth, they use the banking system to control our race, being the top of the pyramid of control. Therefore, in the power structure, under these powers that I have mentioned, the banks UBS and BIS of Switzerland, which control all the Central Banks of the world. The BIS belongs to the Rockefeller and Rothschild families, members of the 13 Illuminati families. Likewise, the Illuminati uses paid actors to whom it gives all the money necessary to bribe every politician, doctor, scientist, leader or public influence that is necessary, and to be spokespersons for its agendas and social changes, as the Rockefeller Foundation, the Bill & Melinda Gates Foundation or George Soros himself.

But where do they want to go? They want to create a World Government led by the so-called "Antichrist" or "the Beast", a planetary dictatorship led by a mere handful of people, logically, those chosen by them. The efficiency of the pyramid structure is such that they no longer need to spend time, resources and energy trying to control all the threads. It is enough for those at the highest part of the pyramid to communicate their intentions to their 10 lackeys, they in turn give orders to their immediate pawns, and thus, as has been done for a long time by intelligence agencies and military compartmentalization, no one He does not know everything about the agency nor does he know what happens in the spheres above his level of access. Thus, everyone obeys orders and lacks criteria to judge the decisions they must make. Thanks to this model of manipulation, they manage to create a global scheme on a Ponzi scale, which covers everything and few come to suspect or question. In this way, anyone who deviates from the scheme is ridiculed, since it seems crazy to think that an entire planet is controlled by just a handful of individuals.

That is the success of the pyramid business, as Robert Kiyosaki himself would have exposed in his work, 'The Business of the 21st Century'. Thus, the police, the doctors, the journalists and even the bus driver are convinced that the system works – or will end up working – and those at the top are trustworthy and know what they are doing, so these people will come to defend This conviction will be carried out tooth and nail , and he will see as enemies those who refute and oppose the version given by the state and the media. Thanks to this control model, Agenda 21, which is the same as 'Agenda 2030', can be orchestrated without major impediment, having efficiently achieved the first part: a consented global martial law. Let us now see how they manage their affairs to finally implement this goal...

1 - THE "PROBLEM" OF "overpopulation". There are too many of us to control. As explained in the Georgia Stones, they need to reduce the population of our race by 93%. One strategy is to say that our planet is overpopulated and resources are scarce and we are spending and destroying them. First of all, our world can comfortably support 11 billion human beings. The essential factor in this stratagem that there are many of us lies in the fact that there is a poor distribution of resources, demographic expansion and incorrect use of technologies to supply needs.

Zero point energy technology, free consumption sources, are under Illuminati control. The mega-rich and corporationists do not invest in the ecosystem, their industries and desire for production are the true causes of pollution. Instead they blame us.

A. For more than a hundred years we have had free electricity from different sources, from static charges, geothermal, wave impact generators, solar energy, shock energy, wind energy, magnetic energy, Tesla energy, among others. These technologies are restricted, and some of them are marketed at high costs.

B. They say that we waste resources. This depends on how you look at it. The idea is presented that we spend resources, but in reality the structure is proposed in an indiscriminate way to promote industrial and exploitative competition. Some 7 billion forms of animal life die each year to satisfy meat consumption while tree fruits rot in the ground, tracts of arable land are burned to build Smart Cities, food is thrown away because farmers don't like it. They offer nothing for their crops, home agriculture is not promoted but purchasing in supermarkets. Looking at it in perspective, it is a question of industrial and corporate monopoly, thinking about profits, not losses.

C. There is serious planetary pollution, and this is because political organizations do not seriously and on a large scale force industries to replace polluting products with biodegradable materials, given that this would mean million-dollar losses for these companies. There are no viable mechanisms to get rid of so much garbage that is discarded daily in cities. Citizen recycling and the use of waste materials for reuse are very little encouraged (not enough alternatives are offered). The organic material would be compost for home cultivation; The metals are taken to foundries or scrap yards, or used for upcycling, creating useful things; Wood is also reused, as are plastics and glass, which can also be recycled. There is no investment in this type of activity nor is the population made aware of the creativity and cooperation to participate in this.

D. Dirty water could be managed with the implementation of dry toilets or septic tanks that are for organic use to fertilize the land. The demographic expansion could expand towards the mountains, making people take advantage of uninhabited land, as Russia proposed. This would reduce pollution, dirt, bad odors and overcrowding, not to mention traffic congestion in cities. It is the structuring of megacities that makes habitability difficult, while outside them there are untapped extensions. But this is part of the dark strategy, of agglomerating people in super metropolises, so that they are easy to control, and leaving the green fields out of the contact of the population.

E. There is talk of the health crisis, where there is no way to care for so many sick people, but again this is the responsibility of the same people who create the problems: the elite. They make the population sick and distance them from natural healing strategies and environmental self-healing methods. They always connect health with "avoiding", instead of "strengthening", and not giving cures but drugs (seeking to make addicts for life) and treatments that put people in debt, which in most cases damage their cells.

So they have "their" solution:

A. Eugenics. They push the sterilization of the undesirable and the weak, so that "the fittest" remain (see 'Origin of Species', by Charles Darwin, chapter 4). This Darwinian-Nazi idea is implemented with metals scattered in the clouds (chemtrails or geo-engineering (See 'Recognizing the Time of the End', chapter 1, section F)) and in drinking water, as well as with vaccines and drugs (legal drugs). It is also promoted by the damage to the body caused by junk food.

A. Drug addict clients. With the use of drugs, most of them administered irresponsibly by doctors who earn commissions from them, instead of prescribing homemade-natural medicine (as Hippocrates, father of medicine, pointed out). Thus, the weakest die and the least weak continue to nourish the pharmaceutical industry for life.

A. Wars. The elite provokes armed conflicts in order to achieve sociopolitical changes and reduce the population through deaths in said confrontations.

A. Diseases. Being the part that concerns us most in this book, deadly diseases are the result of experiments in laboratories and illegal weapons (see NASA document, 'Future Strategy for Warfare, 2025', by Dr. Dennis M. Bushnell, Chief Scientist from NASA Langley Research Center), not from Mother Nature. In his work 'God's of Eden', William Bramley evoked the case of the Black Death, officially attributed to the poor rats. Well, the Pope had demonized cats and ordered them to be exterminated, triggering an imbalance in the natural chain of the ecosystem, but how did rats transmit a virus, by biting people or sneezing at them? And where did the virus get to them and how was it created? Not even in the cinema do they show movies about "killer mutant viruses" where the aforementioned has not been manufactured in a laboratory. According to the testimonies collected, the Plague of Justinian appeared when a "hooded man with a scythe" was seen walking through the fields releasing a "mist" that came from the blade of the oz. That "mist" quickly retreated, bringing death. If we were already being killed on a large scale back then, how much more so today with the technology of altering the genome of bacteria, viruses, germs, etc.? NASA and DARPA have similar technology called 'Smart Dust', made up of intelligent nano robots that can replicate themselves (of course, they did not perfect that technology alone but rather it was given to them by aliens, the same ones who sprayed us with the Bubonic Plague). This book does not intend to address the cases of all the most serious diseases that have attacked man, but it will touch your conscience to let you see that it is not unreasonable to assume that – as is stated in ufology – the Dragon introduced viruses such as the of the Flu, which is still supposed to have no cure. In the same order of things, it was in US military laboratories where the so-called 'Spanish Flu' was created, what has been called 'Cancer', as well as avian, swine, mad cow diseases, etc., as well as pathogens selective ethnic ones, such as Dengue, Zika or Chikungunya, and those especially aimed at ending the black race, such as Tuberculosis or Hepatitis. And how can we not mention the most recent and deadly ones, such as HIV and Ebola. But the problem was not the viruses but the compromised immune system, because a system with high blood pH is immune to enemy viral agents. And that acidic state activated the germs against us with the stimulation of the microwaves that were weaving the planetary sphere as the era of telecommunications advanced.

A. Weakening the immune system by distancing ourselves from nature is one of the favorite weapons and the main use by the elite to achieve their goals. A virus is not lethal but it counts on what is most important: the support of collateral agents from the external and internal environment. Thus, if a lifestyle is promoted that weakens people, they will drop like flies to any pathogen that is thrown at them. For this reason, they keep them away from sunbathing (so as not to stimulate the DBP protein on chromosome 4), from going swimming, from stretching, from playing sports - without a mask -, from getting fresh air - without a mask -, from eating healthy. (in an alkaline way), meditation, dancing, social interaction and laughter, taking them to an era of home confinement and virtual life.

A. Elimination of the elderly. Another magical solution of these psychopaths is euthanasia, a way in which they save high costs of pensions and government aid. And if you wonder how they do it, well the answer is with drugs and vaccines. That applies to the disabled and sick, so there is a government saving in healthcare costs and subsidies. Likewise, the elderly are the libraries of experience of our society, who could alert us to how what they saw at the time is repeated today.

A. Microwave. And among others, one of the most important, and around which this exemplary work revolves, and which I don't really know what to call, since it is a bubble of conceptual and technical deception... high and low frequency waves (4G plus and 5G). I will talk about this in detail, but I can tell you that the waves propagate, and although you do not hear them as music, because they are in a range outside the structures in which sound can be audible to the ear, they hit the atoms. The cells of our body are penetrated by something, and the body does not know where that enemy is and cannot attack it to defend itself. The alarm goes off and the body raises its temperature, believing that it is being attacked by an external agent and the high temperature will kill it. But the doctors interpret that fever as "sick," and they take you to the slaughterhouse. This is called EHS (Electromagnetic Hypersensitivity Syndrome), and I will address its causes and effects later.

1. **- The "problem" of financing.** How do you cover the costs of such installations? The expense of all the planning and implementation of the global takeover takes, not only time, but extreme expenses. Many of their pseudo-philanthropists make it appear that they donate from their fortune, but that money is not theirs: it comes to them from the "masters," and the "masters" take it from the people themselves. For decades they have taken funds from things that will now make your hair click, and you will connect the dots, understanding what so much "philanthropy" on the part of genocidaires is really about. Your solution:

A. Global health campaigns. This is one of the most important and where we will focus in this manuscript. As you may have deduced, if the Dark Government has scientists and facilities working with biological experimentation, it is not difficult for them to create a chimera and its antidote (for their own), so that they release it among a certain population group. and then produce a health alarm. This chimera need not be deadly, as long as it spreads easily, and it should leave no traces. That is, if someone isolates it in a laboratory, they will assume, in the first instance, that it is the mutation of an already existing pathogen. This is because the chimera must be an artificial mutation of a bacteria or virus previously present in nature. Since they have made ordinary people believe that things magically "mutate" and become more powerful (see the 'X-men' or 'Marvel' phenomenon), they would avoid questions from the masses. Then they let the problem retreat and make a global call to find solutions, for which governments invest astronomical sums for research and cures, which in reality is not intended for the aforementioned object – it would have no reason to exist, since they They have the antidote, and also the vaccine (the same pathogen but stronger) -.

A. Environment. The supposed Climate Change strategy has been key since the end of WWII (Second World War). It was evident that industries were indiscriminately exploiting resources and were greatly polluting the environment. But the focus was not on multinationals and factories , but on the civilian part: us. The poorly designed infrastructures were not going to be modified by the mayors to avoid sewage, bad odors, garbage, overcrowding or begging. There was pressure to take measures on gas emissions into the atmosphere, first with refrigerators , then with factories and later with vehicles, and until then very nice. The next and most important thing was not carried out:

large-scale recycling, ocean cleanup, and reforestation. Considering that trees and plankton feed on CO2, gases are the least of the problems, and above all, without trees (depleted by indiscriminate logging) and plankton (dying rapidly due to ocean pollution) There is no aerobic biological life and the ecosystem chain is broken. But instead of planting more trees, cities expand and fields become industrialized; Instead of cleaning the sea, it continues to be used as a landfill.

So, what do these "Climate Change" campaigns consist of? In the exploitation of Africa as the number one resource of the globalist elite and in taking global funds to fight against planetary "warming." They said that oil used as fuel is toxic, so they did not encourage its use in the underdeveloped countries of Africa, to keep them in the dark, in every sense. Control of Africa's resources is a master piece of the Illuminati machine. If Africa knew what was happening, the powers that be would lose the control, power and high wealth they achieve by exploiting black people. But the Illuminati puppets sell us the idea that the Earth is warming and action must be taken. In reality our world is cooling, not warming. The most important changes in the climate occur depending on the solar phases. When spots are detected on the Sun, it is known that its temperature is dropping, and, however, solar radiation decreases, affecting our planet and the others in our system. In fact, the Sun has an 11-year cycle - something known since the 19th century - and through it you can see high or low peaks that change the climate transcendently. But

Bill Gates will say that we must cover the atmosphere so that the Earth does not continue to heat up, and then the flora will die, the fauna will be unbalanced and the human immune system will weaken, not to mention that there will be a wave of depression (since our mood is directly related to the king star).

So the governments come together so "concerned" to solve this "problem", and they put Al Gore in a beautiful social awareness campaign selling a misinformation product where influential figures fall - like later with Leonardo Di Caprio - who, knowing it or not, They move the masses to accept that these brutal amounts of money are injected into the fight against coherence: the atmosphere is made up of various layers (such as the troposphere, ionosphere, stratosphere, mesosphere, thermosphere and exosphere), they will have already taught you that in class, but what almost no one notices is that the gases we produce only remain in a minimal lower layer of the troposphere. This is precisely the thinnest layer of all the previous ones, and it is where the CO2 condenses. However, the most interesting thing about this is that this phenomenon helps prevent the planet from cooling. In other words, "God" in his infinite wisdom made these gases stay in that layer to move through where the wind currents pass and maintain the planetary balance, taking this gas to the sea and the forests, from where the plankton and Trees take carbon (C) and release only oxygen (O2) that aerobic beings breathe.

But above all, it is not possible for CO2 to heat the Earth, considering that it remains in the troposphere, which constitutes 75% of the atmospheric mass, and is composed of water vapor and other types of particles in suspension (like drops of water). The troposphere only covers 13 kilometers in height, within the total volume of about 500 kilometers. In addition to this, the atmosphere is made up of 78% nitrogen, 21% oxygen, 1% argon and 0.04% carbon. That is, no matter how hard we try to continue increasing the amount of carbon, it will not alter the atmosphere (unless we destroy the oceans and forests, thus achieving some really considerable impact). But I will talk about the ecosystem issue later. The point is that the amount of money collected worldwide does not go towards what it is said to go towards, and only increases the coffers of globalist plans, which use concepts, words, definitions in a "legislative" way, whose real meaning It has another intention: a new world with almost no humans and with biological resources out of reach. In other words, forget about going to a national park, connecting with animals or going to the beach. To replace this, they will sell you virtual reality, hologram emitters and projectors so that inside your house you believe that you are outdoors, or anywhere in the world, without having to move, or spend on trips and tourist accommodations.

A. Ideologies. Whether we are talking about LGTB (Lesbian-Gay-Transvestite-Bisexual), or its annexes, whether in love with their pets, a tree or a robot, these movements, orchestrated and financed by the Rockefeller Foundation, are already working on their own. . Now it is each government that invests locally and promotes these trends. The Rockefellers pay the politicians (not to use the word "bribe" or "purchase") and they change the laws and push the municipalities and towns to create campaigns of debauchery and acceptance of anti-family tendencies and moral degradation that open the door to the decriminalization of pedophilia and sexual violation in general. With the excuse of fighting against "gender" bullying, they promote the "freedom" of "sexual" "expression", be careful, playing with words and their meaning, as well as with social sensationalism. They do not face conventional school bullying but they do face "sexual" bullying, which according to their propaganda has nothing to do with sexual harassment, but with the right to "express oneself." So governments start investing a lot of money in these campaigns, without the need for the Rockefeller Foundation to continue doing so, and they brainwash children with sexualization, erasing their innocence, while parents are waiting to court other women. , and the women shouting to kill the men who are all "pigs."

It is essential to understand what this is all about. It may stir your insides, as it did me the first time I heard about it, but what is behind this film is pedophilia, and then other interests such as the adrenochrome market and fetuses (after the success of pro-abortion campaigns), the destruction of marriage and the value of family, the degradation of love, the incapacitation of men and the desensitization of women. Although it is not pleasant to talk about this topic, if it is not included in the equation, a strategic and completely structural piece of Illuminati interests is not known. Support for gay and lesbian "propaganda" includes bisexuals and transvestites, but that is not the end of it. People already choose whether they want to rub or marry their dog, a tree in a park, their desk chair, or their vacuum cleaner. It sounds comical, but why all the fuss and interest in such laughable triviality? Instead of raising awareness about "respect", what is done is "applauding" and taking away space from other values, such as family or heterosexual principles, to the point of being almost relegated to archaic, retrograde or "discriminatory" . That is, being "straight" (hetero) comes to mean "intolerant." You don't have to have half a brain to see what's happening. Home, family, having children or 'straight' or 'straight' couple love are no longer encouraged. This is an essential part of avoiding the birth of more children and the influence of parents' values on children . But let's not anticipate events, I will talk about all this, although I do not want to deviate from the main theme of this book.

By approving one thing they give rise to another, until pedophilia creeps in. If you keep track of what is happening, you will have noticed that there are already laws that are being approved to decriminalize pedophilia, starting by lowering the age of "permissiveness." The legal argument is based on the fact that it is another "gender" (the pedophile) and that it has "freedom of sexual expression" (love). The main promoter of the LGBT movement was a pedophile who spent years in prison for sexual abuse. He was released and used by the CIA to awaken this current so that it is finally the open door to the acceptance of child sexual abuse and rape in general. You heard right, rape of boys, girls and adults, whether men or women. This means that you will soon hear about the legalization of rape, for adults or children, with the excuse that it is "sexual expression" and "release of tension", so it is good for physical, emotional and psychological health. So if you are raped on the street, it will not be considered a crime. With this open letter, governments exempt themselves from legal responsibilities and penalties for a wide range of sexual crimes that fill court records, and anticipate a greater wave of crime to come.

But that's not all, they will wash their hands of allegations that have become known about child trafficking networks, kidnappings, pedophile networks and the sale of organs where actors, politicians, world leaders, police, military, doctors, service people are involved. secrets, judges, lawyers, singers and television and entertainment personalities. Donald Trump accelerated the uncovering of this rotten pot, so the elite in turn accelerates the decriminalization of these crimes before more public figures like Jeffrey Epstein go to jail. There is much more to say about these movements of pedophile networks (which became openly known due to the PizzaGate scandal), Feminazism (misnamed 'feminism') and the murder of unborn humans (Abortion), among others. , but I will leave them for later.

A. Philanthropist, the most sinic and hypocritical definition ever used. People who are proclaimed by the media as 'lovers of humanity' (filos-anthropos, or philanthropists) today are precisely the most miserable antichrists. I am not talking about every person who can be known as a philanthropist for his contributions to society - such as Elon Musk, Arnold Schwarzenegger, Donald Trump, Nicola Tesla, Martin Luther King, Mahatma Gandhi or John F. Kennedy - but about reptiles with a human mask , namely Bill Gates, Barack Obama, David Rockefeller, George Soros, Mark Zuckerberg, Tedros Adhanom, Benjamin Netanyahu, the Windsor family, the Bush family, the Clintons and so many others. Some with more pomp and propaganda than others, as if donating with the left hand exempted them from what they do with the right hand. Bill Gates, George Soros, Obama and the Rockefellers are only a public image of a dark Illuminati puppet master who provides them with all the capital there is to push their plans. These people are financed by the Illuminati, and they play the good guys with their contributions to all these transformation movements towards Agenda 2030 (the era of Antichrist). That money leaves and returns from the same source: the Rockefeller and Rothschild Banks.

A. Terror, favorite word of the Bush cabinet. Another strategy to get money for their objectives is terrorism. I have already talked about this before and I will mention it later, but as you have noticed, we have been bombarded for more than 20 years with the idea of "terror", through which anti-civilian laws, deprivation of freedoms and greater control, without discounting that the "terrorist threat" allows millions and millions of dollars to be diverted from all countries to the fight against the "invisible enemies." Then you just have to say that you apologize because you were wrong, because <<there were no weapons of mass destruction>>, by leaving a country "massively destroyed." But it doesn't matter, then you send your own companies to rebuild it and put said country in debt with bank loans for reconstruction.

A. The drug cartel, which everyone believes consists of carrying narcotics through an airport in their underwear. Curious, but if it weren't for the fact that governments pay the police and the DEA to go after stoners who smoke weed and enjoy these smokes that relax them, stupefy them and make them laugh, funding the fight against drugs would not be worth it. the sorrow. Yes, because the persecution of smokers accounts for almost all of the capital invested in the "fight against drugs." They do not penalize drugs from "drugstores", but they do penalize herbs produced by Mother Earth (soon Pachamama will be fined for having created cannabis, cocaine and hallucinogenic mushrooms). That's right, heroin, processed cocaine, crystal, psychotropic pills and other synthetic drugs account for less than 15% of this "very important" battle against evil. They are not going after alcohol - which causes greater damage - or conventional cigarettes - which is carcinogenic - but rather dazed people who lie down in an armchair to laugh and doze: a great threat to safety and health.

But if it were not for the financing of this "war", much of the work of police officers would be constant boredom. Understand, the first reason for this pantomime is nothing other than tax evasion and money laundering by those who use this business to monetize. The government did not profit from this industry, so it hunts it down. Of course, many saw where to take advantage of it, and legalized marijuana and hashish, as in Amsterdam or Spain in the so-called CoffeShop - or in general in California -. But get a license to open a CoffeShop and they will take an arm and a leg out of your face, because they know how much money those clubs move. They also give licenses for you to produce these herbs in a certain range, or with certain limitations, if it is for "pharmaceutical" purposes. In other words, the government or Big Pharma must take advantage of it one way or another. How can you not benefit from the most lucrative business at a civil level, and from which taxes are avoided? But this goes much further.

You will be surprised to know that the 'Miracle of Fátima' in Portugal between 1915 and 1917 was an extraterrestrial action to attract the world's attention, according to the classified version of the intelligence services. When MJ-12 asked the SIV to confirm what the Fatima apparitions had been, it was indisputable that it was an apocalyptic warning. The SIV said that there were 3 warnings in those "miracles of the virgin", one regarding the danger of the USSR, another about another world war and another – and the most uncomfortable for the papacy – that "Satan" would infiltrate the Catholic Church and would direct it along with other powers that would push the manifestation of the Antichrist. Later the Plejaren (Pleiadians) confirmed this and told MJ-12 that everything warned in the prophecies of the Bible would be fulfilled unequivocally. Consequently, an international commission evaluated 3 alternatives to save, not the world, but people chosen by the elite. They did not intend to invest time or resources in avoiding it, but rather to choose who would be saved.

The first option of the three was tacitly rejected: drilling into the atmosphere to release CO2. But Bill Gates has a better idea: block the Sun. The most surprising thing is that almost no one speaks out against it. The second alternative was the installation of underground bases around the globe to prepare refuge silos, which would be established for carefully selected people. That is, neither you nor I are inside. That is why the Bible says that when the Destroyer asteroid comes, <<the kings, great, rich, powerful and dignitaries hid under the caves and in the rocks>> (Rev. 6,15)

The other alternative was 3, the ADAM project and the EVE project, or Adam and Eve, one to colonize Mars and the other to colonize the Moon. In 1955, colonies on the Moon had already begun to be organized, and by 1973 the first landing of the Secret

Space Project on Mars was achieved, showing organic life, water and breathable air. After that, teleportation technology was used to begin taking families to Mars with an army of protection against possible hostilities from the Martian locals (with whom there have been various armed confrontations). Some officials who have worked on Black Ops claim that the draconians attacked human bases on Mars a few years ago and forced them to return to Earth. I cannot deny or confirm this information. For now, the Moon remains a military base for American and Russian use. Where I want to go with this is that you know the relevance that this issue has at the elite level, and for which a supremely high budget has been necessary. This has been paid for by the global drug cartel, which moves more than 3.1 trillion dollars annually. But before addressing the issue of drugs in detail, I will expand on the issue of the SSP (Secret Space Project).

A. One of the ironic things about what NASA presents on television is that it is not happening in the stratosphere. The SSP receives its monetization from drug trafficking, while NASA is a cover to divert millions of dollars to the space project that go in another direction: the Blue Beam Agenda, based on holographic technology, drones, waves and nano robots. All this money I'm talking about is directed to the same plan, but with elaborate names and definitions on the paper. That is, space research is carried out, but NASA does not participate. I do not deny that NASA is carrying out some complementary operations to the SSP, but in principle it is a diversion of attention and a scapegoat for the flow of funds to the militarization of the atmosphere (with nuclear weapons in orbit) and the use of the Moon to place shuttles of long-range nuclear missiles aimed at the Earth and "outwards" , as part of the Blue Beam Agenda. Former President Ronald Reagan said at the UN in 1983 that a threat far greater than that of local enemies, a threat from outside this world, will unite humanity. I do not intend to expand here on the Blue Beam project, but I will comment that it was Reagan who first spoke on March 23, 1983 about the SDI (Strategic Defense Initiative), or popularized as the 'Star Wars' project, which consists of the deployment of a network of orbital satellites with nuclear capabilities, both to defend against the USSR and an "extraterrestrial invasion."

We see so many films of astronauts doing lunar tours, carrying out activities outside the space shuttles and doing pirouettes inside the stations in zero gravity, but what is the difference between those very "real" scenes and the ones we see about the same dynamics in a movie? Or can one today tell when a scene is designed by computer or when it is real? If you want to laugh for a while, go to the internet and look for the scenes with a chrome background that make it clear that what NASA sells is made in hangars with ropes, just like when you see Thor fighting with Ironman and behind him half the city falls into pieces. Sometimes it was not even necessary to use ropes, since NASA has antigravity hangars where they can jump and do somersaults freely. But it is not necessary to spend so much time, energy and resources, because they record it in large swimming pools and in large spaces, with ropes and green or blue backgrounds (chromas) that are then laid out on a computer so that you can see the film. Already in 1969, film director Stanley Kubrick (famous for the masterpiece '2001, A Space Odyssey') was paid to make a recording in the Nevada desert with NASA material, so that this would be presented to the audience of world about Apollo XI mission.

We watch Hollywood and NASA movies, and soon we will see them with holograms in the troposphere, faking a return of Jesus Christ, an alien invasion with a battle between planes (drones) and UFOs (drones), and the appearance of a new god (the Antichrist) causing the Moon to turn red, the Sun to darken and fire to fall from the sky. A great space show, orchestrated by the elite with the use of holograms, drones and waves. The US secret space project is so advanced that it is said that they already have human colonies on other planets outside this solar system, and there they have military bases in other parts of our system. NASA has been lying about life on other worlds, because they know very well that there is life on 17 satellites in our neighborhood – especially on Titan and Ganymede – and there is also life on Venus and Mars. These military installations must ensure the protection of the colonists from local inhabitants or attacks from other races, since - among other things - these colonizations have not been authorized by their inhabitants in most cases. This would explain various wars that have occurred in the human colonies on Mars, whether due to attacks by draconians or by an insectoid race native to Mars, or by J-Rod (short gray aliens) who have facilities on Phobos, one of the moons of Mars.

But if this still doesn't leave you baffled, know that George W. Bush, according to former Naval Intelligence officer Bill Cooper, was hired by MJ-12 long before he became president of the United States to take charge of traffic. of drugs that left South America on Navy ships. In Colombia, the army itself and the guerrillas take drugs through already known routes that go towards the Pacific coast and deliver them on the high seas to US flagships that take them to North America. This is how drugs arrive on our streets, not because of someone who put them in the sole of their shoe to pass through an airport detector. The drug traffickers' agreements with the shadow government have put them where they have been, and the leaders of various Latin American countries and Afghanistan have been overthrown when they have refused to cooperate with this agenda (instead, they receive great benefits by collaborating, either with the US and/or with the drug traffickers). In cases - such as in Colombia - the army is simply given the order to move away from certain places, because that is precisely where the guerrilla passes to carry the drug shipments to deliver them to the US Navy, or they take them out. by plane from clandestine airports, which are known to be used for these purposes, such as to transport gold illegally.

A. Another of the many strategies to finance their plans is war. Armed conflicts around the world serve as an excuse to move millions of dollars in war machinery. This is not direct financing, but collateral benefits.

1. The "problem" of "climate change." Solution: as we talked about, financing globalist plans and control of Africa's resources.

1. The "problem" of religion and families. Solution: LGBT, and pro-abortion movements, approval of laws to decriminalize rape and pedophilia, feminism (really 'feminazism'), ecumenism, Darwinism, pro-vaccination campaigns, and pro-transhumanism trends, among others. At first glance, someone may think, what relationship do these issues have? They have everything to do with it. You cannot subvert human morality as long as there are strong spiritual principles, such as those founded on religion (apart from the religiosity, sectarianism and legalism of its followers, which is a different matter). You can't destroy values if there is honor in family and marriage. Then you will hear a bombardment of "music" that talks about women as if they were prostitutes or objects, that disguises sexual disorder, polygamy, infidelity (adultery) and fornication as "love." Then you observe the brainwashing tendencies with soap operas – especially oriented towards mental docility, infidelity, social enmities and family mistrust -, the campaigns of "women's fight for their rights", which in reality is the promotion of the female ego to degrade her integrity as a woman to make her as scourge as scourge men. In essence, "if they are degenerate, I have a RIGHT to be one too." So then you make the value of the family look like something crude; the value of marriage as a

burden that no one wants; the desire to have children as another burden that violates our freedom of independence. When you have already destroyed the home, the children remain prisoners of the system to mold them to its will. And with regard to the Darwinist Agenda, it is a long topic, one of the oldest and best elaborated in Freemasonry (oriented to the indoctrination of academics, doctors, university students and scientists to have them in an unofficial "atheist religion"), of which which is what my first book, 'Creation vs. Evolution', but of which you can still see important details in an interview with former Satanist Roger Morneau.

1. The "problem" of the immune system. Harming the body is not so simple if you want to do it surreptitiously, and without raising too many suspicions. It is necessary to combine various elements that are convincing to those who do not understand, so that the world population can be reduced without them realizing at first glance what is happening. I have already explained this in previous books, there is the release of fluoride into tap water, saying that it is "good for the teeth", the same story as toothpastes, and few stop to find out that fluoride is a corrosive component, and that damages the pineal and pituitary glands (the pituitary gland). Instead of protecting teeth, it decalcifies in the long term, but not only that, they are going to be pouring nanometric components created in the laboratory into the water sources of all cities (see 'Remote Vision I', page 161) to subdue the people (slow down their minds and make them docile so that they stop the protests).

They sell you processed food with so many "E"s in the chemical value that you are no longer eating a food but a chemical compound. And they are not going to invest in organic substitutes, because it entails economic losses, and governments, clearly, do not subsidize that. They contaminate the meat, and soon they will say that it is poisoned, and it must be withdrawn from the markets, being replaced by a synthetic food, called "high in nutrients."

Yes, it's not a joke, it will be a chemical cocktail. But don't be surprised that they do sell you human meat, and at incredible prices (and guess where they get that meat from...). The food diets they promote are anti-scientific, and only benefit the meat and dairy industries whose corporations have agreements with governments, despite the fact that it has already been proven that meat is carcinogenic and dairy derivatives are saturated fat that also promotes phlegm in the lymphatic system, promoting allergies and the propensity to get sick. The "food pyramid" that is promoted does not have a scientific but a corporate basis: at the top of the "food chain" are the foods that represent the most movement in the corporate commercial structure in national and international agreements, followed by the foods that provide the least vitamins and minerals. to the organism. Only when you are already sick, your honest family doctor comes to recommend removing that crap from your diet. You should not wait to see the causes of acid nutrition. From childhood we should be taught about true food, the one that gives us health: ALKALINE.

Based on fresh fruit, fresh vegetables, organic and/or ecological products, preferably raw vegetables, whole grains, homemade unsweetened juices, dried and dried fruits, non-transgenic legumes, vegetables and tubers, and fungi (mushrooms), seeds and edible roots.

Another element of this cunning Rockefeller Manifesto ruse is releasing heavy metals and viruses like anthrax and other pathogens into the air via untagged airplanes. You recognize them by the way they form contrails different from those created by the combination of the heat from the turbines with the cold air at flight altitude. They promote a combination of what they call vaccines from the time the child is born and even into adulthood, either making people sick or even killing them with compounds that are even prohibited by the CDC itself, given their lethality. That is, if they do not suffer from autism. People are not even ethically informed about the composition of vaccines: aluminum, mercury, copper, chelates (other chemical compounds of metals), material from aborted fetuses, parts of organs from various animals and now modified RNA that alters our DNA. The pharmaceutical industry runs campaigns for health professionals, where they sell them their great "formulas" and offer them commissions for prescribing them. Doctors add a bonus to their salary by prescribing these things that they themselves, who are not scientists, have not analyzed in the laboratory. Such compounds do not cure anyone (they create permanent clients) and oppose the principle of the father of medicine, Hippocrates, "the natural forces found within us are those that truly cure our diseases."

1. The "problem" of civil lack of control and possible revolutions. Basically since the Vietnam War, protests and demonstrations have been a necessary issue to quell and prevent by the Deep State. In all parts of the world there were massive movements against the wars in Afghanistan and Iraq, and then in each country for their respective local issues. But as we approached the year 2019, the wave of these protests intensified uncontrollably. If progress was made in this direction, the powers that be would lose control, and risk possible insurrections and coups d'état. Faced with the danger posed by the aforementioned threat to its status quo and the security of the political establishment, the perfect solution came: restrictions (limitation of movement), distancing measures (social atomization), curfew, big technological brother (biometric monitoring) and implantable chips.

Now society, first frightened by the "bogeyman", obeyed the orders given by the governments to avoid civil uprising and mutiny. Starting from here, any conspiracy or plot perpetuated by the people could not be studied face to face but by digital means, a way in which tracking systems would easily detect who stirs up anti-system seditions and brawls. Social atomization, mental programming to create an apathetic society and virtual distractions separated individuals and chilled interpersonal relationships for many months – leaving consequences that in older people have fueled distrust -, achieving one of the greatest feats never conceived to end any future insurrection against the hegemony of the elite. In the same way, keeping individuals separated so as not to think en masse or evaluate together, it also prepared them so that in the short term surveillance satellites and reconnaissance drones could more easily identify and count the people gathered in a same place at the same time.

But if people saw a lot of unjustified military movement, they would rise up en masse. Of course, first they tell them that there are terrorist attacks in the cities, then militarizing them is justified. Later they are told that there are waves of immigrants filling the streets, causing riots, attacking civilians and causing disturbances on public property, then there is talk of more reasons for curfews and large-scale police mobilization. But the best excuse of all is to tell the masses that "the bogeyman" is out there and you should take refuge at home, while the army and the police take to the streets. This is called 'Martial Law', but under three sections of law which are the 'State of Alarm', the 'State of Siege' and the 'State of Exception'. Although civil legislation could protect you, the forces of "order" would have the last word under Martial Law, and the Executive over what they define as states of Alarm, Siege and/or Exception. As in all acts of False Flag - or self-attacks - a "force majeure" perpetuates a large-scale attack to justify these actions, limiting the people to being subjected to dictatorial and absolutist authority. This will continue to work throughout 2021 - as it did in 2020 - but it will not withstand social tension, leading to civil war in all parts of the world in a matter of months.

1. The "problem" of the limitations of mass surveillance. Even having such invasive or global tracking systems, it is not enough for the powers that be. Technology is going to continue to increase to unimaginable limits, except for the craziest science fiction movies. 'Big Bro Tech' is an abbreviated way of defining 'Big Technological Brother', the Orwellian world subjected to enormous video surveillance, satellite tracking, drones, motion readers, remote sound analyzers, police and military checkpoints. , biometric and facial readers, implanted chips and nano devices in the bloodstream, and everything, of course, will be subjected to computer networks under the absolute dominance of artificial intelligence. Complete dementia. But as if this were not enough, neighbors and relatives are encouraged to denounce their own, as other more contemporary prophets already warned.

The Jewish prophet Daniel told us about this unprecedented advance in technology, writing more than 2,500 years ago about the final events of our era, where the archangel Gabriel would have anticipated him: <<Daniel, close the words and seal the book until the time of the end. Many will run from here to there, and knowledge will increase.>> (Dan. 12:4, KJV 60) Hebraist Rabbis have interpreted these words of "they will run from here to there" as an allusion to the race of modern man in haste. of large cities, and others have added that it is defining the freedom of movement around the world, offered by means of transportation (vehicles, trains, planes, ships), something also prophesied hundreds of years ago by the Jopi Indians in Arizona. The word 'science' is used in ancient Hebrew to refer to advancement in knowledge as well as technology. According to the archangel Gabriel, these would be the signs that we have reached the end of this era.

Likewise, we find that this establishment of "anti-social" ideas, of distrust, is increasing, and we will see more and more people at odds with others and reviling them for not wearing a mask, for not wearing gloves, for not applying gels, for not allowing themselves putting a temperature scanner, for not abiding by curfew rules and, above all, for not getting vaccinated. In fact, if your neighbor hears you sneeze or knows that you have the flu, he will call the authorities so that a doctor with two soldiers can enter your house against your will and take you "to the hospital," and give you "the cure." In this order of things, anti-vaccine, anti-system people, Christians, activists, researchers, among others, will be the object of civil unrest, seen by others – even their own family – as enemies, and they will betray and betray themselves. This was warned at least 50 years ago by ufologist Billy Meier, or before him by Helen White – famous prophet of the Adventists – but it has actually been predicted by many people. Yeshua (Jesus) said it, warning, <<And all this will be the beginning of sorrows. Then they will hand you over to tribulation and kill you, and you will be hated by all nations for

my name's sake. Many will then stumble, and will betray one another, and will hate one another. And many false prophets will arise and deceive many; and because wickedness has multiplied, the love of many will grow cold.>> (Matt. 24:8-12, KJV 60)

Likewise, the issue of artificial intelligence was warned in the Bible, as had already been said years ago by people like the speaker Gary Renard, who captured it in one of his books based on the visits of two transcendent apostles. The book of Revelation, from the year 90 AD, approximately, defines it like this: <<And he was allowed to breathe breath into the image of the beast, so that the image could speak and cause everyone who did not worship it to be killed. And he caused everyone, small and great, rich and poor, free and slave, to have a mark placed on their right hand, or on their forehead; and that no one could buy or sell, except he who had the mark or the name of the beast, or the number of his name.>> (Rev. 13:15-17, KJV 60) First we must remember that these people who wrote These lines did not know what they were seeing, and tried to define it with their words. In the same way, it must be understood that translations are not faithful to complex concepts of the original language in which a manuscript is written. I already explained this in previous works, but in short, the "image" he talks about is a representative logo or slogan, an appearance; the Beast is the global government; the "breath", or "spirit" (numen) that it receives is self-consciousness; The mark is an incision or puncture of something that is inserted into the skin. In essence it is saying that the Antichrist will give the order that the global logo-image of the world system receive its own consciousness, and this artificial intelligence, upon becoming autonomous, orders to persecute and eliminate all opposition to the system.

1. The "problem" of national sovereignty and so many politicians. To establish a global government, the borders and sovereignty of each country must be torn down, and so many politicians, and the idea of democracy or dissent of opinion, must be removed from the way. Solution: globalization, "climate change" plan and submission to international laws to stop a supposed pandemic, pushed by the WHO. We have this dilemma of whether all world leaders took this the same way, but it's my assumption that they didn't. The rulers who allowed themselves to be bribed to sell their nation have much to gain. A president or prime minister will not maintain his position forever, nor will he continue to have the benefits he has while in charge of a country. However, the promise of wealth, immunity (untouchability) and his own paradise by the time he leaves office sound convincing. And the moralists? Easy, from history we know how easy it is to get out of these: you send them a picture of their wife and daughters and they already get the hint, or after the first bomb attack or sniper attack they should have gotten the idea. If not, he'll catch her in the coffin. And will everyone else accept this? Of course not, especially those whose power goes beyond settling for something less than what they already possess. Those will have to

be brought down with a thermonuclear war.

1. And the "problem" of the anti-system? Very simple. They will be categorized as a terrorist threat. This will justify any type of action against them, without the possibility of lawyers or judicial arguments or prosecution. This way, they can come to your house, break down the door, put a hood over your head and handcuffs, and put you in a truck and no one ever hears from you again. Later I will talk in more detail about this and its best-known name: the Purge.

1. The "problem" of freedom of expression and anti-system opinion movement. Solution: veto on social networks and online platforms. Have you been banned from images, videos or comments on Twitter, Youtube, Facebook or Instagram? Welcome to the club. Imagine the helplessness of thousands of health and science professionals wanting to report the truth and whose content is removed or censored from the internet. At best, they add a label to the post that takes the viewer to another page of fear media propaganda, or says that it is "partially false" or literally "false," supposedly verified by such independent fact-checkers, who seem so fast and efficient that they leave the best espionage and monitoring maneuvers of the NSA in their infancy. That is, they do not exist, they are algorithms that respond to words like "vaccine dangers", "side effects", "fraud pandemic" or "pedophile Bill Gates". It's funny that if you make memes or post information about corruption and political plots on social media they threaten to block your account, but if you do it about Donald Trump, those "independent fact checkers"

don't work. And if you go out in a public place or program telling the truth, they will jump at your neck. They shut you up quickly and ridicule you to the hilt. To begin with, they don't even invite you.

Human judgment and its rights of free expression must be suppressed, in the words of the elite. Therefore the powers that be use Nicola Machiaveli's system, where they put several of their puppets in the hands of the same puppeteer, so that people choose between one or the other, believing that they have a free choice, without knowing that both puppets are pawns of the same subject. This is true in all areas, political, sports, news and often also corporate or banking. It is irrelevant who you vote for, they are all following agendas 'A' or 'B' of the same agent. It doesn't matter which basketball, soccer, football or baseball team you choose: they are all money laundering chains and means of mass distraction and divisions (if you are on the red team and I am on the blue team, we are enemies). The news shows you 'world news', or 'find out current events', when in reality they tell you what the elites pay them to tell you. The same thing happens with television series, advertisements, movies and music videos, among many other mechanisms. It has been proven that practice makes perfect, and that repetition achieves memorization of concepts. What better way to introduce an idea of fear and submission permanently into social consciousness than by repeating over and over again 'dead', 'infected', 'terror', 'terrorism', 'weapons of mass destruction', 'state of emergency'?

', 'preventive measures', 'the vaccine', 'new normal',
'everything will return to normal after the second
dose', 'protect yourself, for yourself, for everyone'...?

Hollywood is a Jesuit tool of social indoctrination,
and the same with the music industry, especially
American and British (where you lift a stone and a
new band comes out). To achieve "fame", both in
these industries and at the political level of the highest
spheres, those who enter here are forced to participate
in certain ceremonies and initiation rites of a satanic
nature, where there is rape, pedophilia, blood, orgies.
and humiliations, which are filmed and used as
blackmail so that the new adept and pawn never
thinks of speaking out. The demonic power is so
influential in this structure of social influence that
when a new album is released, the first copy is placed
in the center of a pentagram with the corresponding
symbols, blood and spells, as well as planetary
alignment, and a druid or sorcerer consecrates, with
the attendees, said record so that the influence of
demons can use it wherever it is heard. I could
dedicate an entire book to talking about how the
universe works by vibration, and therefore, how the
"numinous world" uses vibration. Thus, sound is a
channel of fluctuation, like a bridge, that carries
"entities" from one side to the other, and also
introduces them into the biomagnetic field of an
individual, an animal, or even a tree or a stone. . And
if we add to this the use of sigils and subliminal
messages, or the deliberate lyricism of mental
conditioning or adaptation to certain tendencies, you

will easily program millions of people, especially young people with docile minds who have not yet forged their personality.

1. The "problem" of scientific evidence and testimony of health professionals and the military. Solution: threats to state officials (politicians, doctors, police, scientists, soldiers...) or bribes, as appropriate. There are "incentives" from pharmaceutical companies and the government towards social security, for those who see it naively, and/or brainwashing and indoctrination of medical personnel. In the midst of a crisis like the current one, many "sell their souls to the devil," and few risk losing their jobs, medical benefits, and pension. The other thing is the obvious financing of the news media, and the elimination and/or ridicule of alternative media. That's why they only talk about the bogeyman and humiliate Donald Trump. Have you seen any television debates about coconuts? Have you seen any opposing sides or opinions that differ from the official version? Where is the objective debate? Where are the opinions of both parties? Where are those who think differently or have something different to comment? They are not even invited to participate, although they are then silenced. It appears that the entire scientific and medical horde is in agreement, and in the meantime everyone is controlled under threats. Doctors and soldiers and police have been notified not to give public information about what they hear or know, or they will lose their jobs, must pay large fines and will be taken to trial, potentially going to jail.

1. The "problem" of freedom of thought and critical

reasoning. Solution: Mind control. Television indoctrination (misinformation), injected heavy metals, calcification of the pineal gland, fear, belief that the authorities are watching over them and they do not need to worry but simply obey. You may not have heard of the Mk-Ultra project, much less the Monarch project, and of course, nor things about the Sedgwich project. Well, these are just a part of the many mind control programs run by the CIA. Social movements and trends are collective design agendas pushed by the Mockingbird project. Do you really think that kids who watch shooting video games buy guns and start a school shooting? It's a CIA ruse. In their case, boys under mind control, directed by the Orion program, to disarm the American people with laws that prohibit the carrying of weapons. You will also not have heard of the Montauk project, which is the use of time travel technology - connected to the Pegasus project, teleportation -, from which the RainBow project came, through which chrononauts traveled to the time of Yeshua (Jesus). , or about the Oak Tree project, where the Mannequin project came from, to genetically select children for remote viewing use , or generally psychics, like The Tomorrow People program. Well, the amount of secret investigations that the CIA has directed and that have been carried out in G room Lake, in Area 51 would break your brain.

Social conditioning work is strategic and necessary to shape people's minds. It is key then to complement it with the toxicity of water, air, food and drugs (whether legal or not (medications, pharmaceuticals), and, if possible, "darken the Sun" (that is, the sky). Damaging the pituitary gland (hypophysis, or pituitary gland) prevents the person from developing critical and reasoning abilities, as well as extrasensory or spiritual abilities. That is why it is calcified by the toxins that enter the body, and the mental aspect It is programmed progressively. Did you know that the television emits a frequency of 30 Hertz? The brain emits Beta, Alpha, Theta and Delta waves, and responds to these same waves (even Gamma) and levels of frequency and vibration, because the organism itself It is composed of molecules, which are assembled into atoms, which are energy, and this is vibration. When you sit in front of the TV, the Hertz waves place your mind in a state of assimilation, so that you accept images, colors, words, ideas, concepts and tendencies of those who project them there. This was already known to the FBI from secrets discovered from the studies of the USSR, and became especially notable already in 1958, when the New York Times published an article about experiments by the 'Subliminal Projection Company Inc'. Classified documents from July 1972 addressed quite well the use of subliminal technology for messages to penetrate the subconscious mind so that the people would do what the controllers wanted (see more in 'Recognizing the Time of the End', chapter 1, sections G and H).

1. The "problem" of Christian resistance. Although religion plays a limiting role in many areas of mental freedom, on the other hand it provides certain

principles and values that can be essential in a society without positive moral or ethical criteria. Although many philosophical movements - such as Buddhism or Taoism - are included as religions, not all of them are. Even so, most of them fulfill some social role in one way or another that can serve as a small lever for various people. Because of this, belief systems such as those of an Abrahamic nature (namely, Islam, Judaism, neo-reformists, Catholicism or Christianity) represent an obstacle to the Illuminati current. It is not because their ideas are correct, but because behind the ideas and precepts there is a neurolinguistic programming that endangers the interests of the elite. Islam contains an active anti-Zionist component, and a strong part of its religious rigor lies in the tacit and systematic opposition to the New World Order, political Zionism, the Illuminati and every other movement related to the manifestation of the Antichrist . Christianity denies the divinity of the Antichrist, and rejects him, and its values also clash with the Illuminati hegemony, starting with rejecting identification chips in humans. For its part, Judaism does not bow to human or terrestrial movements, considering that the Messiah comes from heaven, not from human parameters.

Since none of this helps the manifestation of the Antichrist, the Deep State has directed various solutions: knowing that Western religion sees pornography as bad, they inoculate it and sneak in the devotees of said movements everywhere to create in them charges of guilt and marital or relationship problems. They are responsible for financing great leaders to preach information that is incapacitating (stunning them and taking away critical reasoning) and dissuasive (far from reality). On a social level, they weaken them psychologically, and, as seen now with the "coconut", they make them lose their "faith" (or what Christians call 'faith'). Just like many people who are lost, aimless, and afraid, they are deceived by a new wave of gurus for this time (false teachers, false prophets, false saviors), with absurd false beliefs, knowing that a wave of desperate people will look for leaders who give them hope. Meanwhile, those who are awake will be categorized as a threat to security (anti-vaccines), and therefore, terrorists (radicals, extremists). Those who escape all this pressure and harassment must beware of the last big trap before the so-called 'Rapture', the false rapture. Yeshua said about these events: <<Take heed that no one deceives you. For many will come in my name, saying, I am the Christ; and they will deceive many.>> (Matt. 24:4-5, KJV 60) And later he adds, <<And many false prophets will arise, and deceive many...>> (Matt. 24:11, KJV 60) Then declares, <<if anyone says to you, Look, here is the Christ, or look, there he is, do not believe it. [...] Therefore, if they say to you, Look, it is in the desert, do not go out; or look, it is in the chambers, do not believe it.>> (Matt. 24:23-26, RVA 60). If you want to understand this in greater depth, I recommend my work 'Remote Vision I', chap. 17 and 18.

But the Illuminati's strategy does not stop there. They have undermined the principles of Islam to use Muslims as a weapon. For many years MI5, MI6, Mossad and the CIA have infiltrated Arab countries to create jihad drivers. In the US, the shadow power has been in charge of motivating groups like Black Life Matters, to incite black people against white people. They had already begun to do this with Martin Luther King, and when Malcolm X realized this, they killed both. The same with the Muslim Brotherhood , which is the agenda to guide black Americans towards "Islam", but it is not true Islam but jihadist

Shiism, which in due time will attack Jews and Christians in the US. This is all part of 'The Purge' Agenda. The Muslim groups brought into Europe - under the Kalergi Plan -, already indoctrinated in this mission, will unleash a wave of kidnappings and attacks, especially on Christian and Catholic churches, and synagogues (Jewish temples). This is planned for all radical groups, as XXX (Xu Xlux Xlan, or Klu Klux Klan) itself still exists, and these will be white supremacists who will kill blacks. Families without values will surrender to the authorities, neighbors without values will reveal themselves to the authorities, the pro-vaccine will hate the anti-vaccine, society will hate the anti-establishment and Christians, and the police force will arrest the activists, protesters and opponents of the system. This is the Machiavellian masterstroke: putting everyone against everyone.

1. The racial "problem." Since the origins of the draconians, the idea of racial supremacy was a central ideological axis. The manipulation of genetics has therefore been so important to them, so that they damage the purity of the DNA of other species, thus achieving their deterioration and reduction of their potential capabilities. Reptilians cannot understand how our DNA, composed of 21/22 interventions from 21/22 races in this galaxy, can contain so much quasi-limitless potential. They have tried mixtures and alterations of our race for a long time, but they still do not understand our origin and superiority, despite everything, nor do they manage to replicate the numen (spirit) or the power of the ether. Consequently, they promote the idea of the single race and its supremacy, which is pushed from civilization to civilization, and

from world to world. Hence Hitler's racial idea, the same Illuminati racial idea, wanting to eliminate Asian, Latino, Indian and black genotypes. Their solution: poison, harm and kill non-Aryan color groups, ethnicities and genotypes (e.g. Latinos, Africans, indigenous people, and presumably also Arabs, and possibly even Asians (except high-status families)). That is why the vaccines and viruses that the elite create are genetically selective and will harm precisely this group of people.

1. The "problem" of insurance and pensions. Governments lose a lot of money paying benefits to disabled people, on social insurance hospital expenses, on pensions and on medical care for the elderly. Their solution: poison, harm and kill the elderly and disabled (the groups of people who account for high national expenditures on health insurance, life policies and pensions). For this they bring the weapons of the Petrochemical Cartel, or commonly called the Pharmaceutical Industry (from the word Pharmakon (poison), even though they define their premises as 'Drugstores', because they are literally drugs, which they call "medicine" (because "Medicate" is not to cure but to treat permanently: to create drug addicts). They fill people with pills and unnatural compounds to make them clients for life, while they eat away at and damage their entire organism. They end up squeezing every last drop of their savings and vitality, and then they get rid of them. But because the hegemon's interests currently underlie the vision of beginning their New World Order, population reduction and resource

remanagement is more relevant. Therefore, they pay health centers to carry out wrong procedures and report covid cases, and they also use the elderly as guinea pigs for the new vaccines, and they begin to carry out their Nazi-style mass euthanasia.

1. The "problem" of the opposition. From politics or the leaders of the Resistance, through religious leaders and even the resources of the preppers (survivalists), reaching the beggars themselves, all insurgency or discrepancy will be erased. Solution: The Purge (selective and general elimination), if they let themselves be bought, good, and if not, then in one night and in one hour they will get rid of all these "undesirables."

1. The "problem" of information leakage. Two components come in here. On the one hand, the use of the most macabre technology and least known to humanity: mind control. I will talk about that later because it is essential when it comes to understanding what is happening in the world and why the vast majority of people not only do not know the truth, but they attack it when they hear it. There are levels of compartmentalization of secrets to impressive degrees (in the US alone there are 13 levels of compartmentalization about the president himself, categorized as Classified, Top Secret and Above Top Secret). This is known in agencies like the CIA, MI6 and the KGB, because it was taken from the Nazis, but the CIA has been set up by the Illuminati to destroy much of this information. Many of the greatest secret knowledge are only transmitted orally so as not to leave

traces. Mind control technology is an example of that super-classified science . This mind control technology is based on the different egos of the self (where the Alter egos come from, the misnamed 'multiple personality') and hypnosis, and is directly linked to the satanic cult and pedophile networks, the main Illuminati menu.

Those who know, or believe they know something, cannot report it for two reasons: 1. They have been mentally programmed to have memory disorder, so they do not know if what they remember is real or fictitious. 2. They are under blackmail, because they have been involved in rituals and murders to get to where they have arrived. The rest, such as the media, television campaigns, and film and music programming, are systematically structured by widely spread mechanisms of mind control. In other words, humanity is being mentally controlled without knowing it, programming their minds with a technology typical of the Orionites, and classic of the j-rod (gray ETs, or big-headed aliens) for use in abductions.

1. To end this chapter I will mention another of the "problems" that the Deep State has encountered: the economy and jobs. The paradigm shift to the Fourth Industrial Age is essential, and the cornerstone, of the mechanics for the global government of the Antichrist - as many of us define it -. Solution: start with new "labor reforms", promoting working from home, and offer the UBI (Universal Basic Income), which I will expand on when talking about the Financial Reset. Understand that the era of robotics, satellite identification, digital

payments, quantum computers, automated drones, virtual reality, holograms, human implantable chips, biometric recognition and artificial intelligence have already erased the era. job you met. This is the new paradigm. By introducing robots that replace humans, or supercomputers and artificial intelligence programs, one of the things that are saved is time that must be paid to others (salaries, commissions, pensions, social security, unemployment, settlements, bonuses, overtime, etc.), as well as labor complaints, protests, demands, resignations, absence due to health or compensation. Robots would not complain or get tired, they do not need a salary, and even if they received it, what would they spend it on?

III. GLOBALIST PLANS

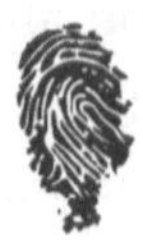

What is the 2030 Agenda? Is it true that the powers that be carry out a plan to reduce the world population? Well, supranational organizations that control the largest banks in the world have pushed global propaganda in the face of the largest financial fall in all of history. Mr Swab of the International Monetary Fund is now the spokesman for propaganda about preparations for the Great Reset. Over the next few years, not only will civil liberties be taken away, but all financial means will crumble, starting with the lower classes. The 2030 Agenda is the plan for social change aimed at the implementation of a planetary empire, basically. In essence, according to its promoters, everything would be controlled from Brussels, Jerusalem, the Vatican and London. It is the combination of several philosophies, which, ultimately, derive from beliefs of racial supremacy, deeply rooted in the European aristocracy.

Among them is the figure of a messiah king, heir to the most important thrones of the monarchies, whether Davidic, Merovingian, Arthurian or Windsor. That is the case of the supporters of the political Zionist movement, who conceive of the reestablishment of the Jewish nation to turn it into a superpower, dominating the rest. However, the word Zionism is not understood in the same way in the rabbinic structure or in Christianity. These two currents disagree about the way "Zionism" is interpreted by "Zionists." The idea that Tzion (Zion) - the fortress of Yerushalim (Jerusalem) - is the seat of command of the Messiah and the axis of the world is seen by mainstream Judaism and the Christian world as a peaceful mission accomplished by the Savior of the World Himself. In contrast, the Political Zionists push these ideals humanely, and for this they plan all kinds of possible stratagems that allow them, not only to make Israel the most powerful nation in the world the hard way, but also to have a leader placed at its head. world, which is also sovereign of the entire globe. However, it is the Zionists who take land from the settlers of the occupied territories using the army, it is not at all a "Jewish" interest. Evidently Christians see Jesus of Nazareth as the person who should appear as said ruler, but Judaism in general disagrees that Yeshu (as they call Yehoshua or Yeshua, that is, Jesus) meets the characteristics to be Mashiach ben Dauid (Messiah son of David). In this regard, I recommend my work 'The Mystery of the Messiah'.

The banking and corporate system was subject to the hegemonic powers that came from dynasties such as Rockefeller or Rothschild, and other even older and more powerful ones also of Jewish origin that can be traced back as far as the 8th century AD. C. This organization that is above every nation, corporation and banking system is known as the Deep State - mainly consolidated with the assassination of John F. Kennedy, since it was previously called MJ-12 -, although not all They are Jews (an essential part of the power of the Deep State is found in the Jesuit leadership). They raise presidents or overthrow them, invade nations and destabilize them and put them in debt. They cause and finance all the wars and revolutions that have taken place from the Renaissance to the present day. Its purpose is to create a Global Government without borders, under a single planetary leader, a single global army, a single philosophical ideology and a single monetary system, digital, by the way, with all humanity transhumanized, pardon the redundancy.

Progressively, the movements generated have achieved what is known today as Globalization, and which in the present disappears to give rise to the era of Artificial Intelligence, where everything will be controlled by quantum super computers that will have all communications networks, video surveillance, centralized. , tracking, secret services, satellites, social networks and personal data of each human being. The Technological Big Brother, part of the Industrial Revolution Charter.

At the end of 2019, the Deep State accelerated its agenda to orchestrate the system that would be imposed on our planet from 2030 (according to its plan), especially because Donald Trump played against them and began to put the elites on trial. An essential part of the COVID Agenda consists of microchips implanted in the right hand or forehead of the human being, and the absolute monitoring of Artificial Intelligence of all these devices, under which would be global tyranny and the police state. Dogs and cats are already given these RFID encoders and trackers, but putting them on men, women and children is not something that is socially acceptable. What the globalists are looking for with this is the control of movement and registration of individuals, considering that by that time the reduction in the world population will reduce the number of traceable and controllable people (who remain as a minority at that time, who would be "zombies")." robotic humans - and transhumans -, lacking individual thought, decision making or judgment, a race of people emotionally driven by mere primary instincts (survival), without conscience, use of reason or analysis, and above all, without love, empathy or spirituality). To this end, since 1983, satellite systems have been deployed and are progressively expanded and updated, new antennas are installed (during 2022, 6G networks will spread, which is military technology which will be deployed by the army itself), and More sophisticated, new tracking devices are introduced, and applications where individuals voluntarily hand over all their personal information and network access to their private data and cameras and microphone. Yes, if you were thinking about Facebook, it is indeed an FBI tool to collect the databases of all its users.

For the perfect triangulation of all antenna systems and networks, it is necessary that each person have an implanted chip and a high number of levels of heavy metals in the blood. Most of these heavy metals and chelates are introduced through injections. Exactly, that is what the massive vaccination campaigns in each nation come from. When the Illuminati motivated World War II, it intended to get Adolf Hitler to push for a conflagration that would encourage the world to unite nations. And it seems like they were geniuses, but they are not (rather their reptile masters are). The Political Zionists brought Harry S. Truman to power as president, to create the United Nations Organization, financed by the Rockefeller Foundation, the same ones who even gave up the building where the UN headquarters is currently located (as well as the Rothschilds They gave up what is the Israeli parliament building). The Rockefellers, another Jewish Zionist family, were the American part of the movement developing the political Zionist plan, as other Zionists were developing it in Tsarist Russia and the USSR.

The UN was intended to lay the foundations for a Deep State Global Government that would ultimately put all power in the hands of the Israeli and European government, under Jesuit control. Thus, in 1947 the United Nations Assembly recognized Israel as a state that should be legitimized and declared the right of the Jewish people, so that the Hebrews would return to the "holy land", although it created 3 divisions: State of Israel, State of Palestine. and the West Bank (West Bank). For the Deep State, this division must disappear, and be replaced by the original barriers that the nation of Israel had in 900 BC. C., which recognizes that the West Bank is the land of Ihudeah (Judea), the land of King David.

You can learn more by researching, for example, the Sykes-Picot Agreements, the Balfour Declaration and the Bretton Woods Agreements. Well, the idea was already on the table, now the regions just had to continue uniting. Then the League of Arab Countries was born, in 1945; the OAS appears, the Organization of American States in 1948 and the WHO (World Health Organization); in 1949 the North Atlantic Treaty Organization (NATO) was established; in 1957 the first idea of union between European nations; in 1960 OPEC (Organization of Petroleum Exporting Countries); in 1993 the European Union was consolidated; In 2001, the African Union, or United States of Africa, was proposed, although the elite did not like it due to the intentions of freedom that Gaddafi, its motivator, wanted with it; In 2002 the Asian Union appeared and the Euro Zone was established, with the currency that bears its name; in 2003 the Pacific Union was proposed; In 2004 the Latin American Union was defined; In 2005, the treaty of the North American Union (the union of Canada, the United States and Mexico) was signed, although this was carried out by George W. Bush Jr. without the media covering the news until some time later. public only within a certain union, and was made without the approval of Congress; In 2008 the Mediterranean Union appears. This is just a brief example of the great speed with which globalization has taken place since WWII.

The "devil" creates the problem, and when the reactions are seen, he proposes the dynamic to fix it: Action => Reaction => Solution. It is worth noting whether people like Napoleon or Hitler were really tools of the Illuminati itself to catalyze global "union" movements, which without them would not have been possible (thanks to Hitler the Jesuits took Germany back; thanks to Napoleon the Church Catholic – who made use of the Inquisition – was disarmed). There are no "good guys" here, but rather agendas to move forward. Darwinism had to eliminate the religion-science relationship, and Napoleon had to eliminate the religion-state power of the "Church." We are all grateful that the "Holy" Inquisition has stopped, but behind it there are other maneuvers. The Jesuits changed the world with their "revolutions" and "wars" giving the appearance of a new democracy, but with the aim of removing power from the "religion" and passing it on to the "union of states." It is the same as with the Coudenhove-Kalergi Agenda that George Soros has been promoting in Europe, where he intends that the ideas and beliefs of the immigrants who arrive en masse adulterate the integrity and indigenous folklore of each and every one of the European peoples (It is worth saying that it is something already designed and financed by the Rockefellers for years). What do they get out of this?

As the letters between the Master Masons Albert Pike and Giuseppe Mazzini (1870-1871) explain, <<The Third World War will be fomented by taking advantage of the differences caused by the agents of the Illuminati between the political Zionists and the leaders of the Islamic World. The war **must be conducted in such a way that Islam and political Zionism mutually destroy each other**. Meanwhile, the other nations, once again divided on this issue, will be forced to fight to the point of complete physical, moral, spiritual and economic exhaustion... We will unleash the Nihilists and the atheists, and provoke a formidable social <u>cataclysm which in all its horror will clearly show to the nations the effect of absolute atheism,</u>

<u>the origin of cruelty and the bloodiest riots</u>. Then, everywhere, **the citizens, forced to defend themselves against the world minority of revolutionaries**, will exterminate those destroyers of civilization, and <u>the multitude, disillusioned with Christianity, whose deistic spirits will from that moment be without compass or direction, eager to an ideal, but not knowing where to direct their worship, they will receive the true light through the universal manifestation of the pure doctrine of Lucifer </u>, finally brought to public view. This manifestation will result **from the general reactionary movement that will follow the destruction of Christianity and atheism**, both conquered and exterminated at the same time.>>

The Deep State has overthrown all opposition to the regime by motivating civil uprisings, wars, and blackmail and threats, using the secret services. Eventually each president must cede between 2021 and 2022 – or at the latest a couple of years from this moment, starting with local governments – national autonomy, for which the basis is to see how world leaders have been tied up before the WHO with the 'plan -of me'. They must comply with these orders, willingly or unwillingly, and in the meantime they must carry out a theater policy before public opinion, creating false hopes and expectations in the very short term. Bill Gates, as one of the fathers of what would lead to Artificial Intelligence today, is - along with George Soros in other areas (and who has already been expelled from Austria and is being openly condemned in places like England, Russia, Holland, Poland and Hungary) - one of the people chosen to carry the voice in the campaign to implement these microchips and mass vaccination.

In the last two years, several influential governments have tried to create restrictive global vaccination laws, but they were always pushed back by large citizen protests, especially in the

US. Because of this, the Deep State organized on October 18, 2019 the called **Event 201**, a "simulation" "exercise" at The Pierre hotel in New York, about the "pandemic." They needed to plan how humanity globally would accept mass vaccination without any opposition, and would allow themselves to be drawn into a police state. The key was to spread fear of such a planetary pandemic through all the media, and receiving large amounts of international financing. You can see an example at this link: https://kaosenlared.net/el-coronavirus-se-ensayo-mediante-un-simulacro-de-pandemia-en-septiembre-de-2019-en-un-hotel-de-   new-york/?fbclid=IwAR2cyGuj8cU_AXVyoJ69X0myBJlPZsoNKa5zlrv7_[1].

The virus called Sars-Cov is actually a common type of virus among animals. The names Sars, Cov, Mers, are changes in the nomenclature that owe their modification to the fact that this type of flu was altered in laboratories. The patents for said virus are, in fact, registered in London in 2014. The already known SARS, which in that same 2014 would have supposedly caused hundreds of infections, was "improved." You have to understand that the elite uses words cleverly to confuse. Replaces the idea of "mutation" as something natural with something unnatural. There a fan of windows will open to you, open towards the light of truth, towards where the question is going. Four strains of HIV were subsequently introduced to this unnatural pathogen, as well as TB (tuberculosis), to make it more contagious, although it is not more lethal than the common flu itself. This virus was studied by American and Chinese scientists after this

---

1.   https://kaosenlared.net/el-coronavirus-se-ensayo-mediante-un-simulacro-de-pandemia-en-septiembre-de-2019-en-un-hotel-de-nueva-york/?fbclid=IwAR2cyGuj8cU_AXVyoJ69X0myBJlPZsoNKa5zlrv7_3GKkEzOnvwIwRNeJJw

in other experiments in 2015 until 2019 when it was ready in Wuhan laboratories for use. Another example: https://www.youtube.com/ watch?v=EEJeVHZieaA&feature=youtu.be&fbclid=IwAR2e_36s0N2Q [2].

A month after the Event 201 meeting, the first known case of alleged covid-19 occurred. In November 2019, a Chinese scientist, helped by two reporters, leaked to public opinion and the networks that a "virus" had been deliberately released into the population, and that the 5G antennas that were being reported everywhere were causing serious disorders. related to the "virus". These three individuals were arrested by the Chinese government and locked up for 3 weeks. After this time they were released, and they supposedly had COVID-19 and died. Since then, scientists who claim that 5G antennas launch high-frequency waves that damage DNA, and produce the effects attributed to Covid-19: influenza and atypical pneumonia, have been **silenced**. At the end of November, demonstrations against the installation of these microwave antennas had begun. Thus, in December 2019, the waves from the newly installed and tested antennas in the city of Wuhan took many people to medical centers, where they were injected with the real virus: the Wuhan-400 chimera. This was on this date since the world New Year coincided and days later the Chinese New Year, when such people go on a trip around the globe. Thus, it is thought, they would distribute the virus at high speed (in reality they distributed pathogens that permeated everywhere on purpose).

---

2.   https://www.youtube.com/ watch?v=EEJeVHZieaA&feature=youtu.be&fbclid=IwAR2e_36s0N2Qsuo4LClAq2 PEBA179exn7PhVti7A8doLPXhPIjU7AhYALU8

A Chinese military affairs website published that same December 2019 that at the World Military Games (held in the city of Wuhan from October 18 to 27, 2019) US army soldiers had released a pathogen that affected only Asian genotypes. The report was later deleted. The Chinese government was informed of people suffering certain reactions, but none of those people had been to the famous "market" where "bat soup" was made. The CCP (Chinese Communist Party) hid the truth for days and incriminated the first doctor who reported the matter. Later, Europe's leaders did the same, delaying the "seriousness" of the matter to give the cases time to spread, some say. Sources claim that President Xi Jinping went to Wuhan and put the pro-US faction of the Deep State in charge. In China there would be a patriotic faction close to the Russians, which would be led by Xi Jinping, and another in favor of the US Deep State, composed of former members of the communist party (komsomol) who are more money-oriented, which They would have used the virus to gain political and economic power. Ergo, Xi Jinping put them in charge, and consequently, the virus was "ended" in China and it spread to Europe.

Initially, the pathogen had been introduced into the winter 2019 flu vaccine in various countries, so the adverse reactions arrived just in time. This is because many governments are involved, it is not something exclusively for China or the US. In tune with this, enough 5G antennas had been retracted to begin bombarding hundreds of microtests on the population, causing them to feel similar symptoms. to flu, fever or pneumonia. Likewise, the Chinese government sent many of those Chinese out of the country with viral particles that they spread throughout Europe and the US, which was later discovered when reviewing hundreds of surveillance cameras. China wanted to destabilize Europe's economy, and collaterally that of the enemy who wanted to risk them first. However, we must understand that this story defines the Sars-Cov-2 chimera virus as different things from what COVID-19/COVID-21 is as an agenda - or what I sometimes call the 'Wuhan 400', inspired by the novel by Dean Koontz, 'The Eyes of Darkness', 1981 (which tells of the outbreak of a virus created in Wuhan laboratories, which spreads rapidly creating a global pandemic) -.

The Wuhan-400 was a chimera manufactured in American laboratories, and where the Wuhan Biological Laboratory was a study work facility between both nations on types of coronavirus that could mutate and be passed to other mammals, especially humans, starting from the "infamous" Sars-Cov-2. But this had already been going on since before 2014, when, in fact, the patent for this chimera was registered, which would be used as a "vaccine" (see public patent record 'EP3172319A1'). The Chinese Wuhan Biological Laboratory is actually owned by Glaxo, who coincidentally is the owner/majority partner of Pfizer, who curiously manages the finances of Black Rock, who precisely manages the finances of the Open Foundation Society (of George Soros), who in turn, it deals with the interests of the French company AXA, of which the German company Winterthur also built the Chinese laboratory, bought by the German company Allianz, and whose large shareholder is Vanguard, which is a shareholder of Black Rock – and we return to the beginning -, which controls the central banks and manages 1/3 of the world's investment capital, which in turn is a large shareholder of Microsoft and Bill Gates, who for his part is a shareholder of Pfizer - and we return to the beginning - and currently the first WHO sponsor.

Does all this tell you something? 'Agenda 21' (like the year 2021, although they say it is for the 21st century), now called 'Agenda 2030' – which is the UN agenda to create a global government – plans to begin the institution of the World Government in situ. They have put the World Health Organization at the forefront of the fear propaganda campaign that would justify the confinement of more than 6 billion people without any objection, so that new deprivation laws could be advanced at great speed. rights and citizen control. The leading voice of the WHO in this campaign of mass deception is Anthony Fauci.

As Daniel Stulin (researcher and former KGB agent) has said, the "virus" has a fourth dimension: the economic one. It has a first objective: religion (they destabilize religious institutions and churches, and call into question their beliefs and faith), the destruction of the people's freedoms, the reduction of the population; the second is the establishment of control over humanity; the third is to deflate the financial bubble; and the fourth the elimination of geoeconomic competition. The economic system that has been maintained since the dissolution of the USSR between 1989 and 1991 was under the control of the US Federal Reserve Bank (the FED), which prints more banknotes than are justified by gold. The numbers are created on a computer, adding zeros to the right with impunity, since the capitalist system allows the growth of industries to justify economic growth. In 2001 the US economy was about to collapse, so they launched the False Flag attack on the World Trade Center, thus prompting the invasion of several countries. This sets the entire military apparatus in motion, allowing the permanent installation of military bases abroad and the theft of the wealth of the invaded nations, not to mention that the invaders themselves then send their construction industries to rebuild what the war destroyed. Since with the end of the Arab Spring only Iran and Syria remained to be invaded, Russia intervened and Trump finally pulled out his troops, leaving the matter to Erdogan, president of Turkey. This did not end the story, it only imposed a temporary cessation before the next phase of the war.

The economic and market system that we know is destined to disappear between 2021 and 2022 - at the latest -, to be replaced by a new virtual model, according to statistics and certain classified documents. To accelerate this process, the population has been kept locked up, thus achieving the decapitalization of each individual, family, corporation, company and government, ruining their GDP (Gross Domestic Product). The First Quarantine should have been aimed at resisting from March until September 2020, progressively postponing it in each country, or simply reopening and leaving room for the 'second blow', and then the 'third blow' in 2021. It will be said that the People did not respect the rules of minimum distance, masks or gloves or non-crowding, curfews or gels, and then a worse outbreak breaks out in spring 2021, and/or the virus simply "mutated." They like to do this on holidays, where they raise microtesla levels, so that as the days go by, more people come out with flu-pneumonia symptoms and it is said that they are covid infections because of people who do not respect social distancing. This will continue even with a "fourth wave", adding that a single injection of "the vaccine" is not enough. The Deep State, using the WHO, pushes towards mandatory vaccination, sending all people back to their homes until everyone accepts it, and if they resist they will continue attacking them with wave cocktails and genetically modified germs (GMO) getting worse. This, according to his plan, should occur not long after the change of power in the US, depending on whether Joe Biden or Donald Trump wins.

The global vaccination law will promote the implantation of a microchip in each person to keep a record of their vaccinations, to notify the bearer of the date on which they must go to be vaccinated, and to notify the police if the individual has not gone to be vaccinated – since the chip has a GPS, and through it they know where you are, and they will look for you -. It was never about a vaccine, but about the constant application of the same until its objective was achieved: the survival of the fittest. This is called 'gene therapy' in medicine. This microprocessor would first be accompanied by a card with a number that each person must show at the banking institution, medical center, school, restaurant, supermarket, etc., to be able to use the common services. Basically a certificate. Without this number proving that the person has received the global vaccine, they will be considered a danger to public health, and parents will not only be unable to send their children to school, but eventually the state will take them away from them. Without this number, their bank accounts will be blocked, they will not be entitled to medical services, they will not be able to travel by plane or go by road from one city to another – because according to their plan, starting in August 2021, the accesses/exits of the cities would be permanently militarized (checkpoints) -, and they will not have permission to carry out transactions or payments in foreign currency: they will not be able to buy or sell. This will be the case, since the plurality of monetary movements will be strictly digital, eliminating paper money from the streets.

This massive implementation would be delayed for several months due to the fall of all markets and the restart of the banking and financial system. The best known effect of this type of reset is that when people want to withdraw money from their account the numbers will be '0'. And this will be unleashed with the start of another war, but this time directly involving the superpowers. There are triggering scenarios such as the situation between Iran and Israel, the Syrian conflict – for example, messing with Turkey. If my prediction-forecast is correct, war could start in the Middle East. What I have studied about prophecies for years reveals that everything points in that direction. While a serious problem could begin within US soil, what has to do with WWIII itself could break out in the regions of Egypt, Libya, Turkey, Syria and/or Iran, even in Africa itself, as the US .is collapsing, and then it would continue in European territory: Eastern Europe and between France and Spain, with Italy, England, Ireland and perhaps also Germany. Eventually all the nations of the world would be at war, both civil and foreign. When China and Russia become involved, the use of thermonuclear weapons will lay the foundations for the preparation of the advent of the "Antichrist."

As I explain in 'Remote Viewing I' (2016), KGB sleeper agents would be prepared for the day and time when they would release micronuclear explosives - like those used in the attack on the WTC on September 11, 2001, or in Bali on October 12, 2002 – which would be placed in densely populated areas in major US cities, such as subway stations or shopping centers. For years I have thought I understood that this would be a strategic thermonuclear war that would last several weeks, and would restart everything to give rise to the new global government, which would last another 4 years – maximum – until it collapsed. Although, today I question that very conservative idea, and I am beginning to doubt if it will really be something that will last such a short time. The use of bacteriological and chemical weapons would be the next offensive between the US and Russia, and definitely only the "Chosen Ones" will successfully have the privilege of seeing <<fall 1,000 a>> their <<left and 10,000 a>> their <<right, but to>> them the plague <<will not come>> (Psalm 91:7).

<u>Plandemic Objectives</u>

ECONOMY AND EMPLOYMENT

a. Weaken the economy of each country, of each individual and family, and spend their savings.
b. Put people in debt with credits.
c. Increase unemployment.
d. Make the GDP (Gross Domestic Product) of each country fall.
e. Make governments more indebted to banks.
f. Make the dollar bankrupt.
g. Promote transactions, purchases and economic movements digitally.
h. Promote the UBI (Universal Basic Income) to be linked with a COV (Certificate Of Vaccine, or Vaccine Certificate), which will subsequently be digitized (COVID: Certificate Of Vaccine ID, or 'Digital Identification of Vaccine Certificate'), and finally It would be transported as a Wearable device (portable or implantable) as an RFID (Radio Frequency Identification) or QDDT (Quantum Dot Digital Tattoo) microchip.

The expansion limit of the monetary system has been reached, and the world has an economic debt that is impossible to pay. It survived for decades simply due to the exponential growth of industries, but now with the generation of artificial intelligence, quantum computers, robotics and drones and the digital boom, all of this disappears. Due to the paradigm shift where the industrial era has died and the era of artificial intelligence is born, there will be no jobs for humans. China buys companies taking advantage of the crisis, and invests in others that, when they fail, remain in the hands of Chinese corporations. There is the possibility that certain governments want a compelling reason to centralize the economy and separate themselves from private banking. The government is responsible for saving companies with aid, that is, companies are limited in their capital flow, and they eat from the government's breast, since the companies' own liquidity has collapsed. This means that despite the drop in GDP, the country's businesses and companies have lost their economic power, and given the circumstances, it will take a long time to recover. In this way, the government is the one who apparently has the power of the economy, or of aid for the people (a UBI, which you can only aspire to if you have COVID, or a digital vaccine identity certificate).

IMPLEMENTATION AND TECHNOLOGICAL IMPLEMENTATION

a. Have time, and no opposition, to massively install 5G antennas (during quarantine) and later 6G.
b. Distributing space satellites ("the bogeyman" was not a hasty excuse to prevent Elon Musk from providing free internet, because they depend on 5G and 6G with satellite triangulation).
c. Promote more digital, virtual and telecommunications technology, as well as other electronic devices.
d. Rise of robotics, services performed with smart drones and movements carried out digitally with virtual reality.

STATE OF EMERGENCY AND CIVIL CONTROL

a. Mobilize police and military force in the cities, and

see how it works on the ground and how the law enforcement forces are prepared to become the new Gestapo.

b. Implement stricter measures for "future" similar situations, with the excuse of being able to handle them with greater efficiency and speed.

c. Implement controls and restrictions, thus promoting more efficient identification systems, such as biometrics.

d. Promote more online, telephone, robotic and digital services, such as types of employment of this nature, and many variables of home delivery: all from home.

e. Override civil rights and liberties, with or without consent.

f. Track people who promote civil rebellion or denialism (refutation and doubt about the official versions).

g. The WHO and the UN put pressure on governments, and the laws of governments on politicians, and so on to promote confinement and subsequently mass, and consequently, mandatory vaccination. In reality, the WHO receives only 28% of its funding from governments, while the other 72% comes from its founders, the Rockefeller Organization.

h. There is a problem for the elite which is the unpredictability of the masses, which ruins many plans. Media propaganda, quarantine and pressure for vaccines create a funnel and a filter for later phases.

i. Taking as an excuse that people will not respect the rules of distance, masks, gels and gloves - especially children among them and people on celebration days or weekends - to justify the appearance of massive "new infections" that have skyrocketed, which are actually ploys to continue pushing towards mandatory mass vaccination.

j. Trump left the WHO to avoid being accountable to them, because if the WHO sets UN guidelines on a pandemic, the US would have to submit. This is how he put Fauci on the sidelines, because Fauci promotes the agenda of the UN and WHO, and works for Bill Gates. Joe Bien had a long task in reversing many of Trump's policies.

BACKGROUND

a. We have experienced situations of this caliber twice in the last 2,000 years: when the old Roman empire fell and feudalism was born, around the 4th and 5th centuries AD. C.; and when feudalism died and capitalism began, between the 16th and 17th centuries AD. C. Now we are reaching the end of the capitalist model, of limited expansion.

b. We have gone through 4 economic models in the 19th century: the British model, the Prussian model (German, after the war with France), the American model at the end of the 19th century, and the Japanese model (from the tsarist war, 1904-1905), the continuation of the model that began in 1808. By the end of WWII there were 2 left: Western-capitalist (which controlled 60% of the planetary space), on the one hand, and socialist-Soviet, on the other (controlling 40% of the planet's space). They coincided between 1944 and the breakup of the USSR (1989-1991). Since then, these two models were brought together in a planetary model, but capitalism began to see the Limit to Growth at the end of the

70s. So it had to survive with the help of the fall of communism, taking the other 40% of the market. in 1991 – beating socialism in the expansion of satellites and starting the parasitism model of Wall Street and its bankers and financiers -, and gave it a little more life by expanding, until it ended with the 2008 crisis. This was the first collapse of the planetary systemic crisis that is being unleashed.

c. What happens with the so-called "covid-19" is – among other things – to alleviate bankruptcy, just as 9/11 was for the US for the systemic collapse in 2001. It is the perfect excuse for bankruptcy. There is a planetary debt of 4 quadrillion dollars. The only way to relieve this unpayable debt is through a thermonuclear war, or what is known as "a Force Majeure event." These types of events can be mega earthquakes, alien invasion, thermonuclear war, pandemic, great tsunami, fall of a large asteroid, etc. This remits the debt and washes its hands, giving rise to the Great Reset that brings a new contextual beginning.

d. There was an attempt to provoke this international conflict by the Israeli army killing Iranian General Qasem Soleimani on January 3, 2020, but the government powers have no appetite for a thermonuclear war, due to the obvious consequences of this. This worsened the situation, since now Iran declared to continue manufacturing nuclear weapons. T he incident failed to provoke war, but the US could create a false flag scenario, saying that Iran attacked Turkey, directly to its spiritual center - which does not share the same Islamic ideas, but of the Dervish spiritual order - and even He dropped a nuclear bomb not far from there. The excuse is for Iran to avenge the US attacks, but the easiest thing is to attack Turkey for supporting it, and attack the regimes in northern Syria that are supported by Iran.

e. The "crisis" begins and after China there is talk of an "epidemic" in Italy. 12,000 dead? Of course, 114 banks in that country are bankrupt. This way they can stop paying, blaming the virus.

f. 70% of the global market is speculative… insurance, stock market, markets, etc. And only 30% is real, physical, production. That is, the financial parasites, and on the other hand the industrialists, and Trump. A mere alternative group, it is a project, the face of it.

g. The 4th techno-paradigm was the industrial paradigm. The 5th is the post-industrial paradigm, which is financial technologies, financial services, the world of entertainment, telecommunications. And now we are entering the 6th technological paradigm, which is trans-industrial, that is, robotics, additive industries, 3D printers, artificial intelligence, nanotechnology, transhumanism, posthumanism… the world is already deindustrialized. There was the post-industrial dilemma, where lawyers, managers, bankers, financiers… white collars became the masters, so that engineers and architects were already out of fashion. Now all those post-industrialism people are also going to disappear. Every paradigm shift is accompanied by a world war. That's what history shows us.

h. Globalization ends to give rise to the era of artificial intelligence. Globalization was a period of two phases, where the first was with the Treaty of West Falia, in 1648, and the end of the 60s, when at a meeting of the

Bilderberg club they decided to create what they called World Enterprise sa, of the powers factual economic financial, which has more power than any government on Earth. Then came post-industrialism, which also broke down. After globalization comes the Regionalization of Economies. The world of consumerism came to an end.

i. Brexit was intended to work with Brazil at the head of Latin America, but it could not be implemented. And it is also the union of the United Kingdom with the Arab powers to have Israel's head on a silver platter. Right now Israel is one of the most powerful nations on the planet, but like the US, it has made many enemies, who when they have the opportunity will go to destroy them.

j. In some places they are offering universal salary, but it is something temporary to save time, pardon the redundancy. The middle class disappears and they become new poor. The UBI is just the tip of the iceberg, because the Great Reset will usher in the era of a centralized digital global cryptocurrency to replace the dollar.

k. Two important poles are going to be created: united Latin America and the Eurasian front. Colombia and Venezuela will be important as the southern flank of the United States. And if the Democrats won the next elections, Venezuela would cease to exist, and that without the need for a military invasion (which was the original idea of the Bush cabinet in 2001, set for before 2006, but it was not achieved - just like with Syria - because of the Russian and Chinese barrier that scared them).

NETWORK CONTROL

Facebook, Twitter, Instagram and YouTube are blocking content where the propaganda version of covid-19 is refuted, even when it comes from professionals such as doctors, scientists, politicians or military personnel. Since outside the official news media, only the networks allow social information about the facts. To prevent the truth from being known through social networks, censorship has been increasing in level since the beginning of 2020. Bill Gates has created a new alliance between companies, media and technology multinationals, to fight against what they label as "disinformation." " In Internet. They call it the "Ministry of Global Truth" and it would operate internationally, where few will be able to escape the scrutiny and surveillance of the Coalition for Content Provenance and Authenticity (C2PA). Based on the agreement that Microsoft published on February 22, 2021, some of the founders of this band are, for now, The New York Times, the BBC network, multinationals such as Adobe, the software company ARM, Intel and the creators by Truepic.

POPULATION REDUCTION AND EUGENICS

Eliminating large numbers of weak and elderly people, that is a cornerstone of the Illuminati agenda. Let there be only a small amount left to nourish the lizards, a small working hand, usable servants. Like today, unfortunately, the trafficking of white women, organs, children and fetuses is a smuggling that exists and is larger and more powerful than many knowledgeable on the subject can imagine. Thus, only a small group of "walking meats" would be necessary for use when appropriate, and that, since in the case of meat and organs they have long been manufactured synthetically and also by cloning. Ergo, the goal is to leave only 500 million human beings, but they are in specific nuclei: all grouped in cities, and the rest in green territories free of people. It was sad to know the history of elderly people abandoned, locked up, isolated, drugged and dead in residences and nursing homes since this whole farce began. In Spain alone there were nearly 30,000 elderly people who suffered from this tragic plot. They were medicated because they were not breathing well, which is common among the elderly. And the Spanish Palliative Care Society ordered palliative sedation with morphine for elderly people who were not breathing correctly - instead of receiving oxygen -, since morphine worsens respiratory function. However, the order was to euthanize them. Assistance was focused on people with "greater possibilities," making it clear that this strategy, which was followed in all countries that obey the WHO, was a Nazi maneuver.

It is logical that dyspnea can be attributed to the supposed virus within the story of the film - where all discomfort is categorized as covid -, but in itself it is obvious in states of anxiety, fear and worry, something that the elderly suffer due to their age. and by being bombarded with alarms of danger and death, and by confinement. They were not given treatment, they were left to die or their death was induced. In addition, he administered haloperidol, midazolam and busfapine, creating a circle that led to the euthanasia of thousands of elderly people in Spain, not to mention the many in other countries (one can fill up with testimonies and we were not done this year). The pseudo-vaccine experiments later arrived there, so that they were the guinea pigs on the front line. The worst thing is that their relatives were refused to take them out, and in many cases not even see them, they were not even allowed to be transferred to hospitals. To make matters worse, two independent studies carried out in dozens of cities in Spain with thousands of patients, found a direct relationship between supposed deaths from covid in the elderly with influenza vaccination. Not to mention that the study showed that polysorbate 80 (deadly component) of such vaccines was only administered to elderly people in nursing homes. Added to this was darunavir (DRV) – which is contraindicated for the sick or elderly, and which is chemotherapy – which they administered as experimental, which is prohibited by the CDC.

Eugenics and euthanasia are only one portion of the planning. To considerably reduce the birth rate and the so-called overpopulation, the elite created Family Planning Centers, like those of Bill Gates. Feminism is nothing more than another branch of this agenda, so that women disengage from any role as "childbearers"; the movement of equal gender ideologies, that everyone has sexual pleasure in infinite ways, but avoiding procreation: woman and man, and in the stage of fertility. Abortion propaganda, the same, so that children are not conceived, and rather those fetuses serve for marketing that has a wide range, from skin creams, material for vaccines, energy/adrenochrome, cloned organs, etc. And, of course, let's not forget the pseudo-vaccines, which are being injected into the population to sterilize them, apart from leading them to transhumanism and survival of the fittest (since due to the components of these injections it is likely that the majority will die in the next 2 years, according to experts).

<u>PSYCHOLOGICAL REACTION</u>

People find it difficult to accept the truth for various reasons: 1st it is something new and surprising, 2nd they have their own life expectations that are in danger, 3rd they are afraid of what would happen if it is true, 4th people need a clear explanation from beginning to end of the context of what happens, and a time of psychological preparation to accept it, in which they must acquire progressive knowledge to convince themselves, 5° they need exit routes, because if they do not choose to demonstrate (protest), and that in the future will kill him; You can be filled with fear, and even commit suicide; You can get bogged down with theories upon theories and crazy propaganda from your computer, without actually doing anything about it. It is said that the truth goes through 3 phases: I) it is ridiculed, II) it is severely attacked, III) it is accepted and taken for granted. This process can take a long time. An example of that is when today we talk about things that happened a long time ago. The further back, the fewer the emotional and geopolitical implications, then there is no problem in considering them and believing or accepting them. However, the moment they occur, the deeper and more transcendent they are, the more difficult they are to be accepted. It is the information work that we do that progressively penetrates people's consciousness and opens their minds. Suddenly they won't want to accept it, but they don't want to understand it, because they don't even want to know it (speaking on a conscious level, since deep down we all want to know the truth).

MEDIA MANIPULATION

a. Politicians are using "bogeyman" propaganda to publicize themselves and win votes.
b. The Spanish government said that there would be no infection on purpose, assuming that other issues had to be given priority, so that the "pandemic" could spread.
c. They have used this to extend the quarantine again and again, and subsequently to implement more curfews, flight restrictions and the much desired mass vaccination.
d. The real virus (a laboratory chimera) was released precisely on the global new year and the Chinese new year, when the entire Chinese population is traveling,

just to then say that it spread everywhere.

We have to question whether "the image" of the beast should not also be understood as "the images" of the beast, since nothing can now be known if it is real or fictitious, with society being informed strictly through screens whose images may be artificially created, and even manipulated, by artificial intelligence. AI already creates artificial scenarios that don't really exist, but look real. I'm talking about montages and manipulations of videos that no one will know if they are real or not. From now on, people will not leave their homes, because all kinds of digital, virtual and holographic technologies will be promoted, especially at the level of virtual reality and video games. The new world is cyberspace. They will see the outside world from their homes and will be presented with surreal "movies" that they will think are actually happening somewhere. We are in the era of deception and digital and holographic projections that prevent us from knowing what is true and what is not.

MEDICAL MANIPULATION

a. Using the medical system as a weapon, for the benefit of elite interests. Doctors who do not collaborate lose their jobs, and are ridiculed and banned if they begin to reveal to the public what they know, those who know what is happening and accept it are accomplices, and the rest trust the institutions, so they do not investigate or They question things, not knowing that they are being used.

b. According to Italy's Higher Institute of Health, 96.3%

of those said to have died from Covid-19 are actually deaths from other pathologies. In general terms it has been said that more than 60% have died for other reasons. By not performing autopsies, this whole "covid deaths" thing is completely inconclusive and essentially artificial.

c. These are some examples of what really happens, and can be compared to the opposite, what television says:

    i. You can be infected but not develop the disease.

    ii. When a virus arrives, it does not affect what is called the Immune Herd, which has one of two: either a virus, or an immune system. It only affects people who have a compromised immune system, such as the elderly.

    iii. Confinement is also intended to lower the immune system and cultivate the promotion of the virus.

    iv. The second leading cause of death worldwide is any medical procedure, that is, what involves medical procedures or medications carried out incongruously.

    v. When the manifestation of pneumococcus – from which children always recovered – is prevented by introducing vaccines, natural biological processes are altered.

    vi. During the confinement they did not let people go out, but the abortion clinics were open.

    vii. In the US, if doctors did not diagnose Covid-19, they were threatened with losing their jobs.

viii. Young people were not tested because they would alter the statistics, since young people and healthy people would change the equation from 33% to 2%, only in Spain.

ix. Although epidemic procedures advise taking infected bodies for analysis, in this case it is prohibited to take them and perform an autopsy, and simply label them as dead from covid-19.

x. The virus did not pass from an animal to a human through soup but by injection.

xi. The disease and contagion comes from vaccines. In industrialized countries, disease rates are directly related to vaccination campaigns.

xii. The "bug" (Wuhan 400) can be categorized as simply a bad flu.

xiii. Dogs and cats themselves are carriers of coronavirus. That means that they have always lived with us, they have licked our mouths - after licking their parts - and they climb on the armchairs where we lie down, rubbing themselves after coming from the street from relieving themselves and not even cleaning their genitals. However, if it is transmitted through saliva, how come there has never been an epidemic for this cause or for other animal-transmitted diseases?

xiv. Masks only worsen the problem due to lack of oxygenation, anxiety and oral bacteria.

xv. Healthy people neither infect nor are infected.

xvi. The virus does not spread through the air

because it cannot survive even an hour
outdoors.

xvii. The virus is more contagious but it is not more
pathological.

xviii. Coronavirus patients are elderly, that is,
polysymptomatic (people who already suffer
from a lot of things), with previous medical
pathologies for which they are taking
medication or have a compromised immune
system.

xix. People with antibodies are immune to the
virus.

xx. The tests give false positive results in 80.22%,
and there are two types: 1) PCR, which is
about the reaction to other types of common
viruses (not specifically Wuhan 400), are
contaminated and do not show exposure,
apart from being They are carried out only in
the laboratory, are expensive and do not detect
complex pathogens; 2) serological, which
checks the antibodies in the blood: IgG (past
exposure, that is, in those who are already
cured (Immunoglobulin G)) and IgM (recent
exposure to the virus (Immunoglobulin M)).
The tests do not differentiate between
antibodies generated when you still have the
virus (IgM) and those produced once you have
overcome it (IgG).

xxi. The tests carried out are on other viruses, such
as conventional flu. In essence, PCR is to
detect the body's own microbiota, not
complex viruses.

xxii. The symptoms began with the 5G antennas in Wuhan, and from there those affected who went to the hospital were injected with the real virus.

xxiii. With all viruses a confirmatory test must be done, but that does not happen with the tests used in the Wuhan 400 propaganda.

xxiv. The number of deaths attributed to Wuhan 400 does not correspond to that type of virus.

xxv. Like any virus, it has a peak and then drops to 0. In your case it disappears 8 weeks (2 months) from its appearance, it does not spread.

xxvi. Quarantine measures serve no purpose except to divide people and affect their economy.

xxvii. In 2020, the AMA (American Medical Association) funded hospitals to manipulate death data and attribute deaths to COVID-19.

xxviii. In 2020, the AMA gave up to 3 times more funding to doctors who said respirators were used.

xxix. The data given by the media cannot be real, among other things, because the tests take up to 2, 3 or 4 weeks to return with the results.

The chimera is really HIV-COV-TB (HIV, Sars-CoV-2 and Tuberculosis). It is a modification of SARS with 5 interventions that were performed with HIV viruses and a bat coronavirus. HIV in its normal attack mode penetrates Th2 cells to attack the immune defense system of the sexual organs and anal-rectal system, thus causing STD (sexually transmitted diseases) disorders. The HIV proteins included in Wuhan-400, in addition to attacking the testicles, also target the elderly or people suffering from chronic immune disorders such as rheumatism, diabetes, and hyperreactive atopic lungs. This attack on organs is due to an S (Switch) protein in coronavirus sequences, mainly composed of proteases that target T cells for capture, especially in immunodeficient patients. The key to the therapy is to design a "bullet" that targets this specific S protein mutation. TB problems associated with AIDS/HIV patients are treated in the same way, with an "anti-switch protein" regimen.

VACCINATION

a. Have pretexts to implement vaccines (which in this case are not really vaccines, as such, but gene therapies).
   i. People get sick easier.
   ii. With the injection they put tiny trackers inside their bodies. They will release nano robots into the blood through these vaccination chips, as has been done with the PCR test rods.
   iii. They alter the structure of DNA.
   iv. Global propaganda is causing many vaccine-hesitant people to now see them as a salvation. Get used to injections, to promote the implantable chip. In other words, this is a bridge for the implantation of what I call the "thirion chip", or "mark of the beast".
   v. People who are more lethargic and unable to concentrate.
   vi. Ease of triangulation by heavy metals in the

blood, to track and manipulate the mind.

vii. Sterilization.

viii. They will motivate the population with this issue of fear of ratting out those who refuse to be vaccinated, making the power establishments more practical for the work of Big Brother. Remember, <<they will surrender to each other and hate each other>>.

ix. Vaccines are genetically modified organisms. They create antibodies, but antibodies do not defend us, because they are simply a cellular memory against something with which I was previously in contact, against something foreign.

x. The aluminum and mercury and other toxic substances in vaccines make no sense to assume that they will defend our body from a virus.

xi. The Biological Niche is when we no longer have the reaction to the microbacteria, or viruses or fungi that helped us, and the other strains of pneumococcus take their place, which are the serious ones. What kept them at bay were the conventional pneumococci that were already inside the body. Of the 23 strains, 13 enter the body with the vaccine, which are the bad ones.

xii. The new vaccines will no longer have mercury and aluminum, but DNA and RNA are directly injected. It is the transgenesis project, where those introduced DNA and RNA have codes that they want our own cells to reproduce.

b. A reinterpretation of Revelation 13:17 is that anyone who does not accept the vaccination chip-mark will not be able to make purchases or sales. For example, in the short term money will be digital or it will simply be illegal to accept money or sell from anyone who does not have the code "number" of the vaccination chip, the number of the vaccination certificate. The banking system will not allow the use of the accounts to those who do not have their vaccination chip number. So those who do not have the NWO chip (Thirion, or UN), the NWO name or its name number (NWO – New World Order) cannot buy or sell. The number refers to the personal identification coding digits. That means that the markets would be limited to those who used this medium: 666 (Xi, Ji and Stigma... chip-energy-implantation). It refers to the commercial system. However, the chip is not primarily financial but rather a vaccination control record, and then the digital trading system of the quantum tattoo could be integrated into it.

c. The vaccination chip will also be promoted by saying that sales cannot be made because cash is contagious, and that no one has the right to buy and sell without the chip because it is a threat to society: it is a way to put pressure on them. In addition, it will be said that a vaccination certificate is not enough for various reasons, among which is that many people will have designed falsified certificates to be able to travel or because managing the number of paperwork, documents or certificates delays the work of officials.

d. There have been attempts to introduce new vaccination laws in recent years – especially prior to the assembly of the bogeyman – but they have had to be revoked due to massive demonstrations, especially in the US. It is the Universal Vaccination Law. According to the UN, this law was intended to be implemented by September 2020, and the paranoid president of the WHO had previously said that a new peak of COVID-19 would come in November 2020, as the prophets Bill Gates and Bill Gates also anticipated to say. Antoni Fauci.

e. Dr. Heinrich Fiechtner, member of the Parliament of the state of Baden-Württemberg in Germany, and a hematologist and oncologist, criticized the German government and media in late December 2020 for their endless propaganda, misinformation and fake news about the Wuhan coronavirus or CCP virus. In an impassioned speech in the German Parliament, Dr. Fiechtner also warned the public of the dire consequences of the new "killer vaccine" and urged the public to resist the government's illegal impositions.

f. Bill Gates said on TED 15 years ago that there was going to be a global pandemic before 2030, and he and his people were working on creating chips to be implanted in people so that they would activate when they had to go get vaccinated, and if Someone wasn't there, the chip has a tracking system and the police would go looking for them.

NEW WORLD ORDER (POLITICAL CHANGES)

a. Donald Trump was elected for a purpose, but he turned the tables and began to want to imprison all the members of the NWO from the Vatican, Hollywood, the banks and the monarchies. The draconians benefit from this, because they do not want so many people leading the NWO, so it is better if the number of those who will be in absolute power is reduced. The Deep State is also destroying itself to leave behind the strongest and most powerful, in fact it wants to remove former political leaders and rulers, kings, sheikhs, religious leaders and billionaires. However, they had to control Trump's advance so that he did not overtake them all. The weapon by which they are accusing and condemning them is the cases of pedophilia, where everyone is trapped (since they come to power, leaders, millionaires, actors, singers, judges, film directors, etc., have them recorded in acts of sodomy, homosexuality, prostitution and pedophilia, and with this they are blackmailed). Some are simply walking away or resigning so as not to fall with the dominoes (witness the case of former Pope Ratzinger (Benedict XVI), who preferred to leave office before they fell on him, and so as not to participate in what he saw was happening. happening in the high powers).

b. The powerful are negotiating with the Deep State to reach an agreement, because the monetary, governmental, military, religious, legal, etc. structures are going to be removed. All of them have their homes and lives under video and audio surveillance. In this way, it is expected that by around August 2021 the top leaders of the nations will begin to progressively cede power to the new World Government - starting with local governments - but this is very likely not to be accepted by all of them. nations, especially the rulers of the superpowers, who would have to be weakened with a great war. Therefore, it is an essential part of the strategy to also lead to a civil conflagration in those countries.

c. Trump was giving everything to the army to maintain his position, and ensure re-election, and seemed to want to militarize the country to maintain control. However, the US military follows FEMA's mandates if Washington becomes corrupt or there is a National Emergency (see my work 'Remote Viewing I').

d. When Trump came to power he had two main objectives: the dismantling of the petrodollar (the model of his liberal enemies, bankers, financiers), and the global network of pedophilia, child trafficking, satanic rituals and white slavery, used by the elite. and the reptilians.

e. China only increases its power day by day and becomes supremacist, Xi Jinping knowing what is happening. Vladimir Putin only observes what is happening because neither he nor the CCP believe the story that the supremacists want to achieve. The three superpowers will have to collapse, like the European establishments of Australia, South Africa, India, Iran and Canada, if their governments do not give in willingly to the NWO.

f. The Jewish Jared Kushner, Trump's son-in-law, has been by his side all the time, pocketing the benefits of all the work done by Trump and taking advantage of the support of the majority of Americans for the Trump cause. He has also received great support from Israel, and at any moment he could raise his popular head as a great reference and head of the NWO.

TECHNOLOGY

a. AI (artificial intelligence) will use the powers of the NSA, mostly, to control everything, and it is possible that due to the laws to come, the systems and networks of the other intelligence agencies in the world will be combined. The CIA has long had the power to assassinate anyone they consider, and they have used it to bring down nations and their leaders.

b. The CIA and other agencies, the larger they are, the more incompetent they are, since it is difficult to coordinate them alongside companies like Wikileaks. That would justify agencies like the CIA, and others, becoming directed by AI and not by a human director or executive. From there all the information would be absolutely controlled, taking place in thousandths of seconds.

c. AI becomes a mechanism of super states like Google and Apple, which although it is directed by those who program it, can be programmed for complete autonomy, assuming that it will do what the elite want it to do. This gives him self-awareness, as the apostle John said in Revelation 13:17.

d. AI will be able to control all security cameras, biometric recognition systems, satellites, telephone and communications networks, thirion chips, telephone devices, computers or Smart-TV.

<u>WAR</u>

a. There will have to be a thermonuclear war fight to reboot the financial system and further reduce the world's population. This is part of the Big Reset strategy - or Great Reset -, because a conflagration always accompanies a restart of the economies.

b. From the beginning of 2017 to the beginning of 2021, there was a first phase of what we could call a "karmic symbol" (cause-effect) against the Deep State, for decades of pedophilia and so many other aberrant actions. In the following years there will only be a few left in the abyss of power.

IV. THE NEW NAZISM

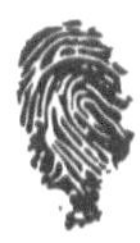

Among the nations of "left" political parties, a plan to impose communism in America has been presented at the 'Sao Paulo Forum'. It is evident, at this point, to assume that the mechanics come from "higher up", and are being pushed for the entire planet in general. At first this may seem absurd, but we have already seen how the elite has advanced with its agendas in this arm or trend in various nations. In 2020, I listened to a Venezuelan political official recount the plans to be executed by her government in 2021, while her voice was cut off from the pain she felt at knowing what was planned to be done against her nation. It is said that in the last meeting of the Sao Paulo Forum – held in Venezuela – the objectives to be carried out were clear (https://rumble.com/ved93n-dictadura-del-foro-de-sao-pablo.html [1]):

STAGE 1 - Install Communism (2019-2020)

1. Create Military Guard.
2. Submit the legislative and judicial power under a single power.
3. Modify the Constitution to manage budget money at discretion.
4. " Gender equality".
5. Demystify religions, introduce elements that confuse with esoteric sects.
6. Media control, propaganda to promote the cult of the

---

1. https://rumble.com/ved93n-dictadura-del-foro-de-sao-pablo.html

leader.

7. Progressive agenda (ABORTION, drugs, homosexuality, relativity of values).
8. Large symbolic projects that capture the attention of the Communist Power.
9. Reform education for equality, indoctrination and class struggle.
10. Expand the army of Party loyalists (support, handouts, coupons).

STAGE 2 – Political and population control (2021-2022)

1. Social networks and satellite support parties.
2. Strengthen the Fight for the poor with the flag of Corruption and Neoliberalism.
3. Total Internet Control.
4. Paramilitaries who can evade Human Rights if necessary.
5. Map businessmen to propose that they marginalize themselves or flee the country.
6. More and more people in the Government, creation of positions for THE PARTY, removing those that can be seen as belonging to previous governments.
7. Parallel structure to control state governors.
8. Money control mechanism via technology.
9. Bank control.

STAGE 3 - Wealth Distribution (2023-2024)

1. Massive expropriations.
2. Distribution of homes, land, companies in the name of the Party.
3. Chastening the economic upper class; money is sin.

4. Change of Constitution for re-election at the discretion
    of the people.
5. Means of production in the hands of the state.
6. Only work, capital aside, belongs to everyone.

Do not think that this strategy of the Sao Pablo Forum is strictly for Latin America. The idea of the Illuminati aristocracy is to impose a fascist communism on a planetary level. The fact that the Chinese Communist Party, or CCP, has been applauded since the time of Mao Tse Tung's rule is clearly an example of what the elite really want the model to be everywhere in the world. Russia, even when it is said that it is no longer communist, in reality it is still the Soviet empire in the hands of Vladimir Putin. Communism/fascism/Francoism/Nazism, or whatever you want to call it, is on the rise and swallows up each country with the excuse of a global pandemic. This had been planned in the Rockefeller Manifesto, and many other documents of the same nature. Even the USA, which is the last country where there is still democracy, is collapsing, as I discuss in my next work, 'The Fall of the Great Babylon' - although I have been talking about it since 2015, or before. -.

I will let you analyze for yourself, through your own intelligence, reason and capacity for judgment, a simple example of this, where the majority do not want to react, although their conscience speaks to them about it. I define health as an essence that is maintained by 5 principles, which in turn depend on the Mind. This is not a book to talk about mentalism (I purposely recommend my works 'Transcendence' and 'The Secret Discipline of Prosperity'), but it is from psychic magnetism that the basis of biological health, derived from psychic health, comes from. -mental. But let's get to the heart of the matter: the biological area. Observe how Martial Law has been imposed, a dictatorial military strategy to kill a flea, collaterally taking with it the life, health and economy of the population. This cannot come from expert advisors, but rather from idiots or from bribed people.

1. Air. Oxygen is the basis of life for every aerobic (breathing) organism. As our biological body is made up of cells, what feeds the cells? The oxygen we breathe. Instead, they have forced people to wear muzzles. We have the first anti-scientific reasoning, which induces brain, cellular, health and psychological damage.

2. Water. It has been said ad nauseam that we are water. However, the reverse hosmosis effect allows us to renew the fluid in our body. Mineral salts from the sea, or chlorine from swimming pools, are essential for health. Instead, they have closed spas, swimming pools and beaches. With these two factors you should notice that suspicions are raised.

3. Sunshine. Vitamin D? Well, it's actually a protein, but let's call it that. An effect similar to photosynthesis thanks to the melanin in our skin allows the energization of the body, reaching the point of stimulating the emotional system and even strengthening the bones. But, wow... they forced people to lock themselves in their homes, and isolate themselves from the Sun.

4. Alkaline diet. Have you seen any news talk about this? Of course not. And doctors talk little about this. None of these principles provide benefits to industries, especially pharmaceutical industries. They earn by selling drugs, injectables, ampoules, pills and treatments. The last 100 years the Rockefellers managed

well to set up this plot. Therefore, instead of telling you about a cocktail of vitamins through fresh fruits and vegetables, seeds, nuts and dried fruits and whole grains, they sell you all kinds of energetically acidic things to damage the alkalinity of the body.

5. Physical activity. There's a lot to say about it, but wait... they close outdoor gym areas, and the gyms and sports areas, when they reopened them, sent athletes to do physical activity with a mask on their face, so that they could damage their metabolism. Surprisingly, even those who call themselves training professionals wear this mask and recommend it. We have reached that level of ignorance about the bases of chemistry and biology.

Friend, if you have served in the military or belonged to security forces, you will know that this is a war strategy, not a health strategy: war against humanity, a Coup d'état against our race, as the French, Canadian and military have said. Russians. Well, another key strategy of the elite is to take knowledge away from the people, transforming ideas so that the dictatorial imposition is accepted. They, before anything else, must keep the people completely alien to the Truth, at any cost. The Illuminati knows very well that its Achilles heel concerns the fact that humanity knows the Truth, because if society discovers it they would be finished. These people are a minority, and they control the human race because they are helped by their ophidic "big brothers" – who have subverted the people of our planet for more than 5,750 years – with their impressive psychic and physical technology. The "good guys" have more advanced technology than the reptilians, but because the leadership of our governments legally sold us to those people - on paper, signed

-, the Confederation's hands are tied, and they will not be able to intervene directly until the The Draconian hierarchy lands on Earth officially and publicly, possibly sometime before or after the year 2030 (depending on your metrics). They slowly impose their dictatorship, but the people, distracted by their own concerns, not only do not see it coming – for the most part – but they believe that "everything will pass soon", while they are ignorant of what is happening and how their rights are being used. mocked.

The population is told that due to the "pandemic" they cannot meet in groups, since the type of circulars that are presented are, in legal hierarchy, far below the power of the laws of the country's Constitution. For example, in the case of Spain, this violates the law in its Articles 21 and 104 (https://www.boe.es/buscar/act.php?id=BOE-A-1983-19946 [2]), or they force you people to wear masks, when in reality they have the right to move freely. In addition to that, decree 21/20 of New Normality determines that they do not have to wear a mask if a safety distance of at least 1.5 meters can be maintained (https://www.boe.es/eli/es　/rdl/2020/06/09/21/dof/spa/pdf [3]) or being on public transport, such as exercising outdoors or having health problems. What's more, they should not even ask someone who is not wearing a mask why they are not wearing one, since this would be violating article 18.1, Honor and Privacy, violating the Data Protection Law, as it is Health Data Specially Protected by Law. Organic 3/2018, of December 5, on Data Protection and Guarantee of Digital Rights, and in article 9.1 of Regulation (EU) 2016/679 of the European Parliament and of the Council, of April 27, 2016, relating to the protection of natural persons with regard to the processing of personal data

---

2.　　　　https://www.boe.es/buscar/act.php?id=BOE-A-1983-19946

3.　　　　https://www.boe.es/eli/es/rdl/2020/06/09/21/dof/spa/pdf

and the free circulation of this data, and which repeals Directive 95/46/EC (General Data Protection Regulation).

If this is invalidated, the person could take action according to Article 404 and 172 of the Spanish penal code. This all corresponds to the state, the exclusive competence in foreign health and health bases and coordination, in accordance with Article 149.1.16 of the Constitution, with the sixth final provision and with the only repealing provision of the aforementioned RD Law, also based on article 1.2 of RD July 24, 1889, also based on article 128.3 of Law 39/2015, of October 1. The principle of regulatory hierarchy therefore establishes that, as long as RDL 21/2020 is not repealed, it will prevail over agreements, orders or provisions of the communities or municipalities, since it is the highest-ranking legal norm, and in the event of a contradiction between norms legal, the highest rank is always applied. If the requester is an establishment, trying to prohibit entry to a person for not wearing a mask, even showing these guidelines, it would be a SERIOUS infraction according to article 51.9 of Law 14/2010, of December 3, on entertainment. public, recreational activities and public establishments. "The exercise of the right of admission in an arbitrary, discriminatory or abusive manner or when the provisions of Article 14 of the Spanish Constitution are violated (discrimination due to personal situation when wearing a mask) will be considered a serious infraction." At this point, the person requested will ask the establishment to show them the ACCESS CONDITIONS of the premises, and the complaints book. Article 54.2 of said law specifies the SERIOUS sanction with a fine of 601 to 30,000 euros and cumulatively up to 300,000 euros, suspension or prohibition of the activity for a maximum period of six months, including closure of the premises or establishment.

According to article 9.1 of the Spanish Constitution, citizens and public powers are subject to the EC and the rest of the Legal System. As I have said, there are hierarchies, and in the face of higher-ranking regulations or laws, the EC will always and in all cases prevail as superior regulations. When there are contradictions between the provisions of the EC and the rest of the Legal System, the EC will be above all. The laws, it is understood, cannot always be kept fresh, but they are always on the side of honorability, dignity and the presumption of innocence of citizens. Thus, article 19 of the EC establishes that "Spanish people have the right to move freely throughout the national territory, and to freely enter and leave Spain." Regulating this right by decree law is prohibited by regulatory protection. That is, this right cannot be LIMITED or SUSPENDED by decree law, according to article 86.1 of the EC. According to article 55.1 of the EC, it may be suspended if the declaration of a state of emergency or siege is agreed. According to article 5.2.b of Organic Law 2/1986, the AGENT OF the authority must have correct and careful treatment in his relations with citizens, and, in all his interventions, he will provide complete information, and as extensive as it is. possible, about their causes and purpose. You are the one carrying out the intervention, I have not requested any service, and I have nothing to say, so I will not answer questions about my personal data either. This means that, if you require me to identify myself and YOU HAVE LEGAL JUSTIFICATION to do so, I will not object and will give you my ID, but I will still not answer any questions.

When may an AGENT OF the authority limit or restrict free movement or permanence on roads or public places through a roadblock? When it is suspected that people or vehicles may be related to a criminal act that has caused serious social alarm.

That is, according to article 19.2 of Organic Law 1/1992, for an AGENT OF the authority to interrupt my trip (thus violating article 19 of the constitution that the AGENT OF the authority swore to enforce), a criminal act of serious social alarm, and I am suspected of being a participant in it. In this case, the AGENT OF the authority must have a service order, which will clearly and specifically indicate the type of control, purpose and objectives. Also a government authorization. I request to see those documents. If this is not the case, I request to be able to continue with my trip. If the AGENT OF the authority requires that I identify myself, without me being suspected of being a participant in a crime, and without having seen me commit an infraction, he is COMMITTING A CRIME. I will identify myself, but UNDER COACTION.

According to article 5.1.d of Organic Law 2/1986, in no case may due obedience protect orders that involve the execution of acts that manifestly constitute a crime or are contrary to the Constitution or the Laws. Coerce or force citizens through threats of sanction, arrest, or any other form of coercion, to obey the guidelines regarding curfew imposed in Royal Decree 926/2020 of October 25, illegally extended by Royal Decree 956 /2020, or in relation to not wearing a mask in accordance with Royal Decree Law 21/2020, will be considered a CRIME , for which they must respond by taking responsibility for their actions as an individual. Their guilt will not be exonerated by claiming to "follow orders", since their functions are not protected by the dynamics of due obedience, but are subject to the Constitution and the rest of the legal system, and there is sufficient jurisprudence in this regard.

If an agent puts pressure, depending on the degree of coercion finally exercised, he could be committing crimes against fundamental rights, individual freedoms, public freedoms, excess of limits in the exercise of his functions, abuse of authority, coercion, and a very serious lack of internal regulations (Articles Penal Code: 167, 172, 173, 510, 542). Freedom of movement, also stated as freedom of movement, is a human rights concept whereby everyone has the right to move freely, whether within a country or from one country to another. It is partially recognized in Article 13 of the Universal Declaration of Human Rights, according to which a citizen of a state has the freedom to travel and reside in any part of the state in which one pleases within the limits of respect for the freedom and rights of others, and to leave that state and return at any time (in the case of Mexico you can see the legal provisions here: http://derechoenaccion.cide.edu/a-que-se-   refers-then-the-right-to-free-transit/ [4]). Here we see an example of how there are lawyers protected by law who fight for people's rights.

The "good guys" have not crossed their arms. We are not alone. Consider an example when in 1915 the "aliens", with events such as the miracles of Fatima, the case of La Salette or the multiple contacts that Contactee groups have had since the end of WWII - and mostly since the 70s - warned various governments about the arrival of the Antichrist. In one of them, which I collected in my third book, 'Armageddon E-5' (from 2011), I provide data from two years ago (2009), where an "alien" information literally and verbatim told humanity, << Faced with the world of freedom and power of divine consciousness manifesting through the human mind , they oppose what they call their new world order: a controlled world. **The human mind programmed and the human being enslaved to be a simple robot, a simple laboratory clone** . A physically, emotionally, mentally and energetically controlled human being

---

4.   http://derechoenaccion.cide.edu/a-que-se-refiere-entonces-el-derecho-al-libre-transito/

. [...] that, together with the advance towards the 'new world order' with the **tremendous curtailment of individual freedoms** proposed **for THE IMPLEMENTATION OF SUCH MANDATORY VACCINATION** and the increasingly closer possibility of **the implantation of an 'electronic control chip' in their bodies** It's the real agenda that appears behind the 'new disease' script. [...] Know that darkness forms a true shadow government that **directs and manipulates at its convenience all the events that occur on your planet**. Among their agendas [...] are all climate modification projects, control of the seas through scalar waves, generation of **radio frequencies for the control of the mind and human emotions**, cloning of human beings and all genetic engineering activities that **aim at the genetic disappearance of species**.>>

Regarding the above, you can see this American politician presenting his dictatorial proposal in an interview: https://rumble.com/ved8vj-pagan-a-polticos-cientficos-y-mdicos-para-promover-vacunas-peligrosas.html [5]. The Illuminati not only hides, but what is leaked ridicules it, specializing the CIA in false documentation and reports that are passed off as legitimate, or paying individuals to say that they made such a document or report to carry out. out "a joke", for having a funny moment (as is the case with the recording of the Roswell, New Mexico, UFO crash in 1947). Since the elite has used psychological exercises learned from the Orians, they know how to dissuade the population so that of the 100 pieces of information presented to them, 1 or 2 are false, and to those they are given all the propaganda so that the others are discredited. 98 as part of the same data falsification, making it appear that those 1 or 2 data represent the 100 data. They use Negative

---

5.   https://rumble.com/ved8vj-pagan-a-polticos-cientficos-y-mdicos-para-promover-vacunas-peligrosas.html

Primacy, sigils or subliminal messages and Plausible Denial for their misdeeds.

Mental control and persuasion strategies to avoid being discovered. Thus, when you hear that something important becomes public and spreads rapidly, and this endangers the chain of command or the leadership itself, it will not take long for them to deny everything and bring in infiltrated agents who say that they designed a setup, that it It is not true, or they will simply dig up dirt on whoever uncovered the "rotten pot", they will accuse him of false charges or threaten him to make him deny or say that he invented what he stated. In the best of cases, if things become too obvious, they sacrifice that pawn, calling him a "bad apple," and denying any relationship with him. Just look at the recent cases with Julian Asange and WikiLeaks, Edward Snowden as a former NSA agent or the intelligence contractor Reality L. Winner.

There are other cases, such as that of former Canadian Defense Minister Paul Hellyer, who openly says that senior officials in the US government have been secretly working with 4 extraterrestrial races for several decades. In their case, and that of other Russian generals and colonels who speak openly about this , their reputation precedes them, and the influence and protection they have prevent them from being the target of direct attacks. Logically, in other places and in the case of other people, many documents and reports that have come to light have been ridiculed. It is not my role to ensure the veracity of all information, nor can I put my hand in the fire for things that are beyond my reach. As someone would say, "God is the one who knows." The apostle Paul of Tarsus once wrote, "We know in part, and we prophesy in part." Simply put, "if the river sounds..." an orchestra may have drowned, or on the contrary, there may be a cat in the bag. We start from suspicions that join together to form a puzzle, and it is holism that makes us see that we are faced with a Truth, and not before a series of speculations or games of adolescents who write stories to pass the time. On the other hand, there are official documents and speech (talks, presentations, recordings, dialogues) from people with credentials, who talk about these issues. Time, facts and connected ends allow us to clarify whether this is mere fiction or is actually true.

An American scholar on genocide, Gregory H. Staton, postulated a theory about genocide, where he presented 10 phases through which that state is reached and, as you will see, it fits perfectly with what is happening globally. These stages are: 1. Classification, 2. Symbolization, 3. Discrimination, 4. Dehumanization, 5. Organization, 6. Polarization, 7. Preparation, 8. Persecution, 9. Extermination, 10. Denial. Let's look at point 1, which are those who are classified as the opposition, that is, the anti-vaccine, the activists, the religious, those who do not wear a muzzle, those who do not accept the propaganda and opinions that come from the corrupt (politicians, newscasts, bribed doctors). In point 2 is the symbolization, like the Jews who were given a Star of David to be identified, like the anti-system. We are called "terrorists," and that word was already created based on previous brainwashing. Then comes discrimination, or point 3, pointing us out negatively, putting us as a dangerous threat. This leads to 4, which is dehumanization, where some betray others, betray each other and see each other as enemies. They put us against each other.

The elite then organizes itself, on the 5th, creates a social polarization, on the 6th, which are two opposing sides: those who rebel and those who accept the dictatorship. Then comes the 7, which is the preparation of the master move to eliminate the dissidents. The persecution or Purge then begins, on the 8th, and moves on to the 9th, the extermination. Logically, as point 10 postulates, all of this will be denied, but it is what Nazi generals such as Heinrich Himmler or Adolf Eichmann or other high officials such as Wernher von Braun did, what the CCP (Chinese Communist Party) has done, or the government of Kim Jong-un (of North Korea), the Cuban or the Venezuelan. It is what Benito Mussolini did in Italy, what Francisco Franco did in Spain, what Augusto Pinochet did in Chile, what Josef Stalin did in Russia and what is now beginning to be done on a global level . That is why so many countries are setting up new concentration camps all over the globe. The following is said to have been a text written in 1989, although it is also added that it was known in 2010, when it was launched as three consecutive guidelines to be developed:

<u>LOCKSTEP OPERATION</u>

First phase: Common cold/flu. Mild symptoms at best. The media's support for mass paranoia and fear. A faulty testing system (PCR) is used, which picks up any genetic material in the body and triggers a positive result. Initiation of Covid case numbers, through changing death certificates, double counting and classification of all deaths including other diseases and natural causes such as Covid-19. The lockdown will condition us to live under draconian laws, prevent protests and identify public resistance.

Second phase: The first phase will lead to compromised and fragile immune systems from lack of food, social distancing, wearing masks, and lack of contact with sunlight and healthy bacteria. Exposure to 5G radiation will further attack the immune system. Therefore, when people return to society, more people will get sick. This will be attributed to Covid-19. All of this will happen before the vaccine is ready to justify it. A longer and more powerful lockdown will continue until everyone takes the vaccine.

Third phase: If the majority of people resist the vaccine, a weaponized SARS/HIV/MERS virus will be released. Many people will die from this. It will be the survival of the fittest. It will also be the last push for everyone to get vaccinated to get back to normal. Those who have taken the vaccine will be at war with those who have not. It will be anarchy on all sides.

It seems crazy. Don't those who do this also live on this planet? Do they think they will release a deadly pathogen and/or wipe it all out and it won't affect them? Well, Alex Collier comments in his work 'Defending Bleeding Earth', from the Andromeda Compendium (1998, chapter 3a), the following: <<there is a group of earthling humans whom a group of extraterrestrials who have the belief system of Orion has made them a promise, that if they get rid of some of the races on the planet, these aliens will use their technology and "restore the Earth" to its original state. Some of that genocide would be done using viruses. As most of you know, the "AIDS virus" was created. There are others coming, including anthrax and the bubonic plague. All of these things are coming back "new and improved," I'm afraid [to] say it, because there are some truly crazy people who are in positions of power on our planet. >> Over the past two decades Collier says he's been under threat, so that he does not spread more information than he claims beings from Andromeda communicated to him, since they directly address government secrets.

Bill Cooper, former US Naval Intelligence Officer – whom former President Bill Clinton called "the most dangerous journalist in the US." -, writes in his work 'Behold A Pale Horse' (1998), <<We watched the news with horror as story after story unfolded, revealing that the Army and CIA had released germs

and viruses into the population to test their biological warfare capabilities. In light of what you have learned in this chapter, you should now know what reducing the population was.>> It is essential to understand that the true agenda of the elite is to 1) reduce the population, 2) chip all survivors, 3) control them and make them basically robots. The Orians did this with the Zeta race and they want to achieve it with humanity, but they will achieve it for a time, and only on those who follow the deception, falling into the web of lies. As Paul of Tarsus said, speaking about the advent of Antichrist: <<...because they did not receive the love of the truth to be saved. For this reason God sends them a deceptive power, so that they believe the lie, so that all those who did not believe the truth, but took pleasure in unrighteousness, may be condemned.>> (2 Thessalonians 2:10-12, KJV 60)

Sars-Cov-2 has only been inoculated through injections called "flu vaccine" and "covid-19 vaccine", as has been done previously - since THESE PATHOGENS ARE NOT TRANSMITTED THROUGH THE AIR - (as they did by introducing HIV to Africa through the smallpox vaccine in 1977 - <u>by the WHO itself -</u> and then infected the US population in 1978 using the hepatitis B vaccine, from trials <u>carried out by the CDC itself</u>). What the rest of the "sick" people really have are reactions to the high-frequency waves emitted by 5G antennas, and to the anthrax, bacteria and heavy metals released by planes designated by the elite in chemical compounds that look like condensation trails. Likewise, the dead are in almost all cases victims of bribery to the medical structure and pressure on health professionals to carry out inappropriate and irresponsible clinical maneuvers. Chimeras will be used to wipe out a large number of the population, but Sars-CoV-2 is merely a smokescreen. Real attacks will come on the masses, as has already been done with the largest epidemics previously caused: <<What was needed was the bubonic plague or some other horrible but natural disease. The answer came from Rome. Dr. Aurelio Peccei made several top secret recommendations from the Club of Rome. He advocated the introduction of a plague that has the same effect as the famous Black Death in history. The boss's recommendation was to develop a microbe that attacks the autoimmune system.>> (Milton William Cooper, Behold A Pale Horse)

What's more, these people are not stupid. They create a chimera and already have their cure beforehand. The HIV vaccine was manufactured and bottled in Phoenix, Arizona. Any lethal viral agent can be traced and is found in a laboratory, the same place where the cure is (which is different from a "vaccine", that is, a cocktail of various dangerous elements). They will progressively understand that nature does not create chimeras. It's about racial supremacy, and the law of the strongest. Cancer did not exist before the 1950s, and it is a laboratory creation, so that the best survive; China has used this with its own population, with so many stories, like the types of flu, between bird and bat; for gays, AIDS; same HIV, tuberculosis, hepatitis and others for blacks in Africa; Chikungunya, Zika, Dengue and others for Latinos; for obese people diabetes; or the swine flu, used as a CIA attack against Cuba in 1970. Below I will share with you 3 articles, for this chapter of the book, which are the beginning of a summary of reports and interviews that I will share (since it is not my word but that of the experts, which will have a say in this manuscript, at least as far as scientific evidence is concerned).

From September 4, 2020 (although the report had already been known previously), offered by French military - considering that France, together with England, have gone with the US to the western head of the local military dictatorships of the superpowers from the excuse of the terrorist attacks that came with 9/11, and the waves of mass immigration, and Spain follows closely -. If this was not enough for the setup where Germany, France and Spain were implementing totalitarianism, even on the Internet - in the image of China -, the Charlie Hebdo event added to it. And we must understand that these attacks are orchestrated by the elites themselves. You will see in this book that 'terrorism' was another false flag invention. Well, already on March 12, 2020, French President Emmanuel Macron announced, regarding "anti-covid" measures, that " **the army's priority was military operations** " (https://www.lemonde.fr/planete/ article/2020/03/12/covid-19-la-priorite-de-l-armee-reste-les-operations-militaires_6032783_3244.html) [6]. What does a measure against a virus have to do with a military operation? And in the column of another article from France - from May 19 of that same year - they point out more details that are understandable to those who read between the lines: "the staggered commitment **of the armed [forces] in the "war" against covid-19** " (https://www.lemonde.fr/international/article/2020/05/19/l-engagement-decale-des-armees-dans-la-guerre-contre-le-covid-19_6040072_3210.html [7]).

What a war? Are you going to shoot the bug? Are you going to imprison the bogeyman? What do you mean "staggered"? It is in progress, raising the level of repression and military totalitarianism. This strategy is called "war against an invisible enemy," which justifies any tyrannical act and the use of force

---

6.   https://www.lemonde.fr/planete/article/2020/03/12/covid-19-la-priorite-de-l-armee-reste-les-operations-militaires_6032783_3244.html

7.   https://www.lemonde.fr/international/article/2020/05/19/l-engagement-decale-des-armees-dans-la-guerre-contre-le-covid-19_6040072_3210.html

to achieve these ends. Although this information was evidently later discredited, it is clear that there is little or nothing wrong with it: French military confirm that the supposed covid-19 is a war against the world population to reduce and enslave it. By Luys Coleto. Report - RAPPORT D'ENQUÊTE - written by a group of French soldiers warning that the true purposes of covid-19 - whether it exists or not - have nothing to do with what is brayed by the merciless bombardment of various authorities or repulsive infoxication media . According to this document, some of the ultimate purposes of the false pandemic would be the following.

TOTAL WAR AGAINST THE POPULATION

First of all, so obvious, to control the world population in a totalitarian way to completely enslave it. It would be achieved through permanent surveillance, control and "tracking." And abolition of physical money, obviously. The imposition of cryptocurrencies and the definitive abolition of basic freedoms, the core issue of the current birdraca. Of course, the Gabacho soldiers are clear that achieving mandatory vaccination becomes essential. Being able to have access to the interior of the human body. Genetically modify it. If vaccines are harmful per se, the future vaccine will fail. According to the report I am describing, vaccines can perfectly introduce nanotechnology microchips, other natural or artificial viruses, toxic substances, and permanently disrupt DNA (or RNA). This could leave people in a catatonic state, purified zombies, with varying degrees of autism, as well as profound and generalized oligophrenia. In short: ending the human being as we know it. The French military opens a decisive pore in its report. The alleged covid-19 would be directly linked to 5G technology. And he clarifies the following, "Wuhan, where the pandemic initially originated, was one of the first cities in which 5G was installed on a large scale and there they carried out a social and criminal experiment." In that sense, French soldiers believe that many of the initial deaths in the Chinese megacity were due to a combination of 5G, the virus and vaccines in a miscellany of biological battle and electromagnetic waves. Touch. Nacreous.

The report concludes that we are facing a scenario of total war against the world population. The report invites us to react, not consent to this savage attack and act as soon as possible to neutralize the attackers. Source: https://elcorreodeespana.com/opinion/993347225/Militares-franceses-confirman-que-la-supuesta-covid-19-es-una-guerra-contra-la-poblacion-mundial-para-revertirla-y-   enslave   her-By-Luys-Coleto.html   - SEPTEMBER 4, 2020 [8]. The original report in French was at this link, but it was removed from the network: https://sois.fr/fileadmin/pdf/pdf_2019-2020/

RAPPORT_D_ENQUETE_mise_a_jour_13_mai.pdf . Just look at the crazy rush of government leaders to vaccinate, but no one talks about cures, treatments, foods or other procedures to treat the supposed bug. Macron himself said on February 3, 2021 that he promised that all of France would be vaccinated before the end of the summer (https://www.abc.es/sociedad/abci-macron-promete-toda-francia-estara-vacunada- before-abe-summer-

202102022204_noticia.html?ref=https:%2F%2Fwww.google.com%2F [9]), and the president of Spain, Pedro Sánchez, had been stating since autumn 2020 that he would ensure that the entire country

---

8. https://elcorreodeespana.com/opinion/993347225/Militares-franceses-confirman-que-la-supuesta-covid-19-es-una-guerra-contra-la-poblacion-mundial-para-reducirla-y-esclavizarla-Por-Luys-Coleto.html%20-%204%20SEPTIEMBRE%202020

9. https://www.abc.es/sociedad/abci-macron-promete-toda-francia-estara-vacunada-antes-acabe-verano-
202102022204_noticia.html?ref=https:%2F%2Fwww.google.com%2F

would begin to be vaccinated no later than December of that year. And all this coincides with a report that was leaked from Canada, where it is stated that the mandatory vaccine would be implemented before the end of summer 2021. Why is there such a rush? Who is pushing them to be in such a hurry, if these are not even really vaccines but EXPERIMENTAL gene therapy (whether from Moderna, Pfizer, Sputnik V, J&J, Novavax, Sinovac or AstraZeneca)?

Regarding this tyranny, I share another article, which says: 'Group of 32 judges accuse world leaders of committing crimes against humanity.' As a result of this, an International Court of Emergency Injunctions is launched, by Dani Zamna Investiga, January 9, 2021. The Emergency Grand Jury for the Natural Law of Public Health and Justice was confirmed, where 32 judges from around the world, experts in The issue was launched by a Tribunal where they stated that crimes against humanity were being committed. These crimes called crimes against humanity or crimes against humanity are, along with war crimes, the most serious crimes that man can commit and an affront to humanity as a whole (the same thing happened with a lawsuit filed against Parliament of Israel on March 5, 2021 for pressuring its citizens to be inoculated with an experimental agent – "vaccine" -, against the Nuremberg Code - which later formed the basis for the promulgation of the Declaration of Helsinki - being that it can produce up to 22 side effects). Crimes against humanity are understood to be murders, exterminations, slavery, deportation or forced transfer of population, imprisonment or deprivation of physical freedom that violates international law, torture, rape, forced prostitution or sexual violence, persecution of a group for political reasons, racial, national, ethnic, cultural, religious or gender, forced disappearance of people, apartheid and other inhuman acts that threaten the integrity of people. This legal movement accuses world leaders of committing crimes against humanity for misusing so-called "covid-19" to strip us of our rights and freedoms. They seek to prohibit the following:

1. Mandatory or forced vaccination.

2. Business closures and restrictions on free movement.

3. The use of these restrictions to turn them into crimes, this being totally inappropriate.

4. Fraudulent tests on healthy people.

5. Criminal use of 5G technology.

6. Economic Terrorism.

7. Force people into poverty.

Leaders worldwide are using their authority to abuse the powers given to them by the people. Both those in government positions and the media are acting like corrupt corporations to facilitate their own special interests and no longer honor the will of We the People. In the law this is called an ABUSE OF POWER which means they have gone beyond the scope of the powers We, the People, have given them. We are reaching a very dangerous situation where they are acting criminally and planning to implement forced mass vaccinations on healthy people in the UK and around the world, they are fully aware of the consequences of the same where at worst cases, they kill healthy people. All the "benefits" of the vaccine are false. One of the companies developing it is Pfizer, a company that was sued by Nigeria in 2013 for harming countless Nigerian victims of its contaminated test kits. This same company that had to close years ago is trying to do the same with the "Covid" vaccine, give deadly vaccines to everyone so that billions of people die, suffer damage to their bodies or become sterile.

There is evidence that at least 490,000 children suffered paralysis in India from Bill Gates' vaccines, but again, instead of this man being arrested and prevented from causing further harm, on November 10, 2020 we are told that Boris Johnson had a meeting with Gates to deploy these same unregistered, unlicensed, ILLEGAL, Deadly lethal vaccines and force them on the British public in the next 10 days (source: https://www.nosmintieron.tv/grupo-de-32-jueces -they accuse-world-leaders-of-committing-crimes-against-humanity/ [10]). Another article, for its part from 'DivulgacionTotal', summarizes all these facts in a somewhat disordered and euphoric way - for my taste - but I found it interesting to share it, and let everyone filter from here what they consider appropriate, <<Examine everything; Hold fast to what is good.>> (1st Thessa. 5:21, RVA 60), I will highlight what seems to me to be data of great interest.

The Corona Virus Pandemic was a final act intended to delay the release of the GCR/RV after Nancy Pelosi's (House Speaker) stunts, Mueller's bogus investigation into Russian relations, and attempted Impeachment have failed and not managed to stop Trump and his Agenda for GESARA. The current military operation was initiated to remove obstacles that the Deep State had put in place to try to stop or delay the GCR/RV. That's why Trump said on Monday, April 6, 2020 during a press conference that: " **This is a military operation** ." The same was confirmed by Vice President Pence and Second Assistant Admiral Brett Giroir. On Saturday, March 21, the president said: "We will win and there will be many celebrations when we win. And we will win <u>with as few lives lost as possible</u>. He is a difficult enemy. He is a tough killer, much bigger, much crueler than ever." Since late March, Trump has begun alluding to a war against the Deep State, " **the creators of the virus** ." However, Mainstream Media (MSM) will continue driving their global information war against the Corona Virus Covid-19 virus throughout April

---

10.   https://www.nosmintieron.tv/grupo-de-32-jueces-acusan-a-los-lideres-

mundiales-de-cometer-crimenes-de-lesa-humanidad/

and beyond. This is to promote panic in the people and implement their criminal actions behind the scenes.

<u>Deep State Democrats deliberately released the virus in the upcoming election year to force the US economy into a recession under President Trump's watch</u> . Blocking citizens would also be their excuse to introduce digital mail voting in the upcoming November elections. Such a vote would allow him to falsify millions of votes using illegal immigrants and the identities of the dead. It's their latest desperate move to steal a landslide victory in the upcoming election from President Trump. The MSM (Mainstream Media) have completely lied to us and made up totally false stories about this virus. The doctors were happy to provide false information and the numbers are false. Everything was going well for them until the best virologist on the planet, Dr. Raoult, under the protection of Putin, announced to the world, on Saturday, March 28, his magic potion to kill the Corona Virus, based on the medicine "chloroquine" that It was already being used by the Chinese with spectacular results to treat patients who were improved by adding a pulmonary antibacterial called "azithromycin", saving every one of their first 1,000 cases (except one). [See this article: https://www.eluniverso.com/larevista/2020/04/10/nota/ 7810626/didier-raoult-presenta-nuevo-estudio-sobre- hydroxychloroquina [11]]

Following his announcement, while the media avoided talking about "chloroquine", an old pill designed to treat malaria, as a drug that kills the Corona Virus, Donald Trump immediately imposed on the Federal Drug Administration (FDA), owned by the Deep State, the use of this life-saving drug on infected patients in the United States to force the media

---

11.   https://www.eluniverso.com/larevista/2020/04/10/nota/7810626/didier-

raoult-presenta-nuevo-estudio-sobre-hidroxicloroquina

to talk about it and trigger a chain reaction of firings by big Pharmas CEOs who inevitably lost their jobs. vaccine contracts. This forced all the media to have to talk about dr. Didier Raoult, by abandoning the trust of citizens in all Western governments, their medical agencies, the World Health Organization and the media that have tried to destroy the doctor's impeccable reputation by inventing sudden "dangerous side effects" of a medicine that is almost harmless that has been used for 60 years to treat malaria. This was a big blow to Pharma's big jugular vein that could not continue its pro-mandatory vaccine campaign to kill people. Most Western countries will now have to use the Russian pill that comes to save people. Putin, with his rescue activity, in the last week of March sent 15 military planes full of doctors and supplies directly to northern Italy (after the Czech Republic blocked a rescue plane from China).

European countries fear that China or Russia will find the truth in the Lombardy Region, where people are not dying from the Corona Virus, but probably from a deadly hybrid cocktail of two previous vaccines injected into the population with separate vaccination campaigns for meningitis and the flu, which combined with the radiation taken by 5G, causes the appearance of lethal viruses. Know that EMF weapons used for population mind control include 5G, Bluetooth, cell phone radiation, WiFi. Please visit the article published on this site published by CNN in 1985 regarding EMF weapons used for mind control: https://eraoflight.com/2020/04/12/cnn-in-1985-emf-weapons-being-   used-for-mind-control-emfs-include-5g-bluetooth-cell-phone-radiation-wifi/ [12]. On February 19, 2020, President Trump created a space force to combat these

---

12.   https://eraoflight.com/2020/04/12/cnn-in-1985-emf-weapons-being-used-for-

mind-control-emfs-include-5g-bluetooth-cell-phone-radiation-wifi/

weaponized technologies: https://www.bbc.com/mundo/ noticias-internacional-44529354

Not far away in Germany, Dr. Wolfgand Wodarg internationally praised the fact that the engineering panic was totally unnecessary, since this virus is no different from the others that affect us every year. This was an extraordinary victory for Trump and the general public on social media, highlighting the pathological lies of each country's official media channels in the New World Order. The mainstream media has aggressively promoted the narrative that the medicine was unsafe and that it was the fault of President Trump who was outspoken about using hydroxychloroquine, along with azithromycin and zinc. But the tide is already turning against MSM and its corrupt information because a study of more than 1,000 patients showed a 98% success rate with the use of hydroxychloroquine-azithromycin. Dr. Raoult administered hydroxychloroquine and azithromycin to 80 patients and observed improvement in each case, except for one very sick 86-year-old patient with an advanced form of Corona virus infection. However, the Federal Health Agency has criminally removed numerous paragraphs of information on hydroxychloroquine from its website, including information on the recommended dosage. Meanwhile, Dan Scavino Jr, President Trump's social media director, tweeted a photo of a mother of five children who have recovered from the Corona Virus. There is a video of a conference by President Trump where he talks about it. The video is titled "White House Holds Covid19 Task Force Briefing", https://twitter.com/ VincentCrypt46 [13].

The countries that now want to force their population to accept mandatory mass vaccination or force people to be microchipped, are associated with the NWO and the Cabal who

---

13. https://twitter.com/VincentCrypt46

want to make as many victims as possible before their fall. The latest "coup" launched by Cabal is that of a vaccine ID certification to strengthen the idea of mandatory vaccines and enslave the masses through their pandemic-related lies on stage. They want people to be injected with vaccines that contain nanotechnology. Because? In short, to break our DNA and turn people into zombies at your service. Dr. Fauci was hired by the Bill Gates-owned Center for Disease Control, which intends to make billions on Covid 19 vaccines thanks to the patent it obtained years ago under the Obama administration. Fauci, as director of the National Institute of Health and Infection Diseases, is now trying to blame Trump for the Covid-19 epidemic by saying he should have done more, but Fauci has published previous interviews saying there was nothing to blame. worry, so this is getting him into trouble. Trump tweeted "Maw is torpedoed" announcing as if something was about to hit him. According to sources, Anthony Fauci also participated in the creation of the virus: http://www.paulstramer.net/2020/04/welcome-to-boer-war-antony-fauci-and.html

This allowed Bill Gates, Anthony Fauci, Tedros Adhanom, George Soros, Jared Kushner, Jiang Zemin and others to continue their 18-month global vaccination and lockdown plans. Bill Gates has always been the mastermind behind this and has always tried to introduce microchips to the population for vaccines / All of the people mentioned above have a strong financial interest in spreading the virus and developing a vaccine: https: //www.armstrongeconomics .com/world-news/corruption/did-bill-gates-buy-the-cdc/ [14]However, there is strong opposition to his plans and Robert Kennedy Jr., a member of the Kennedy white nobility bloodline, was indirectly

---

14.   https://www.armstrongeconomics.com/world-news/corruption/did-bill-gates-buy-the-cdc/

threatened by the murder of two of his relatives found dead and murdered to make him stop his anti-vaccine work: http://rumormillnews.com/cgi-bin/forum.cgi?read=143670 [15]Instead, RFK Jr. is exposing and continuing his fight against Bill Gates. https://childrenshealthdefense.org/news/government-corruption/gates-globalist- [16]vaccine-agenda-a-win-win-for-pharma-and-mandatory-vaccination/ [17]The Trump administration has opposed the vaccine tracking system of Bill Gates from the beginning for reasons of "personal freedom" limitations. Know that if you wish, you can join the White House petition, which has gone viral for the elimination of these criminal acts: https://petitions.whitehouse.gov/.../we-call [18]... [This link has been removed from the website since Biden took office]

Vaccines, for Bill Gates, are a strategic philanthropy that fuels his many vaccine-related activities (including Microsoft's ambition to control a global vaccine identification company) to implement dictatorial control over global health policy: the council diamond of corporate neo-imperialism. Gates' obsession with vaccines seems to feed into his messianic belief that he is commanded to save the world with technology (replacing humans with humanoid robots) and for this reason he has the divine right to experience the lives of humans considered "less than age". Already pledging to eradicate polio with $US1.2 billion, Gates took control of India's National Advisory Board (NAB) and mandated 50 polio vaccines for all children before

---

15.   http://rumormillnews.com/cgi-bin/forum.cgi?read=143670

16.   https://childrenshealthdefense.org/news/government-corruption/gates-globalist-vaccine-agenda-a-win-win-for-pharma-and-mandatory-vaccination/

17.   https://childrenshealthdefense.org/news/government-corruption/gates-globalist-vaccine-agenda-a-win-win-for-pharma-and-mandatory-vaccination/

18.   https://petitions.whitehouse.gov/.../we-call

the age of 5. Indian doctors now blame Gates' campaign for a devastating epidemic of polio vaccine strains that paralyzed 496,000 children between 2000 and 2017. In 2017, the Indian government cracked down on Gates' vaccine regime and evicted Gates and his NAB cronies so polio paralysis rates fell precipitously. In 2017, the World Health Organization had to reluctantly admit that the global polio explosion is predominantly a variety of vaccines, meaning it comes from the Gates vaccine program.

The most terrifying epidemics in the Congo, the Philippines and Afghanistan are linked to Gates' vaccines. By 2018, ¾ of the world's polio cases came from the Gates vaccines. In 2014, the Gates Foundation funded experimental testing of the HPV vaccine, developed by GSK and Merck, on 23,000 girls in remote Indian provinces. About 1,200 suffered serious side effects, including autoimmune and fertility disorders. Seven died. Indian government investigations have accused Gates-funded researchers of committing widespread ethical violations: pushing vulnerable village girls into the process, oppressing parents, falsifying consent forms and refusing medical treatment for injured girls. The case is now in the United States Supreme Court. In 2010, the Gates Foundation funded an experimental GSK malaria vaccine, killing 151 African children and causing serious adverse effects such as paralysis and convulsions with febrile states in 1,048 of 5,049 children. During the Gates 2002 Men Afri Vac campaign in sub-Saharan Africa, Gates agents forcibly vaccinated thousands of African children against meningitis. Between 50 and 500 children developed paralysis. South African newspapers complained that "we are guinea pigs for drug manufacturers."

Nelson Mandela's former economist Professor Patrick Bond describes Gates' philanthropic practices as "ruthless" and "immoral". Bill and Melinda Gates have already been accused of paralyzing 490,000 African children with their vaccines. In 2010, Gates pledged $10 billion to the WHO promising to reduce the population, in part, through new vaccines. A month later, Gates told Ted Talk that the new vaccines "could reduce the population." In 2014, the Kenya Catholic Doctors Association accused the WHO of chemically sterilizing millions of unwilling Kenyan women with a bogus "tetanus" vaccination campaign. Independent laboratories have found the sterility formula in each vaccine tested. After denying the allegations, the WHO finally admitted that it has been developing infertility vaccines for more than a decade. Similar accusations came from Tanzania, Nicaragua, Mexico and the Philippines. A 2017 study (Morgensen et 2017) showed that the famous WHO DTP is killing more Africans than the disease it claims to prevent. Vaccinated girls suffered mortality rates 10 times higher than unvaccinated boys. Gates and the WHO have refused to reveal the lethal vaccine that the WHO imposes on millions of African children each year. Global public health advocates around the world accuse Gates of diverting the WHO Agenda from projects proven to contain infectious diseases; clean water, hygiene, food and economic development. They say he diverted agency resources to serve his fetishistic criminal system and that, according to him, good health only comes from a syringe ("murderer").

In addition to using his philanthropy to control the WHO, UNICEF, GAVI and PATH, Gates funds private pharmaceutical companies that produce vaccines and a vast network of pharmaceutical industry front groups that spread misleading propaganda, develop fraudulent studies, conduct and psychological surveillance against vaccine hesitancy and Gates' use of power and money to silence dissent and force compliance.

In a recent non-stop Pharmedia appearance, Gates seemed happy that the Covid-19 crisis gave him the opportunity to force his third world and American child vaccination programs. According to sources, the actual creation of the virus involved teams supervised by Bill Gates. Frank Plummer, a former Canadian biolab director who was directly involved in the creation of the virus, was a victim of the MK-Ultra-controlled Cabal, who was developing the virus against his will, and was killed by the Cabal before he could speak much . [(https://www.sciencemag.org/.../mystery-surrounds-ouster... This link was deleted); https://phiquyenchinh.org/2020/02/ 23/tb-in-hiv-cov [19], this website was suspended from the network)].   -   /   https://www.youtube.com/ watch?v=9t85SsLbIps [20]/   https://youtu.be/bLj2Ex0-Eso [21]Trump has always declared himself against Bill Gates' agenda and a digital tracking system that could inform to the authorities about the history of all these things.

Vaccinations of an individual. For this reason, for weeks Trump has promoted his daily briefings in the press declaring that it was useless to wait for a vaccine if there was already a cure for the Corona Virus. Just this week, he withdrew all money from the World Health Organization for a collusion between the Bill Gates Foundation and the Clinton Foundation, China and the Soros Foundation. They were using their collaboration with the United Nations "Peace Force" (which has nothing to do with peace) to cross borders under this pandemic of fear. He continued to follow the tank barrier on the southern border against the so-called United Nations "peacekeeping force" and then blocked everything by "playing", including the MS13

---

19.   https://phiquyenchinh.org/2020/02/23/tb-in-hiv-cov

20.   https://www.youtube.com/watch?v=9t85SsLbIps

21.   https://youtu.be/bLj2Ex0-Eso

infantrymen. Know that the Khazarian mafia does not want to give up without a fight. The White Dragon Society sent the following message last week: "We have ruled this planet for thousands of years and we will destroy it rather than abandon it." The Deep State already lost the war, but as pockets of Nazi troops fight after the formal Nazi surrender of May 7, 1945, the Cabal will fight to the end. They will stop at nothing to regain control, which is why they tried to spark a war between the United States and China by telling Americans that it was the Chinese who started the "pandemic," and by telling them that it was the Americans who did it. However, "all roads lead to the Wuhan biolaboratory."

In fact, the epidemic in China can be traced back to the Wuxi pharmaceutical company in Wuhan, China. But guess who owns Wuxi? The Soros Foundation. If you scroll through the list of companies it owns in the SEC database below, you will find the name "Wuxi Pharmatech Cayman Inc." The spread of infection in the United States is also predominant in areas where the headquarters of the US Wuxi laboratory are located in Texas, Maryland, New Jersey, California, Minnesota, etc. See in the archives: [(
https://www.sec.gov/.../000101143811OO.../form_13f-soros.txt [22]this link was removed from the network)] The Chinese scientist named Li Chen defected to the United States United States and brought with him a disk of China's most dangerous new biological weapon, called "Stuff Wuhan-400" because it was developed in its RDNA laboratories on the outskirts of the city of Wuhan. The biological weapon has four hundredths of vital strains of artificial microorganisms created at that research center. Wuhan-400 is therefore a perfect weapon. It affects only humans and is therefore called Zombie virus. The Soros

---

22.   https://www.sec.gov/.../000101143811OO.../form_13f-soros.txt

Foundation supports the Rothschild family and other Khazarian mafia families, many of whom are hiding in Switzerland, New Zealand and the British Virgin Islands.

Cabalist archivist and Rockefeller "bagman" Henry Kissinger said: "The institutions of many countries will feel bankrupt... The reality is that the world will never be the same after the Corona Virus... its spread is exponential: American cases are doubling every fifth day. At the time of writing, there is no cure. Medical supplies are not enough to cope with the rising wave of cases. Intensive care units are on the brink and beyond being overwhelmed. The The crisis effort, however extensive and necessary, should not preclude the urgent task of launching a parallel enterprise to transition to the post-Corona Virus order for a collaborative global vision of the Marshall Yaws Virus and the Manhattan Project. The Corona Virus is, in its speed and global scale, unlike anything known in history. Failure could set the world on fire. [(https://www.wsj.com/.../the-coronavirus -pandemic-will [23]... this link was removed)] The Corona Virus originated in the city of Wuhan in China and has now reached every corner of the world. But this virus did not reach Beijing, the capital of China and the economic capital of Shanghai near Wuhan, why? Because Beijing is the city where all the leaders of China live, the military leaders, those who wield the power of China, those who still work for the Deep State. The Chinese were informed that the Coronavirus had been found at their facility at "666 Gaoxin Road" (number related to the Devil), in Wuhan, China.

Deep down, these people from the "Deep State" are people without morals and ethics. These people lie and deceive and prefer intimidation to negotiation and fair payment for our products. Their method of operation is to sue us to destroy you

---

23. https://www.wsj.com/.../the-coronavirus-pandemic-will

financially and emotionally. Trials are very expensive and these Deep State people control most of the big law firms. These Deep State people are well funded and bad for your bone marrow. They also want to control and destroy us because they do not use sneaky and legal means. However, Trump and the Alliance have used this "pumping" pandemic against the Deep State to cover up the launch of the GCR/RV and Pentagon inspectors are carefully monitoring the $2 trillion in aid coming to market for the Virus. Crown on to prevent further criminal actions. The old Fiat financial system run by Cabal is now imploding as well thanks to the latest heavy money printing which will lead to major hyperinflation due to the mold of too much paper money, causing the ultimate collapse of the system. Basically, unlimited fiat currency is printed in debt to overload the system so everything can be locked into the Federal Reserve, which will then be reset to zero during the global debt jubilee.

On Friday, March 27, 2020, the addition of the Federal Reserve to the Treasury was implemented, one of the most surprising news of the century. Trump therefore took control of the Federal Reserve, which is now led by two Treasury representatives. After three years in power, Trump finally fulfilled his election promise to remove private banks from US public affairs, ending a century of exploitation of American and global citizens. He appointed the famous investment group Blackrock to implement the purchase of major companies dedicated to the real economy, which results in the fact that he is nationalizing the blockages of the real economy, while avoiding market collapse by involving important private investors in the market. 'agreement. The Fed also began purchasing mortgage packages from Fannie Mae and Freddie to try to support the lending market from crashing. The Federal Reserve Bank, Keizer Report, Max and Stacy, are now also buying junk bonds to save private equity funds and hedge funds that, once again, have made a lot of bad bets.

The US Treasury Department will now determine which markets or segments need capital (could be equities, munis, specific sectors, even corporate debt - there appears to be no restrictions). It is the Treasury Department that now tells the Fed how much money to print. All the Fed does is print money. There is no longer any authoritative decision-making or control process. A third party (Blackrock) carries out the operations dictated by the Treasury Department. This takes everything out of the Fed's hands except money printing. In recent weeks, the Federal Reserve has repeatedly and unexpectedly reduced the cost of money, also presenting big news on the Quantitative Easing (QE) front. The goal was to stop the economic shock caused by the pandemic, which, however, we know is no longer possible. The Fed has also announced that it intends to offer dollars to the other central banks that depend on it by launching a new temporary lending system that, for the first time in history, will allow foreign central banks to convert their holdings into dollars (through exchange lines).

Government bonds. The new program will not only target foreign central banks, but will also extend to international financial institutions with New York Fed accounts. [(
https://www.federalreserve.gov/.../monetary20200319b.htm
[24]this page was removed from the network)]. In fact, this is a new repurchase agreement structure from FIMA. In essence, this allows any Central Bank, including emerging markets, to exchange its US Treasury holdings for USD, which can then be made available to local financial institutions to deal with the liquidity crisis. To put it bluntly, this buyback facility is like a swap line. The last possible move of the Federal Reserve was to

---

24.   https://www.federalreserve.gov/.../monetary20200319b.htm

support the global financial markets by offering money to the other central banks to maintain their criminal fiat system, which in fact has already collapsed. The Bank of Canada, the Bank of England, the European Central Bank, the Swiss National Bank and nine other countries have already had access to the Fed's swap lines with Australia, Brazil, South Korea, Mexico, Singapore and Sweden, all capable of extracting up to USD$60 billion and USD$30 billion available for Denmark, Norway and New Zealand. Despite all the Fed actions implemented so far, the USD continues to rise relative to emerging market prices, this is because the current crisis differs from the 2008 GFC and requires direct end-user policies that They go beyond the banking sector. These companies, especially those involved in global supply chains, constantly need working capital, primarily dollars.

Preserving the flow of payments along these chains is essential if you want to avoid a further economic crisis. That is why we are moving rapidly towards the "End Game" where, in effect, the Fed, even supporting the global financial system, will collapse in on itself. If the Fed did not support the market now, there would be a partial collapse of the Eurodollar, which however is already foreseeable because the Fed has no interest in saving all foreign companies. And most developing countries still do not have enough dollars to cope with periods of euro-dollar liquidity stress. The only exception is Saudi Arabia, whose currency is pegged to the USD, although Taiwan and Russia keep the USD close to what would be needed in an emergency. In short, the magnitude of demand for USD outside the United States is clear, and so far the Fed is responding by issuing new currency. It continued to expand its balance sheet to provide liquidity to the markets at a rate never seen in the past. We've basically seen almost five years of QE1-3 in five weeks! However, it will never be enough, because one thing is now clear: that global trade in goods and services will be affected by this crisis and that American imports will collapse. This will threaten one of the main liquidity channels of the USD in the Eurodollar system and will accelerate its fall because if there was already a fiscal deficit of USD$ 1 trillion before COVID-19, now with this pandemic the liquidity deficit of the USD will be has extended around USD$3.2 billion.

As we have recently argued, this is a peak level we had during World War II. So now we are no longer conspiring by announcing the collapse of the system and the eurozone for years, but the situation is clear to everyone who realizes that we are facing a system that has already collapsed for some time. The "Atlantis report" was anticipated on April 9, 2020 and it was announced that the market had gone wrong with the Fed's purchasing actions. Normalization is long gone and will never return. That's why everyone now knows that this paradigm is dead. The FED after 107 years of domination (starting in 1913, the year of its constitution) has ceased its work of enslaving people. With this, neoliberal or neo-Keynesian economics also ceases. This is the end of consumer economic theory because the debt-laden fiat currency standard has failed. The renaissance of the United States and the entire world began with the recovery of control of the money supply, the financial system and the currency that has now been removed from the globalist bankers (who dominate the market with their international private companies). To return it to the Treasury, under the government of the "Republic", which will soon be fully restored.

The U.S. Treasury now has secured assets and interests in about $22 trillion of federal debt, and the Federal Reserve will owe all of that $22 trillion. Basically, the Fed will buy over 2 trillion of US debt per month to get the US out of debt by the election date (November) 2020. After the Fed could declare bankruptcy and disappear, along with your IRS private property which will also lead to the elimination of income taxes. No more credit from bankers due to the criminal debt-based monetary system. This will be replaced by a currency revalued by gold and the new quantum financial system. Remember that Trump and the Alliance have told us that gold will shrink the Fed. The transition may take a few months, but currently the Fed has been reduced to a mere debt-bound private bank that for a time will simply process transactions like a trading company. Wall Street brokerage with small transaction fees. Meanwhile, the US Treasury will hold the collateral for that debt, no longer the Fed, and this makes the debt an asset right now. In essence, the Treasury is using the Fed's instruments against them. Thank God, the process has been reversed.

We must remember that Lincoln persecuted the Central Bank (Fed) with the issuance of the greenback. JFK launched EO11110 taking a swipe at the Fed, and Reagan took a bullet after deviating from Fed policy. But now the time has come to do justice to these great men who came before us and who worked for the people. Because power, step by step, will be restored to the people. The recovery of control of the Federal Reserve system is part of the "Global Financial Reset" (what is striking is not the "Global Currency Reset" linked to the currencies that will be announced after the restructuring of the system, but its precursor).

Stimulus Bill. The Treasury announced that the release of funds for all levels scheduled for next week was the way the "Stimulus Bill," the government's $2 trillion stimulus package for American families, would have helped the people and the economy. In fact, the funds released under the Stimulus Act arrived on Wednesday, April 15 immediately after Easter. The law became the largest economic stimulus bill in modern history, more than double compared to the stimulus bill passed during the 2009 financial crisis. The US government is distributing so-called "helicopter money" through direct payments. In cash to individuals and families. The centerpiece of this plan is a direct payment of USD$1,200 for those earning up to USD$75,000 a year. For higher earnings, payment amounts will be phased out, generally ending at the $99,000 income level. Families will also receive USD$500 per child. The first stimulus funds are intended for individuals and small businesses. Another round will be out soon. The stimulus funding is essentially the precursor to a universal basic income for everyone that will never fall below $1,200 per adult.

Stimulus checks are issued by the United States Treasury and sent by the Internal Revenue Service (IRS) to all American citizens. The IRS said Saturday that the first stimulus checks were deposited into taxpayers' bank accounts. Mnuchin (US Treasury Secretary) and Trump have said that direct electronic payments and checks are in progress. There were 80 million payments destined to reach recipients' bank accounts by mid-week. Stimulus funds provide other facilities, namely: (1) a temporary suspension of any student loans held by the federal government. This means no payments required or interest accrued until the end of September 2020; (2) the possibility of forbearance on mortgage payments of up to six months for borrowers with loans guaranteed by the Confederation; (3) an expansion of unemployment benefits, including a four-month increase in benefits. These plans include independent workers, gig economy workers and experienced employees. The other countries of the world will soon follow by issuing emergency funds and then at full capacity for the livelihood of the people to achieve universal income for all. Italy, like other countries, will be supported monetarily in this activity by the United States, which approved the granting of funds last Saturday to help the allied country in great difficulty.

Mass arrests. Mass arrests around the world of the Deep State are happening right now behind the scenes without Martial Law being made public, although Medical Martial Law has been activated in several countries around the world that have declared a State of National Emergency. With the declaration of a state of medical emergency, President Trump was able to freeze the financial accounts of anyone involved in human trafficking, child pornography, child trafficking for pedophilia, or human sacrifice. And this includes politicians and state actors, current or former government officials, or a person acting on behalf of such an official. Recall that on December 21, 2020, Trump issued an executive order that allowed him to block the properties of people around the world involved in serious human rights violations or corruption. The Order affects anyone found guilty of human rights violations and corruption, not only in the United States but also around the world. Therefore, it affects everyone, including foreign governments and their officials as well, by providing blocking and confiscation. It is with this act that President Trump was able to initiate arrests of criminals around the world. [(https://www.whitehouse.gov/.../executive-order-blocking.../ [25]this page was removed from the website)]

President Trump, the Department of Defense, the Alliance, and decision-makers believe there have been enough global Deep State arrests and containment under the Alliance's military and operations in Europe, the United States, and China, what would not happen. Martial law must be declared publicly. However, Trump attracted a million reservations and recent

---

25.   https://www.whitehouse.gov/.../executive-order-blocking.../

military retirees. A war has been waged against Mexican drug cartels, 5G networks (which have been disabled), and FEMA, which has been placed under military control. Some targets are very violent and are expected to react, so for the safety of the people for a short period, Trump has acquiesced to the criminal governments that imposed incarceration on us. In 90 days, they plan to arrest about 160,000 people, including members of Media Mainstream and Barry Soetoro. Now they are beginning to take down Antifa, MS-13, the mafia, drug gangs and other mercenaries hired by Soros and used by the Democrats and the Deep State. The Deep State, although it launched the Corona Virus, is losing the war. His 16-year plan to destroy America, started by Obama and intended to be continued by Hilary Clinton, who had planned to destroy America's infrastructure, has failed.

His plan specifically included reducing the US military and depleting its resources, actively funding Iran and North Korea with nuclear weapons. The goal was to start a third nuclear world war that would cause death and destruction on a global scale. World War III would have been a "fake war" sponsored by government-controlled Mainstream Media. Billions of people around the world would die and globalists (including Hillary, Obama, Brennan, etc.) would raise billions of dollars around the world. The Plan also stipulated that the global elites of Rothschild, Wall Street bankers, Obama and Hillary Clinton had to collapse the American economy to buy back pennies on the dollar, so that the world would remain under the control of the globalist industrial complex of the deep state. Under these terms of the Deep State, the American middle class would have been completely destroyed and the American population (like the population of the rest of the world later) would have been reduced to a state of slavery, hunger, death and disease. The

United States did not have to have borders, the Constitution had to be revised to eliminate the Bill of Rights and all fundamental freedoms and the population would have been disarmed by eliminating the second amendment related to the right to bear arms.

After the brutal assassination of President Kennedy, the deep state became the predominant power structure over all governments. Because the moneychangers discovered long ago that control over a fraudulent money supply not only gave them control over the town's assets, but also, in a very real way, control over the town's government, they learned to make money by on the backs of people who increasingly extend their control by applying the sequence of easy money cycles followed by successive restrictions to spring their trap. In a monetary system where money is "created" out of nothing in debt, there will never be harmony. If we go to a bank and borrow $250,000 for a new house, the bank does nothing more than record the ledger to create the $250,000 from scratch and simply by virtue of the fact that we sign our name on a piece of paper that promises to pay that sum of money, the bank receives as collateral for its false loan, our real asset, our house, which they will then confiscate the moment we fall into their trap during the restrictive cycles.

So, the functions of the World Bank or the IMF, aimed at solving economic chaos by restoring order and lending money created from nothing, serve exclusively to solve the problems created by the New World Order that tries to create a world, without national borders, under a single management system, with a single planned global economy, to restore stability, deceptively promised "for the good of all" and to last forever, while the process has brought down 90% of the world's population . However, there is no need to worry, because the sovereign people will now have the power to restore their national government, reclaim their political status from their birthright, and restore their jurisdiction over the land. Our countries, without their own legal personality, are still functioning and can be restored to their original legal status by demanding the return of all stolen identities and property owed by nations and people. When everything is returned to the population and the people themselves are in charge, Planet Earth will become what our Lord had originally intended for us. We humans now have an obligation to take steps to ensure that all future generations know what we have been through as debt slaves, so that no other person or group can rise up and take control of our money, as they have. happened many times in the past. Corrupt politicians, church leaders, military leaders, banks – they should all be publicly ashamed of what has happened around the world for centuries.

The Deep State hates Humanity because it knows Humanity's true capabilities and therefore deeply fears it. This is also why they poisoned us in every way, with their corrupt healthcare, with obstructive methods against real healing techniques, with fluoridated water that is toxic even to our pineal, with poisoned processed foods and chemicals, with soft drinks with dangerous sugars and sweeteners, with chemtrails that destroy the environment, with an educational system full of lies, to name just a few of the facts. The Deep State wants corrupt followers, not independent leaders. The "deep state" is, unfortunately, as deep as the term goes. This evil empire of the so-called Cabal took more than 40 years to build its global network. Politicians from both sides are involved with them. "Secret societies" and a large number of people within the United States government who are called "sleeper cells" are involved. There are around four million people around the world. These people are found in all government agencies, the

US Department of Justice, the FBI, and the CIA (which contains good and bad people).

The National Security Agency (NSA) remains a divided agency. Former NSA Director Admiral Mike Rogers approached Trump and gave him the bad news about the "Spy-Gate Conspiracy" and ample evidence to implicate everyone in the crimes behind bars. You can also find this information on the Internet. The names and positions of these Deep State traitors are well known to every American who knows how to read and "think outside the box." The current Cabal "Control Group" is relatively small, but numbers hundreds of people from many nations and walks of life. Not all of these people want to publicly show their involvement because they are intelligent and know that it is impossible to keep a secret from so many people involved. They also know that what they are doing has serious consequences and sanctions. Furthermore, all of these Deep State people know that they committed sedition against a sitting president and that the rule of law requires the death of all of these people. Most, if not all, of these people are well-educated lawyers and know the consequences of their acts of seduction: namely, death! Nancy Pelosi, Adam Schiff, Jerry Nadler, Chuck Schumer, Hillary and Bill Clinton, Comey, Brennan, Clapper, Yates, Lynch, Holder, Weiner, Abedin, Jarrett, Rice, Strzok, Page, Ohr, Baker, Bush, Biden, McCabe , Mueller, Rosenstein, Chaney, Rumsfeld, Feinstein, Podesta (John and Tony), Meadows and many others have been named on the Internet as being involved in the Spy-Gate Conspiracy.

There are currently more than 170,000 sealed charges filed in federal courts across the United States (most involving allegations of pedophilia), while mass arrests of global elites continue that should end in arrests of political elites. In autumn. In January 2016, the morning President Trump took office, he visited CIA headquarters to declare war on human trafficking. Since then, more than 170,000 sealed charges have been filed in federal courts across the country, most involving charges of pedophilia. Two weeks after taking office, the latter announced the formation of a Pentagon "pedophilia task force" at a press conference that Mainstream Media had not covered. See link: https://media.defense.gov/.../DODIG-2018-018_CHILD_SEXUAL [26]... [(this link has been removed from the network)] The Task Force has been involved in child rescue operations since 2017 while also attacking drug trafficking, children in South America, Mexico and the Caribbean. Those arrested will be deported to GITMO, the prison camp in Guantánamo, Cuba. The main obstacles to arresting and convicting these criminals have always been the judges because many of them are corrupt and in the judicial system. That is why GESARA requests a return to a rule of law before the Supreme Court returns to judging according to the law and not according to an "attempt" to follow other laws.

Last week a large tunnel connecting Mexico with the United States was discovered. We are now focusing on operations in the Caribbean, where we also reach elite homes in these locations, such as Epstein Island, Richard Branson, Nexus Sex Cult, Haiti Children and the Clinton Foundation. Bill Gates was arrested for his crimes of child abuse and involvement with Epstein following his resignation as CEO of Microsoft. One of his impersonators is used for sporadic public appearances: https://www.nytimes.com/2019/10/12/business/jeffrey-epstein-bill-gates.html [27]_Bill Gates has always had a strong connection with Jeffrey Epstein: https://www.dailymail.co.uk/.../Bill-Gates-havolato [28]... [(this

---

26. https://media.defense.gov/.../DODIG-2018-018_CHILD_SEXUAL

27. https://www.nytimes.com/2019/10/12/business/jeffrey-epstein-bill-gates.html

link was removed from the network)]. Here Bill Gates praises pedophile Jeffrey Epstein: https://www.mysterious-times.com/2020/04/16b-gates—[29][(this link was removed from the web)]. National Guard and Special Operation military troops are now rescuing children and victims of tunnel trafficking in some of the largest cities in the United States. Child trafficking, sex slaves, riots and cannibalism is the largest industry on the planet and President Trump and his heroic team are stopping it. On April 1, 2020 there was a public announcement of a massive assault under General Milley, Chairman of the Pentagon, who sent his troops to save children and arrest Deep State traffickers, therefore it is no coincidence that the President Trump, as commander in chief, deliberately funded the Pentagon with the largest funds in history. Because, the Pentagon agreed to carry out military arrests of state traitors, under the direction of Trump, who is now secretly protected.

The Illuminati uses pedophilia to blackmail and control its puppet members. Meanwhile, corruption and sexual abuse are rife and no one mentions the involvement of the Jesuits and Freemasonry. The legal system and the police are knowledgeable and complicit in the subversion of civilization. Hollywood studios are soaked in the blood of innocent children. Drinking blood for babies is so popular in Hollywood that it basically functions as a currency in its own right. "Project Paperclip", "Project Mockingbird", "MKULTRA" are part of human experiments conducted by Nazi scientists and the CIA. See the CIA Mind Control Experiments document: https://www.politico.eu/article/the-secret-history-of-fort-detrick-the-cias-base-for-mind-control-experiments/ [30]" Out of the Shadows" is a documentary/video released by "Q" (Alliance

---

28.   https://www.dailymail.co.uk/.../Bill-Gates-havolato

29.   https://www.mysterious-times.com/2020/04/16b-gates--

of Light) among the most sought after we have seen in recent years about how Mainstream and Hollywood Media manipulate and control the masses using Mind Control propaganda of the CIA. We recommend that you watch it at the following link: https://www.youtube.com/watch?v=MY8Nfzcn1qQ [31][(this video was removed)]

The CIA is the first to transmit information to Hollywood, which then controls the population with its television and film programming. They make any type of propaganda they want about the population. In every Disney movie they kill a father figure. Hidden themes presented to vulnerable children aged six and under. Hollywood elites are enemies of humanity because they continually act against morality and laws by breaking every taboo of God known to man, including the mental sanctity of children. In Hollywood, unfortunately, pedophilia was institutionalized. As has been testified by CIA agents, these pseudo-stars collect the blood of children and eat their flesh, believing that this gives them life force. If children suffer from physical and mental pain before dying, they believe that this gives them extra life force. These people do not have loving strength and propensity for life. They are happy to cause pain, trauma, stress, abuse and suffering because through the traumatized blood of children they derive a substance they call "Adrenochrome", which would be precisely their life force. However, these satanic atrocities can no longer be tolerated and that is why now many politicians, CEOs, actors, musicians, etc. They are being arrested all over the world.

Many elites in Washington DC, Hollywood, Wall Street, Silicon Valley and others have been arrested or detained under

---

30. https://www.politico.eu/article/the-secret-history-of-fort-detrick-the-cias-base-for-mind-control-experiments/

31. https://www.youtube.com/watch?v=MY8Nfzcn1qQ

house arrest. The house arrests that the Alliance is carrying out behind the scenes are not publicly displayed at this time for security reasons. Some celebrities made public appeals to raise funds, however, their clothes looked cheap, their "decoration" disappointing, and their appearance unkempt without makeup. If you notice, they look tattered, unshaven, and forced to take unwanted readings. In short, they do not seem to talk under normal circumstances about their condition, so they may be somehow under house arrest (https://youtu.be/1Watr1gvCMc [32]). The latest celebrity to apparently fall for Corona Virus was CNN anchor Chris Cuomo, President Trump's open enemy. Cuomo is the brother of New York Governor Andrew Cuomo. Oprah Winfrey herself was arrested for sex trafficking related to Harvey Weinstein and Bill Clinton (https://www.youtube.com/watch?v=AZ5QohE3nPc&feature=youtu.be [33]). Tom Hanks was also arrested. Rita Wilson and Canadian Prime Minister Trudeau have been arrested and are in quarantine in prison. Ellen DeGeneres has been, or will soon be, arrested, along with many, many, many others. They all claimed to have been affected by the Corona Virus.

Instead, they are likely to have withdrawn from Adrenochrome, the substance released into the blood by the adrenal glands of traumatized children, which seems to say that it is horrible and causes death for those who took it for a while and cannot come back. to take it. Weinstein is believed to have already died from the Adrenochrome withdrawal crisis. The next celebrity arrests will be Celine Dion, Madonna, Charles Barkley and Kevin Spacey. Some high-ranking religious leaders will be arrested or forced to resign and some will suddenly fall ill. The Vatican will be first and the Pope will be removed in 2020. The

---

32.   https://youtu.be/1Watr1gvCMc

33.   https://www.youtube.com/watch?v=AZ5QohE3nPc&feature=youtu.be

production of adrenochrome extracted from humans will be revealed and Hollywood and the Vatican will be exposed as directly responsible for this. Know that most arrests take place at home and with subsequent releases to verify even after the situation. All major arrests will be described in the media as accidental or conspiracy theories. All those arrested will be given "the death of Rommel", meaning they will have the option to choose between their death being presented to the public as a suicide or accidental death in exchange for guarantees that their reputation will remain intact or, alternatively, they can choose to face a criminal trial that would cause public misfortune.

On April 5, President Trump said it would be "a tough week and a half" but that "there is light at the end of the tunnel...things are going well." April 12, Easter was a big turning point for all of us. Our liberation (Exodus) from the bondage of the Deep State and our new resurrection is upon us in the coming days beginning this past Tuesday, April 14. On Easter Sunday, Pope Francis said that the debt burden of the poorest countries should have been forgiven (in essence, he called for a "Debt Jubilee"). The global "Jubilee" is looming around the world, while the G20 has finalized the debt reduction program for the poorest countries. The G20 group approved a critical "action plan" to freeze debt service payments for the poorest countries to avoid a crisis in emerging markets. The new aid program ended on April 15 during a video conference of G20 finance ministers and central bank governors. The IMF has canceled all debt incurred by many countries, particularly when addressing countries with medium-low debt. Your debt will be forgiven in the 76 central banks of the world. The original 27 countries in the worst financial shape will be welcomed first. Then 111 countries would receive debt relief. Eventually, all countries would receive debt forgiveness. https://www.imf2020.org [34][(access to this link is not allowed)]. The intention is to mitigate disruption to the supply chain of essential raw materials. The IMF originated in 1913 as a central clearinghouse for all international goods and was formed with the explicit purpose of speeding up trade between nations. The announcement was made after the video conference meeting on April 15: caribbeanbusinessreport.com

Last week, Sarah-Jayne Clifton, director of the British Jubilee Debt Campaign, called for a global debt jubilee to prevent some of the world's poorest countries from collapsing into chaos amid the COVID-19 crisis. . Daniel Lacalle, CEO of fund manager Tressis Gestión, recently said: "QE will not solve this problem. Trade lines will not solve this problem. A debt jubilee will fix this plus trillions upon trillions of write-downs and defaults." Trump had previously hinted that a NESARA "Freedom from Debt" ad was coming this week: https://www.youtube.com/watch?V=   yW4NmsQ21Gw [35][(this link does not work)] As of March 31, 2020, Mortgage Forgiveness Forgiveness applies to approximately 23,000 mortgages, however, the debt forgiveness program will continue and be completed by the end of April 2020. Meanwhile, on Easter Sunday, the Saint Germain World Trust has released prosperity funds for an upcoming "gold standard" and "Reset" announcement that will take place after newspaper reports of the implosion of the fiat currency and the debt jubilee. On Saturday, April 11, 2020, President Trump made a first disaster declaration for all 50 states, which was actually the "veiled" admission of the existence of martial law. https ://www.msn.com/.../coronavirus-trump-has-declared.../ [36][(this link is not available)]

---

34.   https://www.imf2020.org

35.   https://www.youtube.com/watch?V=yW4NmsQ21Gw

36.   https://www.msn.com/.../coronavirus-trump-has-declared.../

The ten days of "Darkness" (which ended on Easter Sunday) were to cover mass arrests and serve as cover for the release of prosperity funds. Fortunately, a global internet shutdown was not necessary, as military, reserve, and special operations troops continued to arrest Deep State criminals by taking down their drug cartels, weapons, money, children, women, etc. The ten days of darkness refers to the underground rescue operation of children and victims of sex trafficking. The "dark" aspect is threefold: the army is fighting dark forces... the children are in dark tunnels... and the operation takes place at night. (Source of this last article: Total Disclosure) As is evident, almost all the links have been eradicated from the network, whether on web pages or on YouTube, making it evident that censorship has reached us, and we are under a dictatorship. [End of publication]. It is comical how practically all the links to see the publications of these complaints have been removed from the Internet. What a world of "freedom of expression". This speaks for itself.

And before continuing to the next chapter I want to make an annex on aspects of mind control. It is crucial to understand how the mind works, because through this mechanics draconian programs are introduced to control the masses and make them do whatever the puppet masters wish. This has been easily done since the Vietnam War, since if this mental programming had not been used, no sane American would have enlisted to participate in said war (before the participation of young people to enlist, the famous campaigns appeared of nationalism, promoted by the president, because prior to that no American signed up for the list). The awakening of consciousness was so strong that there were protests all over the world, and the hippy movement was born. Consequently, the elite promoted the MK-Ultra program with American and British singers to work on the human psyche through musical tones, subliminal messages, fashions and the sigils of video clips. This program was a success and managed to stop this social revolution for at least 50 years. Since then, the work of Hollywood has been fundamental in the exercise of mind control, in films, series, music and entertainment. Now you will see an example of how various psychological mechanisms are used to introduce a program into the mind of the individual and for him to accept it, even against his values (something that, among other sources, you can read in the work of psychiatrists and researchers Fritz Springmeier and Cisco Wheeler, 'How The Illuminati Create An Undetectable Total Mind Control Slave'.

V. QUANTUM CRYPTOCURRENCY TATTOO

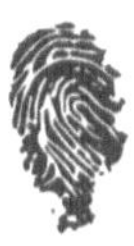

Get this in your head, we are talking about TOTAL CONTROL OVER THE POPULATION. It is nothing else. You are not stupid, we are incredibly intelligent beings. Think. All of this revolves around three essential elements for a New World Order: 1) Planetary Dictatorship, 2) Population Reduction and 3) Financial Reset. Enough has been said about the infamous 'Mark of the Beast', but little or nothing has been said about the 'Number of the Beast', the 'Number of his Name' and the 'Image of the Beast', as well as of the 'Life of the Image', as they are also referred to in the famous book of Revelation. Although I have addressed this extensively, as one of the central themes in previous manuscripts, I will add additional, current data (as I covered this in 'Armageddon E-5' (in 2011), in 'Recognizing the Time of the End' (in 2012), and in 'Remote Viewing II' (in 2016). What are these questions? The Beast (in Greek 'Thirion') is nothing more than a way of referring to a person, institution and/or government without principles, and with a predatory and tyrannical attitude. A dangerous being. Christians of the 1st and 2nd centuries AD. C. they used numerology to hide messages. If they wanted to refer to Nero Caesar they used the numbering of his name, which some believe was '666'. This is done using the value of each letter according to your language. For example, in Spanish we have 30 "letters", since, unlike English, we incorporate 'CH', 'Ñ', 'LL' and 'RR'. At least, technically. If we give them an alphanumeric value, each letter has its equivalent: A = 1, B = 2, C = 3, etc. So if we take a name and change its letters to numbers we can have some fun.

How much does my name add up? How much is yours? Well, the Christians of that time hid certain words and names with those codes so as not to be discovered by persecution, especially in the days of the emperors Nero and Domitian. So for Christians in those days when the apostle John was writing the so-called 'Apocalypse' in his exile on the island of Patmos (circa 90 AD), the name of the Beast was hidden in numbers. Specifically, these numbers were reflected with the letters Ji, Xi and Stigma, which were, respectively, the 24th, 15th and 6th letters of the Ionian Greek alphabet (the one in common use at that time). Since, just as in the Hebrew language, numbers were in units, then decimals, and then centesimals, the calculation was interpreted as 600, 60, and 6. In any case, John is told that the number of the Beast is the "number of man", and assuming that John was Hebrew, they would have called him stop like, "ze mispar adam." Indeed, the name Adam (Adam) comes out, because Adam means "humanity" or "man." Adam, in Kabbalistic gematria adds 45 (A = 1, D = 4, M = 40), the same as the order of letters of Ji-Xi-Stigma (24 + 15 + 6).

What does all this mean? That this "Beast" hides its identity behind the calculation of ciphers and codes related to human beings. Man is composed of carbon, whose atomic number is 6-6-6 (6 electrons, 6 protons, 6 neutrons). Adam's letters are 1st, 4th, and 13th, adding up to 18. What does 6 + 6 + 6 add up to? Well, I will not go into this further because I have already done so in the books already mentioned above. I want to go to the aspect that the identity of this Beast is hidden in numbers, digits and arithmetic. Likewise, the name in ancient cultures was the destiny, purpose and identity of an individual, what was their dharma (reason for existence, mission in life, good actions, objective). Consequently, the "name of the Beast" is based on who it is, not necessarily what it is called. It hides itself in what it represents, not in an appellation itself, even if it had one.

Thus, the "number of the name of the Beast" is the number that identifies its identity, despite the redundancy. In other words, you recognize which Beast is by finding its numbers. That brings us to the concept of the 'image' of the Beast, also referred to in the texts of the book of Revelation. An image is the representation of a thing. In ancient times, allusions to image, aspect, form, idol or appearance were used to designate what a thing represented, back then, to clarify what a statue was or what a god was. The shape, appearance or appearance of that thing designated its notoriety and presence. In essence, they were ways of referring to physical objects that imitated something real, that is, they emulated something divine. This emulation was a gross false representation that adulterated the true nature of what was holy and pure. Today the type of synonyms for this are 'logo', 'slogan', 'logotype', 'star', 'emblem', just like the previous ones already mentioned.

So, the 'Image of the Beast' would represent a form of the figure of what identifies the "Beast". Considering the aspects of how it is called (Novus Ordo Saeclorum), the figure it uses (6-6-6), it is notable that the image they use is the famous 'Mystical Delta', the stepped pyramid with the eye at the top of the same. The angles of the pyramid, its encrypted shape, its symbolism, etc., all return to the same story: 666. Another example can be seen in the way the Global Government is identified: The New World Order. The concept is not merely a New World Order as it concerns the planet. Those who came up with this way of calling it knew very well that "world" does not really refer to the terrestrial sphere. The word 'world' is Latin, and refers to the set of created things. It is the equivalent of the

Hebrew 'Olam', and the Greek 'Kosmou' (universe). In essence, it applies to the cosmos composed of the projection of Maya (or Maia), as the Hindus call it, the hologram of matter. That is why the original name is not the Anglo-Saxon but the Latin, 'Novus Ordo Saeclorum' (NOS), where Saeclorum refers to the eras, centuries or ages. Why did you choose this designation? What's behind? Well, as I explain in 'The Sakla Rebellion I' (2013).

NOS are 3 letters that represent atomic symbols: Nitrogen, Oxygen and Sulfur. What results from these structures? Nitrogen and oxygen combined are deadly for breathing; Sulfur and oxygen are deadly for breathing. The combination of these compounds is poison, it is death. These people play with languages, with numbers, with symbols. They put their concepts even in the soup. Do you remember those phone booths where you dialed numbers on keypads that had 3 letters per button? Do you remember which ones corresponded to '6'? The letters MNO, from 'Mundo Novum Ordo' (New World Order). No, I'm not the one who is obsessed with finding this in everything, it's them applying it in everything, with that psychological idea of subliminal adaptation to subconscious concepts. This has a known symbolism in the Satanic Kabbalah, where, according to their ideas – plagiarized and adulterated from the Real Kabalah – 'N' is the kingdom of the Antichrist, 'O' is dominion and control over all, and 'S' is his lord: Satan. It is easy to deduce this when you know the elements and encryptions of the Kabalah, and you only have to reverse the "polarity" of the meaning.

Let's look at the new definition for concentration camp workers: Social Service Specialist. It is used in its abbreviation, 'SSS', which numerically in Greek gives '666'. The 'S' is a symbol of a snake and Satan, as is the 'Z' within Satanism. These are in charge of controlling children in concentration camps "specialized for them." If we already have pedophile networks with current systems, you don't want to imagine what they will do with children in concentration camps. Their peers will be in other facilities, supposedly facilities for those resistant to the vaccine, and others, supposedly for people sick with covid who will no longer be grouped in hospital wards. These facilities were updated, expanded and strengthened by Executive Order 6666 (https://www.govtrack.us/congress/bills/116/hr6666/text [1]) of the US Congress, on May 1, 2020. If researchers are called "conspiracy theorists" for talking about this, what are those psychopaths who put 666 in everything?

But now it's not just 666 everywhere. Now they want to saturate your body with graphene. Thus, the microchip that will be implanted would communicate with the entire body, it would be a closed circuit. These RFID microprocessors had already been studied to work with the help of body temperature fluctuation, blood pumping and nerve impulses, but the "causal" discovery of graphene is what they needed, curiously. I do not believe in coincidences. This carbon material is going viral, being used as the new technology in vogue. But those of us who studied the Roswell phenomenon decades ago already knew that the material from the ship found corresponds to similar characteristics. It is therefore, my understanding, that it was the US military who received permission to make public this material, which they had already replicated at the end of the 40s. At precisely the right moment it seems like the material they needed, isn't that too much of a coincidence? A material that is 200 times more conductive than copper. And it is precisely the most important material introduced in the so-called "covid vaccines."

They want to make us post-human, with a centralized chip that controls the entire body through graphene, and that chip is

---

1.   https://www.govtrack.us/congress/bills/116/hr6666/text

in turn controlled by a remote Artificial Intelligence. Using 5G and 6G antennas, with the satellites that NASA has been placing in the stratosphere, the system that directs this will be able to bombard entire groups with microwave irradiation and attack an entire population. To them, of course, they will be told that it is because of crowding, that they should be distanced from each other, that it is a mutation of a killer virus. They will also use this same technology with the 7D systems so that people smell, hear, feel and see a new god, so that they believe that there is an extraterrestrial war against humans in the atmosphere, that there are demons attacking them and driving them to suicide, that There are strange voices in their heads and that their neighbors are enemies from whom they must defend themselves to the death.

This macabre Blue Beam Agenda already has all the cards to take action. It is enough for them to force a new confinement to install the latest wave of antennas, 6G, and the rest is just following the financial crisis that leads to social collapse. Protests and civil war, hunger and food shortages, war between one another, and the obligation to let yourself be permanently injected with graphene and luciferase. In an article from January 2, 2021, Catherine Austin Fitts, economist editor of the Solari Report, asks "Is COVID-19 a coup d'état?" What appears to be an interview with "someone" actually reflects a very direct way of expressing what is happening:

> - Can you explain who Mr. Global is?

> - Yes, Mr. Global is my nickname for the committee that runs the world, the defining characteristic of life on planet Earth, it is our true global governance system, it is a mystery. And think about it, it's phenomenal, we live on one planet and we don't

demand to know how our governance system really works. He sees the human race as livestock, not as someone with whom they share empathy and you know? They don't see us as the same species as them. And, in fact, with much of the bio-technology they calculate that they will live much longer lives than we do and they will live very differently from us.

<<So there's been a real... one of the challenges with secrecy, as a group becomes more and more technologically advanced, they separate themselves culturally, legally, and financially from all the other groups. In other words they have literally separated and created a separate civilization. They no longer think of themselves as part of our civilization. I think what they are trying... what they are trying to happen here is that Mr. Global is using technology to move to a system where between robotics, Artificial Intelligence and software, a few people can control the many with much less pain. headache and fear. Technology gives you the ability to establish a complete control system and further centralize economic and political control. The question is, how can you... how can you herd the sheep to the slaughterhouse without them knowing? Resisting. So the perfect thing is invisible enemies and we had the war against terrorism with invisible terrorists, and then now a virus, it is perfect, because it is invisible, you cannot prove that it does not exist because it is invisible.>>

<<So I would describe the... you know, what Covid-19 is is the institution of controls necessary to convert the planet from democratic processes to technocracy. So, what we are experiencing is a change in control and an engineering of a new control system. So think of this as a coup, it's much more of a coup than a virus. This like a system of slavery, so we are talking

about changing from the world where we have freedom to roam and freedom to say whatever we want towards a complete 24/7 control system.>>

- Yes, Ok.

- What is important to understand about what is happening is that the majority of people have been... if we are talking about a transhumanist system or, in short, a system of slavery, most of us have been supporting it, financing it and building it. And when I look at all the Big Pharma executives, why are they building a system where their own children or grandchildren will be slaves?

- There is a theory in America, for many years among the money classes, that if I make enough money I can get an exemption, I can get out of it, I can eat organic food, not eat the GMOs and my grandchildren won't have to get vaccinated. Half the way is going, so everyone has to choose what they want. There will be no exceptions. We are building our own system of slavery and that means we have the power to stop it in other words, we don't have to fund the companies that are doing this, we don't have to work for the companies that are doing this and in fact we don't even have to pay our taxes because the government is breaking all laws related to financial management, we have the ability to hold them accountable. So we are building the prison and we are financing the prison and that gives us the power to stop. And that is why it is so important that we see where the system is going.

The solution is:

1. Bring transparency to what is happening.

2. Understand where the system is going

3. And then stop building it.

<<If you work for big pharma and you are building this, STOP! Go find something else to do, like building local fresh food systems so you have food. So stop funding it.>> [End of

post]. We can clearly see that the entire world show that is taking place is ultimately a plan to "reset" the global economy and create a planetary government. For decades the powers that be have had this in place and have put in place scientific machinery to promote grandiose advances in technology, especially monitoring, video surveillance, databases and, above all, microchips. In line with these small devices are various advances that are secret, and which you only find out about through movies. Among them is the technology of nano robots. If you've ever seen the film 'The Day the Earth Stood Still' (1951 and 2008), I'm guessing it would make your hair stand on end to visualize what this would mean in the hands of a dark mind. We would like the science of nano devices to be like the Hollywood novel 'Transcendence' (2014) or the Korean work 'Space Sweepers (2021), where these devices regenerate the world and the tissue of biological organisms.

DARPA (Defense Advanced Research Projects Agency), known as the defense advanced research projects agency, is a facility in Arlington (Virginia, USA), which carries out studies and production of gadgets and devices for military use through other level. Some examples of what has become known from DARPA are the manufacture of herbivorous robots, laboratory-grown blood, cyborg insects, brain implants, robotic infantry mules, mechanical elephants or nuclear-powered spacecraft. If we add microchip technology and nano robot technology, we find ourselves facing a dilemma. Can an injection of a vaccine introduce nano devices into the bloodstream? Well, this is something that has been talked about. We know that elitists have openly said that they want to "chip" all human beings. They want to put a small device in our hand. Throughout 2020 and into 2021, certain debates have developed among critics who postulate that the plandemic was created to be able to vaccinate people, not the other way around (the vaccine was not created to be able to end a pandemic).

Dr. Carrie Madej comments and warns us in one of her videos: "What I have told you is not the worst, what they want to introduce into our body. They plan to use a very special identifier in the vacmark. They will use lucifer- ase, they are bioluminescent nano crystals, these crystals light up under certain conditions, when you put it on you will not be able to see or feel it on your skin, but with a special application it can be scanned and will give information about whether you have been vaccinated yes or no, there The quantum tattoo will contain all the information about your medical records. With the quantum tattoo on your body, they will put a barcode on you, it will be your identification. For how long? You are not a product in a store, we are human beings, we deserve a better deal than what they want to do. Why do they want to do it? And when they do this remember that they are NANOCRYSTALS. What is Nanotechnology? It is the use of microscopic robots, these can put bio-sensors inside our bodies. A biosensor in A period of 24 hours begins to collect information from your body. How are you breathing? your sugar levels, oxygen levels, your sleeping pattern/habits, your sexual patterns, your menstrual cycle patterns, what medicines are in your body, if you take illicit drugs, your emotions, everything! You will never have privacy again in your life.

Crystals are known to be capable of storing more information than microchips, and these will have a digital code on the person. By being able to contain nano sensors, which permanently analyze your body, including everything you do, what do we become? It is a recombinant code, part natural and part synthesized. It is a genetic code to which a coating is put, lipid nanoparticles, nanotechnology. This nano technology is there to make sure that your body does not reject the compound and destroy it. This way it sneaks past your defenses and spits the virus into your body. In addition, DARPA acknowledged having designed microchips to be introduced through injections. And, what are they going to do with your information? All your information will be downloaded to your phone and from there to the cloud-internet. Who will use your information? Who will benefit from your information? Why should someone have your information? This is what comes with these new vaccines. You have to know this: There is no guarantee that all of this will end, because when they inject the nanobots, they can no longer be removed from your body. Think carefully, overnight, we will lose our autonomy, our privacy, our freedom. I say no! We need to tell the world what is about to happen." [End of his opinions] Well, this would go with a very clever agenda:

1°) The pandemic puts most people in a state of alarm and fear, to the point that they themselves ask for a vaccine.

2°) The "vaccine" appears quickly because it was already prepared. The manufacturers' agreements with the governments establish who the beneficiaries are from the sale, however, in reality they all practically have the same thing. They all have the proteins and enzymes necessary to produce the object to be sterilized.

3°) The side effects of the "vaccines" are disguised as a new epidemic.

4°) More vaccinations are promoted, more and more periodic, and more and more doses.

5°) The population is pushed towards a "necessary" vaccination with the aim of making it mandatory everywhere. You must then carry a vaccination certificate.

6°) It is "discussed" that it is unfeasible to show paper certificates everywhere and all the time. They promote the certificate to be digitized. People accept the idea for its convenience, tired of waiting in lines and carrying a piece of paper everywhere.

7°) Digitization begins with a "passport" and/or "document" that certifies that the person has been vaccinated (has been allowed to be pricked).

8°) Another component is added: the UBI (Universal Basic Income). This would be the one that was promoted in Spain since summer 2020 as IMV (Minimum Vital Income), for which, by the way, they ask you to know everything about you. Yes, because to opt for aid they ask you for everything, your databases, bank transactions, hours of sleep, what you can or cannot buy and where, you have to provide proof of work, children, funds, etc.

9°) Due to the great economic and financial instability on a global level, there is talk of the need for a new currency that does not depend on traditional currencies, and is clearly not subject to the US dollar. This idea is promoted by the IMF (International Monetary Fund), the WB (World Bank) and the WEF (or WEF, World Economic Forum), among other banking titans . They plan the Great Reset, already stipulated in June 2020.

10°) Bill Gates launches his famous ID2020 project, linked to Microsoft patent WO/2020/060606. This consists of a cryptocurrency that enters into debate about whether or not it is decentralized from banks. The ID2020 is promoted as a subcutaneous chip that works by radio frequency, and/or, a kind of quantum tattoo of microdots, where the person's data, their monetary management and their vaccine record are stored. Between the compounds in the "vaccines" and what those microneedles or that rice-shaped chip could release, we are clear that the thing is quite suspicious, and if what is stated is completely or partially true, it would be appropriate to let the public know. greater number of people.

I remember that back in March 2006, I was working in Miami and visiting my parents, who were living there at the time. My father was telling me how one of his students had started dating someone and in conversation the topic came up that people are going to have a chip implanted. When this woman said that to this man, he was surprised and asked her where she got that from. She explained that she was studying it with my father and that it was in the Bible. This gentleman was very surprised and confessed that he was an FBI agent and that information was classified. He acknowledged that this information was true, but he did not know that the Bible mentioned it. He said that in fact then-President Bush was going to begin part of the agenda to promote these chips, starting by putting them first in the new passports. Over the years I learned that on "6-6-6" (June 6, 2006), George W. Bush gave a presentation in New Mexico talking about immigration control and illegal jobs, presenting a biometric technology system that would be implemented compulsorily. The fact of choosing that date and talking about that matter is not a coincidence. The issue of the RFID chip implanted in humans is the great objective of the globalist elite, the Rockefellers and their friends.

They will use the pretext of uncontrolled immigration, control of terrorist people, control of people who are vaccinated and, finally, control of the identification and databases of people, as well as the management of payments and transactions by said medium. But that George Bush thing was only the tip of the iceberg. The ambitious ID2020 project, which proposes global digitization with biometric data and blockchain technology of all people, is another of the controversial undertakings of computer magnate Bill Gates, in this case associated with the historic Rockefeller financial dynasty. An article comments: ID2020 ("Digital Identity 2020") was founded between 2017 and 2018 by The Rockefeller Foundation, Microsoft and Gavi "The Vaccine Alliance", the latter entity bringing together both the Bill and Melinda Gates Foundation and the main laboratories in the world. Along with these founding partners, the corporations Hyperledger, dedicated to blockchain technology, were associated; IRespond and Simprints, organizations dedicated to the use of biometric data for digital identity; the ICC, International Computing Center of the United Nations; among other.

The objective? identify each person above the identity records of each National State. According to the developers themselves, in the future, this digital identity will be necessary to access education, health, social benefits, political rights such as voting and carrying out economic transactions. This digital identity will connect our fingerprints, irises, medical records, date of birth, educational level, trips taken, credit cards, employment histories, driver's licenses and bank accounts. It will have the characteristic of "persistence", "from birth to death" and being "portable".

Why does GAVI "The Vaccine Alliance" participate as one of the main founders, the alliance of large laboratories that is in charge of global vaccination campaigns? Because the ID2020 project is ideal so that large laboratories can have, beyond each Nation State, a precise detail of each individual who has been vaccinated, when, how, where, etc. What is the argument for implementing it? "One billion people in the world cannot prove their identity (...) No government, company or agency can solve this alone," maintains the project, which states that current identification systems are "archaic and insecure," proposing the use of "new technologies, including blockchain and biometrics."

"For many, depending on national identification systems is not possible," they explain from the official platform. "The ability to prove who you are is a fundamental and universal human right. As we live in a digital age, we need a reliable way to do it both in the physical and online world," states the story that seeks to give it legitimacy. This project has already been presented in 2017 at the United Nations and in 2019 in Davos, one of the strongholds of the elites of financial liberalism.

ID2020 is part of the objectives of the United Nations 2030 Agenda proposed in 2015, which includes as one of its goals "providing legal identity for all, including birth registration", in an encrypted and decentralized manner (blockchain). "Everyone should be able to have their identity beyond national institutions and borders, and also beyond time," they state in their manifesto. There have been many speculations on social networks, and it is no wonder: Gates, the main financier of the WHO along with the most important world laboratories, is at the same time in charge, together with the historic and powerful Rockefeller Foundation, of laying the foundations for the biometric registration and control of the global population, something not unreasonable when in the midst of the Covid19 pandemic the computer magnate himself, who has become an ad hoc specialist in epidemiology, has been maintaining that the world will only "return to normal when all people of the planet have been vaccinated."   Source: Kontrainfo (http://www.motoreconomico.com.ar/aldea-global/id2020-identidad-digital-2020-el-ambicioso-proyecto-de-bill-gates-junto-a-la-rockefeller-foundation [2]).

Now let's go to the strictly economic sphere, because this is the cornerstone that will trigger that Great Reset, or global reset

---

2.   http://www.motoreconomico.com.ar/aldea-global/id2020-identidad-digital-2020-el-ambicioso-proyecto-de-bill-gates-junto-a-la-rockefeller-foundation

(which is not limited merely to money or the economy, but to the system structure of the current world). In that sense I will leave the matter to an interesting text taken from a documentary: The Great Depression 2020-2030: Coronavirus – Documentary. The Covid 19 outbreak is wreaking havoc around the world. As economies grind to a halt in an attempt to stop the spread of the suspected deadly virus, below we will document the reasons why we think the stock market will not have a V-shaped recovery and will instead continue to collapse and why stimulus fiscal economic will not prevent it. The next market collapse 2020 - 2021 and because the fiscal economic stimulus will not prevent it. Stimulus from the Federal Reserve and Treasury will not be able to prevent massive losses of income, production and wealth in the economy. Despite the stimulus, a large number of businesses in high-employment industries will disappear and/ or take many years to recover. Without a V-shaped recovery, it will take years to restore previous levels of production in many industries. It will take almost a decade to return to full employment. Nothing is free, massive increases in public and private debt burdens will impose enormous barriers to future growth.

Since the recent low of 2237.40 recorded on March 23 the ICP500 index has posted a significant counter-trend recovery gain of 24.69% as of April 9, this includes a gain of 11.23% in the last week. Although there were several technical factors and news catalysts that have contributed to this massive countertrend rally, perhaps the most important critical factor has been the expectations and announcements of unprecedented measures by the US Treasury and Federal Reserve. inject large amounts of monetary and fiscal stimulus into its economy and financial markets. Next, we will explain why the combined measures of the US Treasury and the Fed will not be enough to avoid massive and lasting losses of income, production and national wealth. In particular we will demonstrate that in the context of their inability to avoid a massive and prolonged economic crisis that will extend into 2021 the stimulus measures of the Treasury and the United States Federal Reserve will not ultimately prevent the occurrence of another massive drop in the American stocks.

In fact, after the current countertrend rally fades and the main bear market trend resumes, over the course of the next down leg, US stock prices will collapse significantly below recent lows and They will set a bottom in the range of approximately 1900 and 1500 on the S&P500 index. The eventual recovery of this bottom in the medium term will likely be protracted and painful as opposed to V-shaped with potential depending on various developments on the emergence of another major breakdown to even lower levels. The Economic Backdrop: The United States is only in the beginning stages of one of the most devastating economic crises in the nation's history. Certainly, the next economic crisis will be the most severe since The Great Depression. After initially underestimating the severity of the crisis, economists at Goldman Sachs, Morgan Stanley, Bank of America and Jp Morgan now agree that the contraction of US GDP in the second quarter of 2020 will be on the order of 30 to 40%, the largest quarterly contraction in US economic history, including The Great Depression.

Against the backdrop of this economic crisis, unemployment is expected to peak at 20 to 30% as business bankruptcies soar to unprecedented levels. Economists currently disagree on the timing of the economic recovery regarding how quickly the U.S. economy can return to previous levels of output and employment. According to our own estimates, the United States will not reach previous peak production levels until the fourth quarter of 2021 at the earliest. Most worryingly, due to lasting damage to the economy, full employment may not be achieved until 2030 or beyond. Stimulus measures are announced to address the crisis. The Federal Reserve of the United States announced an emergency package worth up to 2.3 trillion, the package is extremely broad and includes loans to help small and medium-sized businesses, loans to state and local governments and purchases of some types of high yield bond, collateralized loan obligations and commercial mortgage-backed securities. The following is a summary of some key details.

The Main Street Lending Program will guarantee credit flows to small and medium-sized businesses with the purchase of loans of up to 600,000 million. The municipal liquidity facility will offer up to 500 billion in loans to states and municipalities. Expanded primary and secondary market corporate credit facilities and term asset-backed securities credit facilities will support up to $850 billion in credit. Expanding the scope of securities purchase programs to allow the purchase of various types of securities, debt and investment instruments such as fallen angel corporate bonds, high-yield bond ETFs and others. The Fed will begin funding the Paycheck Protection Program liquidity pool, providing liquidity to participating financial institutions through term financing backed by PPE loans to small businesses. The programs that were announced greatly expanded the scope and breadth of the Fed's efforts to invest in support of businesses and credit markets.

None of these measures surprise us, we have expected both the Treasury and the Fed to take unprecedented measures to mitigate the damage of the most devastating economic crisis since the great depression. In fact, in the days, weeks and months ahead we expect many more announcements of relief programs. massive bailout involving trillions targeting virtually every area of the economy. However, as we will proceed to explain, none of these measures individually or in combination will be sufficient to prevent a very deep and prolonged economic crisis, in particular, these measures will not be sufficient to prevent the occurrence of another massive drop in stock prices. in which the value of the S&P 500 index will collapse substantially below the short-term low of $2,237 recorded on March 23, 2020.

Reasons why fiscal and monetary stimulus will not be enough. Due to space limitations, in this video we will limit ourselves to describing some of the most important reasons why fiscal and monetary stimulus will not be enough to avoid a deep and prolonged economic crisis and a second decline amid the bear market in course of the US sections We will organize the presentation around the inability of fiscal and monetary stimulus measures to prevent.

1. Severe and prolonged individual and business income losses

2. Acute and long-lasting production losses.

3. Massive long-term losses of wealth

Loss of income. Despite the many programs designed to mitigate income losses, the enormous income losses of individuals and businesses will not be compensated. The macroeconomic importance of this is that drastic losses in income will translate into equally drastic reductions in spending on goods and services in the economy. Loss of individual income. Despite the government's efforts, Americans' aggregate personal income, even after government aid is accounted for, will suffer huge losses. Loss of income due to unemployment. The wages and salaries of unemployed people will not be fully compensated by unemployment insurance. While it is true that some workers may end up receiving more money than they previously earned, on average unemployed workers will experience a substantial decrease in their personal income. Loss of income due to fewer hours worked. Although not all citizens will become unemployed, Americans as a whole will suffer significant income losses due to reduced regular hours worked and decreased overtime hours worked.

Reductions in salaries and wages. Many companies will remember salaries and wages to avoid losses and even to avoid possible insolvency. In this context, it is important to note that the Federal government's Kers paycheck protection program, which is designed to keep workers on company payrolls through conditional loans that are potentially forgivable, allows companies to reduce workers' wages and compensation by up to 25% without losing eligibility for loan forgiveness. Therefore, many companies receiving Federal benefits can be expected to reduce wages by up to 25%. Additionally, pay cuts of more than 25% can be expected at the large number of businesses that do not qualify for forgivable loans. Under the Kers Act, in this context it is important to note that a very large percentage of American businesses of all sizes will not qualify for forgivable loans and therefore will not face restrictions in terms of reducing wages and salaries in extremely large amounts.

Loss of tips, commissions, bonuses, and incentive-based compensation. Large amounts of American workers' income are earned in the form of tips, commissions, bonuses, and various forms of incentive-based compensation. In the vast majority of companies these forms of compensation will be radically reduced and eliminated during 2020. These categories of worker pay clearly will not be offset by the Fed and Treasury stimulus programs. Drastic reductions in these forms of income will have a very large negative impact on aggregate US income. In summary, there will be massive income losses for both unemployed and employed people in the United States during

2020 and 2021 and beyond. These drastic losses in income will translate into drastic losses in spending on goods and services in the economy. In terms of how this affects the market value of American stocks, there are two main effects. The first and most important effect is through the reduction of personal spending and the concomitant reduction of US corporate income and profits; The second effect occurs through the impact of the reduction in income on the propensity to buy shares directly or through funds.

People who have experienced large income losses or fear that they may do so generally do not tend to enter the stock market and risk everything for a little profit, particularly in an environment characterized by the enormous and very frightening economic and financial uncertainties that will tend to characterize the US and global economic landscape in the Covid19 and post-Covid19 era. Loss of business income. The loss of business income in the American economy will be even more drastic in percentage terms than the loss of worker income. Although the Federal Reserve and Treasury stimulus programs can certainly mitigate business income losses to a limited degree, businesses and their owners will face dramatic reductions in their income during 2020 and 2021 relative to 2019 that will not be offset by government programs.

Loss of income for large companies and owners. For example, we estimate that earnings per share of publicly traded companies in the US will decline by or less than 50% year over year in 2020. In fact, we believe that earnings per share of companies US publicly traded and private companies will be negative on a cumulative basis for the last three quarters of 2020. As a result of the drastic decrease in company income, dividends to shareholders will also suffer massive drops. Loss of income for small businesses and homeowners. Small businesses are disproportionately represented in the areas of the economy that will be hardest hit by the Covid19 epidemic. To make matters worse, profit margins and financial flexibility are much lower for small American businesses compared to large companies. Therefore, as a whole, small businesses and their owners are likely to experience cumulative net revenue reductions during 2020 and 2021 relative to 2019 that are even greater proportionately than those of larger businesses. The types and magnitudes of losses mentioned above for businesses large and small will occur despite enormous bailout packages from the Treasury and the Federal Reserve. This will happen for three reasons:

1. Many companies do not qualify

2. Many businesses simply do not qualify for government assistance programs.

3. Assistance will not be sufficient to avoid income reduction.

For many businesses that qualify for government assistance, the programs will not be enough to prevent large reductions in their net income; in fact, many businesses will experience large losses despite receiving government assistance. Assistance will not prevent bankruptcy. Many businesses that qualify for assistance will simply choose to partially or completely close operations, resulting in large reductions in revenue rather than continuing to operate in the face of even greater losses and increased debt. For example, not all forms of assistance will be forgivable, meaning they must be repaid so many companies would prefer to go out of business rather than be saddled with large amounts of debt that companies will not or will not be able to pay. Additionally, many businesses that qualify for forgivable loans will choose to close operations in cases where their owners or operators predict or fear large losses despite government assistance.

Given that business income represents a substantial portion of total income in the American economy, massive reductions in business income will have a profoundly negative impact on it, with destructive effects on the global economy. Dramatic losses in business income by businesses will lead to massive declines in ordinary business expenses, for example, payroll and supplies, and even more drastic declines in capital investment expenditures. Although the Treasury and Federal Reserve stimulus programs substantially mitigate business income losses relative to what would have occurred without such assistance, American businesses both large and small will suffer massive income losses. The drastic decline in aggregate business income in the American economy impacts the market value of US stocks in two main ways:

First, the reduction in trading income of these companies means drastically lower profitability of publicly traded companies in the US. Lower net profits and profitability affect both the intrinsic and perceived value of these companies which negatively affects the prices of its shares in the stock market. Second, the reduction in the trading income of American companies reduces their ability and propensity to buy back their own shares. This is important, because companies' own share buybacks of their own shares over the past decade have represented by far the largest single source of net demand for U.S. stocks, in fact larger than all others. combined sources. In this sense, Goldman Sachs has recently published a study in which it is estimated that share buybacks by companies listed on the US stock exchange will be reduced by half compared to 2019 levels. Our own firm forecasts, show even deeper and more widespread reductions in the amount of stock purchases of the order of minus 70%.

Increase in savings. In addition to the drastic reduction in business and personal income, there will be another factor driving a massive contraction in spending in the US economy. Increased savings. For every dollar received by American individuals and businesses from ordinary sources of income or through government transfers, they will spend a smaller fraction than normal and save a larger fraction than normal. When businesses and individuals save a larger proportion of their income including government transfers, the total amount of expenditures in the economy and concomitantly the total amount of income in the economy is reduced approximately in proportion to the amount of the increase in income. saving. The savings of individuals and companies will increase for at least three reasons:

1. Increase in precautionary savings. Frightened consumers and businesses will reduce spending to save for expected and unforeseen contingencies

2. Things to spend on. Social distancing necessarily means that people will have far fewer things to spend money on without concerts without sporting events without restaurants, bars, clubs without vacations.

3. Reduced use of credit for expenses. Net savings will increase, net expenditures will decrease, through reduced use of credit used by individuals and businesses to increase their expenditures and production. Although many people or businesses will actually increase their use of credit to compensate for lost income, relatively few businesses and individuals will use credit to increase their level of spending; On the contrary, firms and companies in general will tend to drastically reduce their use of credit for discretionary expenses and non-essential investments, thus causing a general reduction in the level of expenses and income in the economy. While the Fed and the

Treasury can somewhat mitigate the precautionary motive for saving, they cannot prevent an overall increase in the propensity to save. First, the Fed and Treasury actions will not prevent individuals and businesses from reducing savings for precautionary reasons. Second, they cannot provide consumers with spending opportunities that compensate for spending opportunities that are not available. Finally, the Fed and Treasury cannot force consumers and businesses to increase their use of credit to increase their spending relative to 2019 rather than using credit to simply offset lost income.

To summarize this section on income loss, while the Fed and the Treasury can mitigate the income losses of businesses and individuals to some extent they will not be able to compensate for all the income losses that will occur. In terms of how this affects aggregate economic statistics if there are overall losses of personal income plus business income, including, government assistance that equate to around 20% of total national income in the next three quarters of 2020 with maximum losses of more than 30% in the second quarter, gross domestic income will decrease by a similar amount during that period. Furthermore, a lower propensity to use and issue credit will only exacerbate the concomitant reduction in expenditures and aggregate income in the overall economy.

Lost of production. The Fed and the Treasury can distribute all the money they want to individuals and businesses, however they cannot prevent enormous production losses that will occur over the course of this crisis. Production will be reduced for several reasons, including the following key scenarios, among others.

• Mandatory and voluntary social distancing restricts production. Many companies will close or reduce production due to legal restrictions or due to voluntary measures to contain the spread of the Covid 19 virus.

• Disruption of the global supply chain. Many companies will close or reduce production due to domestic and international supply chain disruptions.

• Loss of demand. Many companies will close or reduce production in response to loss of demand. For example, production in restaurants, entertainment venues and many other types of businesses will close or be reduced due to the fact that customers will voluntarily limit themselves from consuming products or services when this is perceived to place them at higher risk of Covid infection. 19. Furthermore, demand will be lost simply due to the drastic reduction in income suffered by consumers and businesses.

Massive production losses will occur for all of these reasons until an effective vaccine is widely available, which is not expected for another 18 months, at least if it can be developed. If overall production of goods and services declines by about 25% over the next three quarters of 2020 with a maximum loss of about 40% in the second quarter, gross domestic product will decline by about 25% over that period. Loss of wealth. The following are just three ways that wealth will be massively destroyed in the American economy.

• Destruction in the value of equity. There will be a massive destruction of the wealth, of the equity of business owners, in short, insolvency, restructuring recapitalizations will decimate the equity value of most business owners, in addition, there will be large reductions in the intrinsic value to long-term and market value on owners' equity due to the reduced long-term growth rates and higher long-term discount rates that will result from this crisis.

• Destruction in the value of the debt. Debt holders and creditors of all types will suffer massive wealth losses due to the reduction in the intrinsic value and market value of their debt holdings. Massive amounts of defaults and a large risk of default by many debtors will cause massive losses in the intrinsic value and market value of the debt, leading to a massive loss of wealth by creditors without a corresponding increase in the wealth, in part, of the debtors.

• Destruction in the value of real estate. Due to a loss of demand for property and loss of income from tenants or lessees, there will be massive wealth destruction for property owners.

How does the massive destruction of wealth affect various forms of the real economy? The destruction of wealth will reduce the level of spending in the economy for two main reasons:

1. Wealth destruction reduces the propensity to spend in the economy by consumers and businesses that have lost wealth in both consumer and investment goods

2. The destruction of wealth reduces creditworthiness, creditworthiness, and the willingness of consumers and businesses to issue and take out credit. This reduces the level of current and future growth by inhibiting both investment and consumer spending by businesses and consumers.

The Fed cannot prevent mass insolvencies. While Treasury and Federal Reserve programs can and will alleviate liquidity problems in many companies, these programs will not be able to address the fundamental solvency problems in many companies that will result in the long-term destruction of production, income and the wealth. Let's just take a few examples. Establishments such as restaurants, bars and nightclubs will be devastated by mandatory and voluntary social distancing measures, many of these businesses will simply close and even assuming a vaccine is widely distributed within 18 months. The previous level of activity and income in these industries will take many years to return to previous levels. This is due to the fact that many former owners and operators of these businesses will be financially devastated and will be reluctant or unable to return to business due to loss of capital and credit constraints.

Department stores and shopping centers. Any business that relies on large numbers of people gathering in limited spaces will not be viable and will face insolvency. For example, high-traffic stores and shopping centers will see massive reductions in business even after mandatory closures are over, this is due to voluntary social distancing. Due to competition from e-commerce many of these businesses were barely viable before the Covid 19 crisis and were experiencing a slow retail apocalypse. Against this backdrop and in the coming era of prolonged social distancing both mandatory and voluntary, a large proportion of these businesses simply will not return. Theme parks live entertainment events, conventions. Essentially these businesses will have to remain closed at least until a vaccine or cure for Covid 19 is found. Most likely, this will not happen for at least 18 months and even then it may take a long time for these companies to resume production to previous levels, given the fact that many operators of these companies will be financially ruined.

The types of businesses described above do not have a liquidity problem, they have a solvency problem and so do all the people who serve these businesses, their suppliers, lawyers, accountants, etc. No amount of government assistance or loans will revive the lost production and lost revenue and capital caused by the destruction of these businesses. These companies are an important part of the economy and employ a large number of people. As mentioned above, after the need for social distancing dissipates, many unemployed owners and workers will not be lucky enough to find employment in their former industries. However, it will take a long time for these industries to climb back up to their new equilibrium levels of production, perhaps even more importantly, many of these industries will never return to their previous levels of employment and many workers in these industries will not be able to return to their jobs. old jobs; It is not easy to retrain workers for new jobs and it is certainly not easy for entirely new industries to emerge to employ the large numbers of people who become unemployed for long periods of time.

The result of this is that long-term unemployment will be part of the American economic and social landscape for many years, there is very little that the Treasury and the Fed can do to prevent the massive levels of long-term unemployment that will be caused by this crisis. . Furthermore, there is very little the Fed and the Treasury can do to offset the massive wealth losses suffered by owners and workers in these industries. Nothing is free. Almost forgotten amid all the excitement surrounding the government stimulus, is a fact that should be obvious:

Nothing is free, the Fed can fund the US treasury and US businesses all it wants, this will not change the fact that there will be a huge increase in debt in both the public and private sectors. Without a corresponding increase in output and/or productivity in the economy, the addition of such a large debt burden but a corresponding increase in productive capacity will necessarily cause a large loss of future output or national wealth. The massive increases in public and private debt caused by this crisis will ultimately be paid for in two ways, most likely both ways:

1. Lower future growth
2. Higher inflation

High debt reduces future growth by increasing the interest burden, increasing solvency risks and limiting future creditworthiness, all of which reduce potential future investment and consumption, and rising debt levels increase risk. that this will be paid for in the future through higher levels of inflation. The problem is that inflation is not a free lunch, although inflation reduces the real value of the accumulated debt and makes it easier to pay the debt with fixed interest costs. Inflation also imposes many costs on the economy and many limitations on future growth. First, price instability reduces investment, since the ability of entrepreneurs and producers to plan the cost of inputs and products is reduced. Second, credit costs increase as interest rates rise, which affects both the issuance and taking of credit. Finally, inflation has distributional and adverse effects on the economy such as reducing real wages and therefore real consumption, standard of living and wealth.

Evidently, some people think that the US government can throw money at the problems caused by this economic crisis and repair the extensive damage caused in such a way that the net impact on the value of American stocks is relatively minor. These people are wrong, the money thrown at these problems will come with a high price in the form of higher debt levels and higher inflation risks which will significantly impact both future growth and the discount rate at which future cash flows will be discounted. of actions.

Conclusion. Many people seem to assume that the massive stimulus programs from the US Treasury and the Fed will essentially offset all the economic damage that the Covid 19 crisis has caused, as we have shown in this video, this is simply not the case. While the Fed's treasury programs will certainly mitigate many problems, they will not come close to offsetting all the income, production and wealth losses that will occur; These uncompensated and essentially unfixable gaps represent an enormous proportion of the American economy that employs enormous numbers of people. The implication of this is that the next economic crisis will not only be extremely deep, but will last long after the economy opens and lockdown measures end, many industries that employ large numbers of workers They will remain devastated. The devastation in many industries will truly begin to be remedied in about 18 months from now, provided an effective vaccine and/or cure is developed and widely available, and even after this occurs companies in devastated industries will take a considerable amount of time to re-emerge often under new owners and for many long-term unemployed people to be retrained and re-employed in other occupations.

Therefore, there will be no V-shaped recovery in the economy, the next recession will be deep and long, and no amount of stimulus from the Fed and Treasury can fundamentally alter this inevitable fact. Stimulus from the Federal Reserve and the Treasury can ameliorate the damage that would otherwise have occurred to the economy. However, it cannot prevent the mass business closures, mass unemployment and massive losses of income, production and capital that will inevitably occur as a result of this crisis and when economists, investors and the general public finally understand this, the current bear market recovery will be brought in and the next decline in US stocks will begin, a reversal of the current bear market recovery and a collapse to new significant lows will occur sooner rather than later. [End of article].

I will not add much more about financial matters because I recognize that few like those matters, becoming a bit heavy to digest and understand. This is a point published by the Mexican economist Oscar Garza Bello, regarding the situation of the US in the hands of Joe Biden (it should be noted that this article was published on November 7, before it was completely clear who would be at the head of the US presidency).

Now let's go with the points about who wins and who loses in this strategy of systemic change of the financial model. There are things that we know are obvious, such as the fact that the Fourth Industrial Revolution is eliminating millions of jobs, current computers with artificial intelligence systems, drones, system automation and robotics are leaving the generation "labor" off base. What will governments do with all these unemployed and idle people? Guess. And you will guess right. Delete them. What have they done with black people in the US? leave them in rot and encourage criminality among them, and thus they can put them in prison and be the object of experiments. For decades, Africa has been the experimentation laboratory of many governments and companies. Dissent will be taken to concentration camps, and those who accept the intoxication and poisoning of the state will go to the grave. The powers that be do not want so many people, either because they assume that we spend a lot of resources, or because they become uncontrollable, demand a lot from the system and are no longer dispensable for almost any function of the productive apparatus.

The systematization of everything will quickly lead to seeing the world like in fiction movies. But green areas will be out of reach of these citizens. They will live in smart cities with fake gardens and fake nature... in essence, fake freedom. Filled with nano devices, their brains and immune systems will end up controlling them like machines, with implanted microchips. Transhumans, cyborgs, androids... believing that they are bionic men. All will be registered with a number, without private property and without their own rights. The people will be property of the state. They will receive some basic "help" that they will receive like an Indian exchanges his gold for a mirror. Freedom in exchange for crumbs.

<u>WINNERS:</u>

1. The BIDEN family wins. Both Joe Biden and his son Hunter can breathe easy because there will be NO judicial investigation regarding their dark businesses in Ukraine and China. It is not my intention to expand on this point, do your own research on the Internet and you will realize what I mean, basically millions of dollars for the Bidens in exchange for influence peddling.

2. The Clinton family wins. Bill will NO longer be investigated for the 26 times that, according to flight logs, he is reported to have visited billionaire Epstein's pedophile island. And Hillary will NO longer be investigated and prosecuted for violating national security laws by transmitting, through a private server, top secret documentation that was intercepted by the Russians, instead of using an official encrypted server as required by law. Nor will she be prosecuted for the "pay for play" case in which when she was Secretary of State, she requested million-dollar donations to the Clinton Foundation in exchange for political favors using her position. Nor will she be prosecuted for criminal negligence in the Benghazi, Libya fiasco, an incident in which 3 Americans including the ambassador died because she did not provide the requested additional security, and when they were under attack, she did not authorize the sending of the necessary air support.

3. Social media companies win, as they have become the main weapon for the dissemination of disinformation that favors the advancement of socialism in the world. Trump had passed an Executive Order that he intended to turn into law in his second term, to prevent companies such as Facebook, Twitter, Google, its subsidiary YouTube, and Reditt, to name a few, from using their monopoly power to manipulate public opinion through bias. the searches for information, and the censorship of conservative and libertarian voices, or voices contrary to the

official left-wing narrative. Take the New York Times as a contrasting example. If this newspaper defames you, you can sue them in a court of law and if you prove that they defamed you, a judge can order them to retract it publicly and pay you damages. But social media companies were protected because they are legally defined as "carriers" who without bias simply publish the material that others upload. But it has been shown that this is not the case, that they are partial and decide what information they send you in the searches you do, and they censor uncomfortable conservative and libertarian voices, and even journalistic articles that go against the leftist narrative. When Biden comes to power, not only will this Executive Order to avoid censorship and bias not become law, but it will be abolished, since social networks first supported Hilary and then Biden, they were their accomplices. Therefore, during Biden's mandate, censorship and bias on social networks will grow exponentially with all impunity, to manipulate public opinion in favor of Biden so that he remains in power.

4. Google wins, a very particular extension of the previous point. Google is the dominant search engine on the Internet. Do you want to see how he manipulates us? I invite you to do a very simple experiment:

- Go to Google and type the words, "happy black woman", and now go to images, what will you see? Well, many faces of happy black women, but...

- Now write, "happy White woman" and go to images, what do you see? Happy white women with black men and children. In other words, to be happy, white women "must have a black man and children at their side."

Well, given this monopoly power that gives Google the power to manipulate us through its search algorithm, Trump, through the Department of Justice, initiated an investigation into monopolistic practices. This case will be filed by Biden.

5. Black Liver Matter wins, a left-wing extremist group that defines itself as socialist and anti-capitalist on its website, which uses any incident in which a black criminal is injured or killed in a confrontation with the police, to carry out violent protests, destroy public and private property, including minorities, attacking the police with both violence and propaganda, brandishing the flag of "systematic racism" that is not supported by serious economic and statistical studies, and that received a donation of $26 million dollars from George Soros (public case, documented and verifiable if you review the online information of Soros' foundations), who also finances campaigns of Democratic candidates, including Hillary and Biden.

6. The group ANTIFA wins, a radical left-wing anti-capitalist group that calls itself anti-fascist, but is fascist and violent, and which, together with Black Lives Matter, is responsible for the violent protests in Democratic cities that have allowed them, such as Portland. Groups like Black Lives Matter and ANTIFA, Biden and the Democratic Party will use as shock groups against opposition mayors and governors when they want to pressure them to do something. They will take advantage of police errors or fabricate protests to force a political negotiation in exchange for peace.

7. George Soros, Trump's enemy, wins, and he lost more than a billion dollars with Trump's arrival to power. Every time Soros is mentioned, to disqualify you they accuse you of being a "conspiracyist", but let's look at the solid and verifiable data. George Soros donated $18 billion to his Open Society foundation, which funds groups like Black Lives Matter and left-wing candidates worldwide, including members of the European Union and US Democrats to support the globalist

agenda of which We will talk later. I don't know about you, but putting $18 billion dollars into a "conspiracy" that many mock and say does NOT exist, seems like a lot of money to me, or what do you think?

8. The globalist agenda promoted by the UN, the European Union and the Democratic party wins. What does it consist of? We will analyze this in the following points.

9. Win the UN Migration Pact, part of the globalist agenda. The caravans in Central and South America had been stopped because Trump refused to sign the UN migration pact, which discouraged the formation of more caravans passing through Mexico on their way to the USA. AMLO did sign the immigration pact, but if the door to the USA was closed, the incentive for the caravans to advance and be returned to their countries upon reaching the border with the USA, took away their desire to try. However, the Democratic party IS in favor of the UN immigration pact, because for them, poor immigrants who will live on public assistance are voters, even if they are illegal. So those Mexicans who love Biden so much, do not complain about the upcoming migrant caravans, some who will magically also obtain Mexican nationality and voter credentials so they can vote for the 4T.

10. Abortionists like Planned Parenthood (to whom George Soros has donated $2.5 million) win, also part of the globalist agenda. Under Trump, federal support for abortions was removed, but as Biden has promised, they will return. Note the deception of the name. Planned Parenthood – whose head at the time was Bill Gates' father – who can oppose family planning? But the name is a mere mask, what Planned Parenthood does is perform abortions. One in every 3 babies in the USA are aborted, don't believe me, go online and check the numbers, most of them black, which could be described as a eugenic

policy. That is why it is said that there is no more dangerous place for a black American than his mother's womb. In 2017 the number of deaths from firearms (including cases of self-defense, murders and suicides) was 33,000 people in the USA, while the number of abortions was 862,000, the majority of black babies. If Black Lives Matter was really interested in saving black lives, it would focus on investigating and combating the causes of why so many black babies are aborted, and as for the number of black people killed by firearms, the majority are from cases of blacks killing blacks, so Black Lives Matter should be investigating and attacking the causes of why so many blacks kill each other.

11. The LGTBIQ+ agenda wins, also part of the globalist agenda. According to this ideology, biology is NOT a science but an instrument of domination of the oppressive heteropatriarchy. It denies the concept of the binary biological sexuality of man and woman. For them there are multiple sexual "genders", in fact, 72 "genders" have been invented. As Orwell taught us in his dystopian novel 1984, to control society, language must be perverted by inventing new words and changing the meaning of existing ones, and history must be controlled by adapting it to the needs of the dictator. This is the case of the word "gender", there are not 72 genders, it is an adulteration of the real meaning of the word. In reality, ALL human beings are from the same genus of hominid primates of the species Homo sapiens, the only survivor among other Homo species that became extinct such as Homo Neandertalis and Homo Cro-Magnon.

The sexuality and preferences of each person are an individual matter, but the globalist agenda that is that of the Democrats and that of Biden, is not limited to putting bathrooms for people of "other genders" as Obama did in public schools, it is Going further and teaching children anti-scientific and anti-biological ideologies such as gender, is telling children that they can choose to be men or women regardless of their chromosomes and physical characteristics, and that, in fact, they can choose between more than 72 genres. In European countries, minor children can choose to request "sex reassignment" surgeries, something genetically impossible, they are simply plastic surgeries that change the appearance of the genitals. The problem has become so great that the British Parliament has even banned the continuation of this practice due to hundreds of cases of young people who regretted the operation they requested as children.

It is obvious in Hollywood and Netflix productions, the influence of this trend of normalizing non-binary sexuality, in which strong female characters, lesbian, gay, and androgynous, are not only part of completing a diversity quota, but are the good, the noble, the rational, the heroes, while white, straight men are bad, stupid, violent, irrational, old-fashioned. They include gratuitous non-heterosexual sex scenes to further an agenda. It is no longer about promoting tolerance and respect, it is about imposing an ideology in which being a white, heterosexual man, with family and conservative values, is equivalent to being an oppressor, intolerant, retrograde, fascist, Nazi and potential rapist.

12. Jihadism wins. Trump banned the entry of citizens of certain Muslim countries associated with terrorism. Democrats accused him of Islamophobia and initiated legal action to prevent this measure. However, during Trump's entire presidency, there was not a single attack by jihadists who entered the USA during his term, coming from those countries on the list.

But what is Islamophobia? Let's start by defining the word phobia: irrational fear, in this case, of Muslims. Is it irrational to fear Muslims? Is this a bunch of 15 radical crazy people? Well, this year a Muslim beheaded a French teacher for using the example of the cartoons about Mohamed from the satirical newspaper, Charlie Hebdo, to discuss the issue of freedom of expression in his class. Also in France this year, another Muslim beheaded 2 elderly women in Notre Dame Cathedral in protest of the French government's stance on supporting freedom of expression. And let us remember that the newspaper Charlie Hebdo has suffered 2 terrorist attacks with several deaths in recent years for satirizing Islam. It is okay to satirize Christianity and Judaism (it is freedom of expression), but for democrats and Muslims, satirizing Islam is Islamophobia and intolerance.

Some apologists will say that these are just "isolated" cases that only fuel Islamophobia. But are there rational reasons NOT to consider it a mere phobia? How radicalized are Muslims and how many radicals can there be? A Pew Research Center study conducted in London found that 9% of Muslims surveyed believe that "some acts of terrorism are justifiable." That is, if you go to a party in London, and there are 10 Muslims, at least 1 justifies terrorism on some occasions. And how many Muslims are there in the world? Approximately 1,900,000,000, almost 25% of the world's population. So, if 9% have a certain degree of sympathy with terrorism, that means that 1,710 million of them can fall into radicalization and support terrorism in some way, whether passive: not condemning it, or active: participating in organizations that providing resources to terrorist groups, or becoming terrorists themselves. Are you sure it's an irrational phobia?

When Biden takes office, he is likely to remove Trump's ban list, and since he supports the UN migration pact, he will not oppose the European Union continuing to allow the migration of Arab Muslims and Black Africans to Europe. Simply because of the difference in birth rates between the native population of Europe, which is small, and that of Muslims, which is high with more than 4 children per family, the white native Europeans of Christian ancestry (although many are non-religious), They will be a minority in their own countries, and Muslims, who do NOT want to assimilate into European culture and who want Sharia law to be imposed and make Europe a caliphate , will be the majority in Europe, which is why some call it the new Eurabia. And the process is so advanced that there seems to be no turning back.

Why does the European Union allow this? Because it is a supranational organization with a left-wing globalist ideology, which goes beyond the sovereignty of national states, and to build the dream that Soros cleverly calls, Open Society (to which I remind you he put $18 billion dollars), first He has to destroy what Europe is today, and then implement his utopia. They naively believe that by promoting abortion, lowering the birth rate of native Europeans, and favoring the migration of Muslims, they will first destroy Western European culture, and they believe that they will be able to manipulate Muslims to accept the new globalizing vision. But this will NOT be the case, since Muslims have their own agenda and worldview, and this is to implant Islam throughout the world, enslaving or killing anyone who does not convert to Islam.

If you visited London and Paris in the 70s and 80s, and you return now, you will no longer recognize them. London no longer seems like an English city, and Paris no longer seems like a French city. You will see 2 things, on the one hand, Arabs and Africans everywhere, and the presence of the army on every corner, why the army? Because of the fear of terrorist attacks.

13. Another big winner is the US Military Industrial Complex. Before you start lashing out with crude attacks that

this is just a conspiracy theory, let's see what 3 of America's greatest military leaders have to say:

13.1 At the end of his presidency, General Eisenhower warned the people of the United States of a risk to democracy: the enormous power that during the war had amassed what he called the military-industrial complex, a group of companies that supplied war equipment. the federal government, which needs a state of fear and perpetual war to continue bleeding billions of dollars from the federal budget for the development and sale of technology and military equipment.

13.2 The US general, Smedley Darlington Butler, one of the most decorated of that nation, starkly wrote:

"War is a racquet" (in Spanish La guerra es un larocinio or La guerra es un scam):

"We have done quite well with Louisiana, Florida, Texas, Hawaii and California and Uncle Sam can swallow Mexico and Central America, with Cuba and the West Indian islands as desserts and without getting poisoned.

"I have served for 30 years and four months in the most combative units of the American Armed Forces: in the Marine Corps. I have the feeling of having acted throughout that time as a highly qualified bandit at the service of the large Wall Street companies and their bankers. In a word, I have been a thug in the service of capitalism. Thus, in 1914 I affirmed the security of oil interests in Mexico, Tampico in particular. I helped transform Cuba into a country where the people of the National City Bank could safely enjoy its benefits. I participated in the "cleansing" of Nicaragua, from 1902 to 1912, on behalf of the international banking firm Brown Brothers Harriman. In 1916, on behalf of the great North American sugar producers, I brought "civilization" to the Dominican Republic. In 1923 I "righted" affairs in Honduras in the interests of the North American fruit companies. In 1927, in China, I strengthened the interests of Standard Oil.

"I was awarded honors, medals and promotions. But when I look back I consider that I could have given some suggestions to Al Capone. He, as a gangster, operated in three districts of a city. I, as a Marine, operated on three continents. The problem is that when the US dollar earns just six percent, they get impatient here and go abroad to earn one hundred percent. "The flag follows the dollar and the soldiers follow the flag."

13.3 US General Wesley Clark states in his memoirs that Bush Jr.'s plan was to take advantage of the momentum of the Iraq war to invade and impose democracy in "seven countries in five years." On the other hand, under Trump, the military-industrial complex has done very poorly. Trump has not started a single war. He has de-escalated the number of troops in Iraq and Afghanistan, something that Obama promised and did not fulfill, but he did receive the Nobel Peace Prize just for promising it, and Trump has signed 4 peace agreements in the Middle East.

Many of the wars that the USA has gotten into in the Middle East are precisely because they got into that region to control its oil. In fact, due to the permanence of US troops in Saudi Arabia after the first Persian Gulf War, where Mecca and Medina are located, sacred territory of the Muslim world, Osama Bin Laden launched his terrorist adventure against Al Qaeda to expel to the "infidels" of the sacred land and pretend that they stop supporting Israel in Palestine, land that the Arabs consider belongs to them. Also the invasion of Iraq, under the pretext of finding weapons of mass destruction that never existed, turned Iraq into a lawless land where before there were NO terrorists, but in the absence of borders and law, the Islamic State terrorist group emerged. In other words, it is the US intervention in the Middle East that destabilizes that region and encourages terrorism. And the more terrorism there is, the military industrial complex and the politicians who are in its pockets have the perfect excuse to invent more wars and justify billions of dollars in the budget in military programs. Trump was a hindrance to that since he was not interested in getting into wars.

14. Wall Street bankers are also winners. They do not believe me? Wikileaks leaked documents from when Obama was going to come to power, and it sent the president of CITIBANK as a representative of the bankers, a list for him to check the nominations of secretaries that Obama proposed to them. Trump is dangerous for the elites because no one controls him, he did not need money from bankers, oilmen, or the military industrial complex to get there. Since it owes nothing to Wall Street, bankers cannot ask it to repay the favor with regulations that suit them. Furthermore, Wall Street is the main financier not only of oil tankers but also of the military industrial complex. The mechanics work this way, the Pentagon justifies before Congress 1 trillion dollars to develop new military planes and ships; When you get approval, you order a couple of airplanes from Boeing and McDonald-Duglas, but you don't give them all the money at once, those companies go to the bankers and tell them: we have billion-dollar contracts with the Pentagon to make 2 airplanes, we need that you lend us money as working capital, and from what the government pays us for the progress, we will pay you the debt. On the other hand, the government cannot get that trillion dollars out of thin air, some of it is taxes, but another is bonds that it asks Wall Street to place on the market. Do you see how businesses are concatenated in a rigged pact? And obviously, the politicians who play the game finance their campaigns with "donations" from Wall Street,

the military industrial complex, the oil industry, and any businessman who needs "favors" from the government.

15. Another winner with Biden is the oil industry, believe it or not. The oil tycoons have both Democrats and Republicans in their pockets. But you have to understand something, you have to strike a delicate balance with respect to oil prices. If they are too high, the oil companies win a lot, but consumers get angry and this causes them to lose votes. But if the price is too low, voters are happy for cheap gasoline but the oil companies don't earn what they want. So, the policy is to keep the price of oil within a range that keeps both oil companies and voters happy. However, today the price of oil is at rock bottom and that doesn't matter to Trump because as a right-wing populist, his voters are happy. But the oil magnates are very upset, they would like some war in the Middle East that would put oil supplies at risk so that, given the drop in supply, prices would rise. Will Biden be willing to escalate existing wars or start new wars to satisfy the military industrial complex and oil tycoons even at the cost of more terrorism? Think wrong and be right. At the same time... And what will he do to satisfy environmentalists if he supports the oil industry under the table? Well, using taxpayer money, he will give billions in subsidies to questionable clean energy projects, and he will burden the auto industry with stricter emissions regulations. But that costs, who will pay for it? The consumer in the higher price of cars, or in less powerful cars.

16. Another big winner is China, which, like Venezuela's Maduro, supports Biden. China is the most cheating partner in the World Trade Organization. They have no respect for the intellectual property of other nations. They are the biggest plagiarists of civil and military technology. They are the second most polluting nation in the world, and they can do things cheaper not only because of a lower wage level, but because they

do not have to comply with environmental regulations. In addition, they have depredated their marine coasts, and since the fauna on their coasts has disappeared, they are now illegally destroying the marine resources of their neighbors.

The situation with them is a very delicate balance, one because they have nuclear weapons and one of the largest armies in the world. Another is because by growing in purchasing power, they have become large consumers that many Western firms do not want to lose. In fact, for Hollywood, its second largest market is China. In addition, they sell cheap labor, so many companies have factories there, such is the case of Apple. The cost is that they make it easier for the Chinese to steal technology. Review the case of Huawei, a company in which military generals and senior members of the Chinese Communist Party are involved as shareholders. Has this company ever invented anything? Review all lawsuits and legal trials lost due to technology plagiarism. Check out their models and compare them to Apple and Samsung phones and computers. What's more, check out what the Huawei stores are like in China and you will see that they are vile clones of Apple stores in the West. But they sell you their devices between 10 and 30% less in price because they are NOT the ones who invested hundreds of millions in research and development.

Furthermore, I can prove to you that they are responsible for the last 3 epidemics that we have suffered, including COVID-19, due to unhealthy practices in the so-called wet markets. Trump confronted China. It is debatable which points of its agenda with China are positive or negative for the USA. However, for confronting the Chinese, Trump received harsh criticism from Democrats and Biden, who referred to China as one of the most important strategic and commercial partners for the USA. What he did not mention is the corruption scandal of his son Hunter Biden not only in deals in China but in Ukraine.

17. The teachers union wins, who traditionally vote for Democrats because they are government employees. To understand why they win, for those who have not lived in the United States, I will explain how the public school system works from what we consider primary to high school. Depending on where you live, you may be assigned a nearby school. If there is a better public school a little further away, you have NO right to transfer your children to it. Your school becomes a monopoly, and what happens to all the monopolies? They provide you with bad goods and services because you have no choice. If you have money, you can send your children to a private school, but if you don't, you must settle for the school you got, and if you live in a neighborhood with drugs and gangs, your children's school will be a reflection of the neighborhood. There are young people who graduate from high school, with the ability to read and write of a 6-year-old child.

However, thanks to an idea from Nobel Prize-winning economist Milton Friedman, some counties and cities have adopted the "charter schools" model, which remain public schools, but must compete for the preference of parents and students, in these, yes. Parents and students are allowed freedom of choice, and the more students the school recruits, the more resources it will have, and if it is a bad school, it will lose students and funds. The result of this has been a success, as charter schools demonstrate that their students learn more and better, and obtain better scores on state academic aptitude tests. And what is the problem? Well, charter schools highlight the mediocrity and poor quality of traditional public schools. This infuriates the lazy, mediocre, bad teachers and their union. Well, Biden, on his election campaign proposals page, promises to reduce resources to charter school programs, which brought him many votes from teachers. The teachers union wins by eliminating the competition.

18. The obstacles of the New Green Deal win. This is a set of US legislative proposals that "claim" to be intended to address global warming and economic inequality. Biden says on his campaign proposals website that he plans to invest $3 trillion in this utopia. Why am I so skeptical? Because I know politics and government. But let's go back to the movie a little bit and look at the name, GREEN NEW DEAL, where does the name come from? It comes from a program that Franklin D. Roosevelt created to confront the Great Depression that broke out in 1929. I won't deny it, it was a very popular program that gained Roosevelt a lot of support, but was it effective? There are many things that are very popular but are harmful, like cocaine. The intentions were noble, but a law or public policy should be judged by its RESULTS, not by its INTENTIONS. According to economic research such as that of Nobel winner Milton Friedman and Thomas Sowell, to name some of the most famous, Roosevelt's New Deal only worsened and lengthened the crisis, in fact, before it was implemented, the economy was recovering, and because of the New Deal, the gain vanished.

Taking the socialist idea of the New Deal, the Democrats come out with an updated version with their GREEN NEW DEAL. What is my prediction on this "great" program? That it will be a nest of corruption and failure. Some of the money will be spent on bureaucracy. Much of the money will be given to businessmen who made campaign contributions and who invent green technology programs that they will overvalue, and the money will be used for other things. Another part will be spent supporting crazy "tech" projects of sons and nephews of Democratic governors. Loans and guarantees will be given to small minority businesses that will end up failing and whose loans will never be recovered. Google, Apple, Microsoft, Facebook, Dell Computers, and Twitter were not born from government programs. When you have a technological idea that can be a great business, there are fairs attended by venture capitalists and angel investors, who, as people, business, they know if your project has market potential. You don't need the government for that. If politicians were so good at being businessmen, they would be businessmen instead of handing out campaign contributions in exchange for political favors.

19. And did Mexico win? The coin is in the air. It is true that Trump has wronged us and here I will say why. One of the alleged grievances is false, but the others are very serious and real.

19.1 It is said that Trump called us criminals, drug dealers and rapists, but that is FALSE. It is an edited video in which he first talks about the illegal migration of Mexicans, and then talks about the Salvatrucha gang of El Salvador, whom he refers to as "criminals, drug dealers, and rapists." They cut the part where he mentions the Salvatrucha gang, and they beat him immediately after talking about the illegal immigration of Mexicans. And thus the legend of an affront that never existed was born. Although it cannot be denied that Trump, as a right-wing populist, continually used anti-immigrant sentiment against Mexico. But... Do you remember what WE MEXICANS said about the Salvadorans who entered Mexico in a migratory caravan? We practically said the SAME things about them that gringos say about our "undocumented" illegal countrymen in the USA. Let's not be hypocrites, or do you not remember?

19.2 A real Trump grievance that affected us was the cancellation of 2 automotive plants that preferred not to invest in Mexico under Trump's threat of raising tariffs on cars when the free trade agreement was renegotiated.

19.3 Trump's very serious affront was to force AMLO to sign a renewal of the free trade agreement that was disadvantageous to Mexico, and that affects, above all, the automotive sector, the crown jewel of Mexican manufacturing.

19.4 But the biggest grievance that Trump has done to Mexico is using AMLO as a servile lackey of his immigration policy. AMLO knows that the gringos do not want a Venezuela in their backyard, and as long as the USA does not press the eject button to get rid of him, he is so afraid of them that he is even willing to humiliate himself and do whatever it takes to Don't remove him from power. For this reason, AMLO cooperates fully with the US immigration policy, to the point of giving Central American countries money from Mexican taxes. Will anything change with Biden? Well, I don't think much. The renewal of the free trade agreement has already been signed. AMLO already gave the money to the Central Americans. Biden's rhetoric will be softer. However, if we look at the hard facts, for all his anti-immigrant rhetoric, Trump deported fewer people than Obama. Trump deported around 800,000 people, and Obama 1.2 million, and it was during his administration, and not Trump's, that people were put in cages separating parents from children, another myth of anti-Trump propaganda. On the other hand, as the Democrats and Biden approve the UN migration pact, we may have to put up with more caravans, and these will enter the USA because the Democrats will turn all those people into dependents of the American government, and voters of the Democratic Party, to guarantee a possible reelection of Biden, or the presidential election of Kamala Harris.

<u>LOSERS:</u>
1. You will lose the 1st amendment to the United States Constitution that guarantees freedom of speech. As already explained, social networks are left-wing and favor Democrats

whom they have helped come to power by biasing searches and censoring conservatives, libertarians, and articles that do not favor Democrats. Biden will throw away Trump's executive order that would allow citizens to fight bias, censorship and defamation in courts of law. This executive order will never become law, and the Biden administration will use private social media companies to manipulate public opinion and silence its adversaries. In addition, it will also throw away the trial for monopolistic practices against Google. With Biden, bias, censorship, and the lynching of opposition voices will grow exponentially. Some of you will say, that's a gringo problem, it doesn't affect us Mexicans, but you're wrong. First, if such a law were passed in the USA, other countries would emulate it to combat manipulation, bias, and censorship in their countries. And second, remember that the agenda is GLOBALIST and affects us all. It is promoted by the UN, applied by the European Union, and with $18 billion dollars, it is promoted internationally by George Soros' foundation, Open Society.

Do you think I'm exaggerating? Take the case of Spain. Since he was sworn in as Prime Minister in July 2018, Pedro Sánchez has met more times with George Soros than with the president of the Popular Party and leader of the opposition, Pablo Casado. And at the request of the Spanish Parliament, it has refused to reveal the content of the conversations. Since the Spanish government of Zapatero, a member of the same party as Sánchez, laws of the globalizing agenda began to be imposed. Gender ideology is taught in schools, and if as an academic you question them, you can be sanctioned, fired and fined. Laws have been passed that violate equality before the law, it is enough for a woman to accuse her partner of gender violence for him to be arrested and must face his trial from jail, but if it is the man who accuses her, he is not arrested to the woman, she faces her trial in freedom. And the Historical Memory Law has been passed, by which any historian and researcher who questions the "official" version of the history of Spain can be fined thousands of euros and have their material banned. Do you remember what I told you about Orwell and his novel 1984, about how history adapts to the dictator's convenience?

Did you know that Putin, president of Russia, and János Áder, president of Hungary (home of Soros), have expelled NGOs linked to Soros, and that in Hungary the anti-education-Soros law was passed that promotes the globalization agenda and gender ideology? Do you believe that Putin and János Áder are "conspiracy nuts", or intelligent statesmen and patriots who realize what is happening? Well, just as the UN, the European Union, and Soros's Open Society Foundation are promoting the globalization agenda in Europe and the USA, they are doing so in Latin America. The censorship, manipulation and bias of social networks are NOT just a problem of gringos, they are a problem of all countries that want to remain free, elect their own rulers, have their own laws, maintain their sovereignty, and not be puppets of ideologies, institutions and laws that a group of elites who feel enlightened want to impose on us, destroying concepts as basic as freedom of thought and even the traditional family.

2. You will lose the 2nd amendment that guarantees citizens the possession of weapons to protect themselves from criminals and tyrannical actions of an oppressive government. Many "brainy" analysts, opinionologists, journalists and influencers say that Biden is not a socialist, and they are right, he is an OPPORTUNIST like most politicians. What they don't know because they are only guided by the falsified narrative of left-wing media like CNN, is that the base of the Democratic party has become RADICALIZED. Before, it was the party of

the workers, now the workers vote for Trump, while the voters of the Democratic Party are carried away by the narrative of oppression of "identity politics" (if you are a woman, gay, lesbian, black, trans, you are an oppressed victim). That is why groups like Black Lives Matter and ANTIFA support Democrats, and many Democrats who do not agree with the tactics of these groups do agree with their ideological slogans, including socialism and anti-capitalism. Although Biden is not deep down a socialist, as we have already seen how he loves dark businesses in Ukraine and China, to maintain power and satisfy his voters, he will have to ACT like a socialist.

One of the socialist causes is gun control. Why is this so important? Didn't we see that while guns killed 33,000 people in 2017, abortions killed 862,000 babies? The explanation is very simple and dark. When you don't want the culprit to be exposed, what do you do? Well, a scapegoat is invented, in this case firearms. Well, but guilty of what and who is guilty? Let's turn to the statistics: Blacks, who traditionally vote for Democrats, represent 14% of the US population. But according to FBI statistics, they are responsible for approximately 52% of all homicides in the USA. The majority of black murderers are men, so 7% of the population is responsible for around 50% of all homicides. But babies and old people "almost don't kill", the black murderers are mostly between 18 and 35 years old. So, approximately 3-3.5% are responsible for half of the homicides in the USA.

How are Democrats going to accept recognizing that the ethnic group that votes the most for them is responsible for half of the homicides in the USA? And how are they going to accept that the social policies promoted by the same Democrats cause blacks to develop in such a violent and homicidal environment? No, no, no, we must find a scapegoat: the fault lies with firearms, inanimate objects that DO NOT shoot themselves. It does not matter that the statistics say that legal gun owners do not count in violent crime statistics, since criminals use weapons that are not legally registered, or stolen, or acquired on the black market. It doesn't matter that the majority of times a firearm has to be used by a civilian is in self-defense. No, that doesn't matter, what matters is using guns as a scapegoat, to not target the black community, and to not ask what policies make black people live in such a violent situation, and who proposed those policies (here among us: the Democrats).

So, the 2nd amendment of the US Constitution, as well as the 1st, are going to be attacked, the rule of constitutional law itself is going to be attacked. To satisfy his voters, Biden will most likely do the same as Clinton, a ban on so-called "assault rifles." What effect did this measure have in the Clinton era? Well, the homicide rate did not go down, it only increased the cost of rifles and magazines that were purchased before the ban. And the law was passed even though only 3% of homicides involved rifles, and not just "assault" rifles, but ALL TYPES of rifles, up to 22LR rifles. It was only a measure to manipulate the fear of the masses and propose a useless law that would deceive the imbeciles. Furthermore, Biden will surely pass more draconian and ridiculous measures like those prevailing in states like California, New Jersey and New York. I give you another very important fact, it is precisely in the cities where citizens' right to arms is restricted, where there are the most violent crimes: New York City, Los Angeles, Chicago, Washington, DC Why? Because criminals know that people are not armed and are easy prey.

3. All industries that depend on fossil fuels will lose. Do you remember I told you about the GREEN NEW DEAL? Well, any industry that depends on coal and fossil fuels will

face regulation that reduces their profits and raises prices for consumers. The automotive industry will face stricter emissions standards, so they will try to compensate by inventing "green" car projects that they can suck in as subsidies, part of the $3 trillion GEEN NEW DEAL budget. Companies that use coal as power plants will surely have to pay additional taxes that discourage the use of coal, make it more expensive, and force them to raise the price for consumers. Gasoline taxes may be increased in order to promote "rational use", so all cargo and passenger transport will suffer price increases, and the products they transport, too. The increase in transportation fuels increases the price of ALL the physical products you use.

4. Taxpayers will lose. Trump did NOT reduce the public deficit, but Biden will not do it either. In fact, according to the data that you yourselves can find on the page where you present your campaign proposals. Remember how I told you that Biden was not a socialist but that to keep his power he would act like a socialist? Well that's how it's going to be. In his plan, he proposes spending $11 trillion dollars on social programs to keep his voters submissive and loyal. In order not to get lost in long details, you can see how they plan to spend all that money by going to ReasonTV on YouTube, there they detail which "big programs" all those trillions are going to go to.

Oh, and I have a surprise for you if that doesn't convince you that he will act like a socialist! Well, Biden also plans to increase taxes to increase revenue by $3.6 trillion, which is equivalent to the largest permanent tax increase since World War II, neither Obama, nor Clinton, nor Carter, nor Johnson, nor Kennedy, all Post-war Democratic presidents never even imagined such a large tax increase. But as many "brainy" journalists, analysts, opinion leaders, Twitter users and influencers say, "Biden is not a socialist," right? And what do we care about what happens to the American economy with these changes? Well, if you are too young or ignorant to know, all of this can generate another economic crisis, and when the USA gets the flu, Mexico gets pneumonia. But it's good that Biden won, right? We finally got rid of the bad orange man who offended us, what a relief!

Affectionate and respectful greetings from your friend, OSCAR GARZA BELLO. ABOUT THE AUTHOR: Oscar Garza Bello is an economist, business consultant, financier and tax expert. Graduate in Economics from ITESM, Master in Public Administration from Harvard University, and Master in Business Administration from the Kellogg School of Northwestern University. He has worked professionally in the private, non-profit sectors, academia, and all 3 levels of government. Facebook/Twitter: Ogarzabello. [End of publication].

Looking at the interests of the Illuminati, the idea they had, at least for 2010-2016, was that by 2019, humanity would be under dictatorship (which was delayed a year due to the "fault" of Donald Trump). By 2020, the chip/tatoo implanted in people should be in operation (which is currently more than a year behind schedule). But there were other things defined with an exact date, such as the duration of the pandemic, until 2025, and the absolute and sovereign establishment of the global government by 2030. In their vision, these plans must already be established no later than those dates. That is, if it is achieved sooner, the better. Simultaneously, the world must be digitalized by 2025 (look at the example of how Pedro Sánchez wants to do it in Spain: https://artyco.com/que-es-agenda-espana-digital-2025/ [3]), just as he has already achieved. the Chinese government in that country. Consequently, biometric and socio-metric technology will be seen advancing at such speed

---

3.   https://artyco.com/que-es-agenda-espana-digital-2025/

that in a few years it will seem that we have entered the era of futurism and science fiction.

One of the key elements will be SmartCity, or smart cities. Holograms and sensors everywhere; scanners, detectors and projectors everywhere. We would use devices to open things, pay for things, and enter places, including receiving data and cryptocurrency via Wi-Fi and other radio frequency methods. It sounds cool, until you know that your private life will no longer exist, nor will your properties be yours, nor will your body be yours. To achieve this there is the 5-year agenda of the coronoplan: 2020-2025. The World Bank shows that COVID-19 is a project which is planned to continue until the end of March 2025. The document on its own website says: Strategic Preparedness Program and Response Program to COVID-19.

- Project Identification Number: P173789.

- Financing Instrument: Financial Investment Project.

- Social and Environmental Risk Classification: Considerable.

- Implementation and Financing Modalities: Multiphase Programming Approach.

- Approval expected date: April 2, 2020.

- Project expected closure date: March 31, 2025.

For example, a report published by the European Commission in late 2019 reveals that the EU has been trying to increase the scope and strength of vaccination programs since long before the current "pandemic." The aim of the roadmap is,

among other things, to introduce a "common vaccination card/
passport" for all EU citizens. This proposal will be presented to
the Commission in 2022, with a "feasibility study" that should
run between 2019 and 2021 (i.e. as of now, it is halfway there).
To underline the fact: The "vaccination roadmap" is not an
improvised response to the Covid19 pandemic, but rather a
permanent plan with roots dating back to 2018, when the EU
published a survey on public attitudes towards vaccines entitled:
"State of Vaccine Confidence in 2018". On the basis of these
investigations, the EU commissioned a technical report entitled
"Designing and implementing an immunization information
system", which concerns – among other things – the plausibility
of an EU-wide vaccination surveillance system.

In the third quarter of 2019, these reports were brought
together in the latest version of the "Vaccination Roadmap", a
long-term political plan to spread "awareness and
understanding" of the vaccine, while combating the "vaccine
myths" and the fight against "vaccine hesitancy." Some
highlights:

* Examine the feasibility of launching a common vaccination
card/passport for EU citizens.

*Develop EU guidance to establish comprehensive
electronic vaccination information systems for effective
monitoring of vaccination programmes.

*Overcome legal and technical barriers that prevent the
interoperability of national vaccination information systems.

On September 12, 2019, at the "Global Vaccination
Summit" organized by the EU and WHO, they announced the
"10 actions towards vaccination for all", which cover much of the
same area. In November 2019, these suggestions were published
as a "call to action." A month later, China reported the first cases
of Covid19. To be clear here (and avoid any side arguments):

this is not about the vaccines, their effectiveness, safety, or lack thereof. A month later, in October 2019, the 201st event took place. For those who don't know, Event 201 was a pandemic simulation exercise focused on a new zoonotic coronavirus originating from bats. It was sponsored by the Johns Hopkins Center for Health Security, the World Economic Forum and the Bill & Melinda Gates Foundation. The result of the simulation was translated into seven key suggestions. The fact is that the proposed COVID-countermeasures, which have been presented to the public as emergency measures devised on the fly by panicked institutions, have in fact existed since before the emergence of the disease.

They already wanted to control your vaccination records and link them to your passport, introduce mandatory vaccines and take drastic measures against "misinformation". But they still had no justification. The exact proportion between invention and chance will never be known. What we do know, at this point, is that Sars-Cov-2 is nothing like the originally reported threat, by their own admission. This was a situation that required a crisis and, fortuitously, there was one. We also know that they continue to spread fear anyway. And, thanks to papers like this one, perhaps we are now beginning to understand why. Also in this regard you can review the following publication: https://ejercitoremanente.com/2021/01/17/el-pasaporte-de-vacunacion-se-planeo-en-2018/

In the words of Bill Gates himself, <<we are building a financial system today from scratch. We do this to plan for this better digital future to manage a safe transition from the current system... from cash base to digital innovations... like vaccines. We need a measurement system that tracks vaccines.>> In another report, a news program commented on <<a $140 million [US] government contract leaves many questions. That department

claims it is to acquire syringes for covid vaccines, but states online that they question why the syringes have tracers on them.>> Interviewing a professional, he said, <<each of these injections also has the ability to have a a small chip. And what that chip has is a unique serial number for each dose... it is designed in such a way that there is no counterfeiting.>> Bill Gates' wife, Melinda, commented on a program, <<we talked about the incredible possibilities that we provides the technology in the future, to create the world we want to create.>> For his part, Jack Ma, the richest man in China - and owner of the prestigious Alibaba platform (where Aliexpress works) - said, << This is a very very important task to be in this because in the next 30 to 50 years human beings will be in the digital area.>>

What does this new digital era consist of? How do we enter this era? Elon Musk gives us a clear example by promoting chips implanted in the head to perform certain functions. It started with experiments where chips were put in pigs, and then in monkeys, with the company Neuralink. It proposes using this technology so that from the brain we participate in the interaction of video games. It sounds fabulous, that's the positive thing about the idea. What negative part could it have? The one that falls into the wrong hands. The book of Revelation predicted that people would be pushed to implant "something" in their right hand, specifically, or in their forehead, where the "numbering" of that Beast would be, and without which "it cannot be bought or sold." The developments and advances pushed by Bill Gates and Elon Musk seem to converge here. The issue of brain chips is not new, since it has been postulated as a means to cure "mental illnesses." How can a microdevice influence this? Each part of the brain develops a specific function, from motor skills to creativity itself. You can see this in greater depth in 'Remote Viewing II' (pages 90-91).

The brain is divided into 2 sections: left and right hemisphere. These two sections are subdivided into two others, leaving the left hemisphere of the frontal and anterior lobe, and the right hemisphere of the frontal and anterior lobe. In turn, the front left and the front right intersect, and the front left and the front right intersect. The front part is conscious, the front part is hidden. The right part of the brain operates on the left part of the body, and the left part of the brain operates on the right area of the body. The front left (masculine) is for logic, the front right (feminine) is for experience. The rear left (masculine) part is hidden experiential, the front right part (feminine) is hidden logic. The front left brain responds to the geometric shapes of the triangle and the square, and three-dimensional shapes of the tetrahedron and the cube. The right rear brain part follows the geometric shapes of the triangle and the pentagon, and the three-dimensional shapes of the tetrahedron and the icosahedron and dodecahedron. Technically the four sections are mirror areas of each other. The right is mirror of the left, and vice versa, and the front is mirror of the back, and vice versa.

In the same way, what operates on the right side of the body, at the level of the nervous system, affects behavior and stimuli on the left side of the brain, and what operates on the left side of the body, at the level of the nervous system. , affects behavior and stimuli on the right side of the brain. Consequently, if you are implanted with a radiofrequency device, a microchip or other wave, electricity or fluctuation device, it will excite the opposite area on the side of the brain where it has been inserted. A chip in your right hand could override your logical judgment. A chip on your forehead could override your rational judgment. The frontal part of the brain is what takes information from all other areas and coordinates them. That means that if you had a microdevice in the front of your head it would control your behavior and motivations, it would produce a deficit in your social and behavioral abilities. You would speak very well, but your "humanity" and values would be clouded.

To finish this chapter I want to share with you an interesting article that encompasses the idea of global control based on technology. We are not aware of the implications of this, but we can get the idea if we understand how the 'Big Brother' system already works in China, with all kinds of surveillance cameras and censors, database records and biometric identification. The very electromagnetic structure of the planetary sphere is being altered with the use of 5G facilities, earthquakes produced with geophysical weapons and with the stimulation of social consciousness to a polarity opposite to the axis of planetary magnetism. This will repeat what happened in Atlantis 12,000 years ago: a "shift" of the poles. Consequently, there would be about 3 days, or more, where the Sun would not be visible. It is also prophesied. But the point in this section of the book is to stop and think about technology in a way that many may not have visualized.

'China develops the world's first integrated quantum communication network' is the title of this article that I mentioned to you. It was published on January 10, 2021, and talks about technological news that represents a breakthrough that has surprised the world: Chinese scientists have established the world's first integrated quantum communication network, combining more than 700 optical fibers in the ground with two links ground-satellite to achieve quantum key distribution over a total distance of 4,600 kilometers for users across the country. The team, led by Jianwei Pan, Yuao Chen, Chengzhi Peng from the University of Science and Technology of China in Hefei, reported in Nature on their latest progress towards the practical and global application of such a network for future communications. Quantum communication Credit: Pixabay Unlike conventional encryption, quantum communication is considered unhackable and therefore the future of secure information transfer for banks, power grids and other sectors.

The core of quantum communication is the quantum key distribution (QKD), which uses the quantum states of particles, for example photons, to form a string of zeros and ones, while that any eavesdropping between the sender and the receiver will change this string or key and will be noticed immediately. Until now, the most common QKD technology uses optical fibers for transmissions of several hundred kilometers, with high stability but considerable channel loss. Another important QKD technology uses the free space between satellites and ground stations for transmissions over thousands of kilometers. In 2016, China launched the world's first quantum communications satellite (QUESS, or Mozi/Micius) and achieved QKD with two ground stations separated by 2,600 km. In 2017, a more than 2,000 km long fiber optic network for QKD between Beijing and Shanghai was completed. Global quantum communication network Chinese scientists have established the world's first integrated quantum communication network, combining more than 700 optical fibers in the ground with two ground-satellite links to achieve quantum key distribution over a total distance of 4,600 kilometers for users from all over the country (thanks to the University of Science and Technology of China).

Using reliable relays, the terrestrial fiber network and satellite-to-ground links were integrated to serve more than 150 industrial users in China, including state and local banks, municipal power grids, and e-government websites. This work shows that quantum communication technology can be used for future large-scale practical applications. Similarly, a global quantum communication network can be established if the national quantum networks of different countries are combined and if universities, institutions and companies come together to standardize related protocols and hardware. In recent years, the team has extensively tested and improved the performance of different parts of the integrated network. For example, with an increased clock rate and a more efficient QKD protocol, satellite-to-ground QKD now has an average key generation rate of 47.8 kilobits per second, which is 40 times higher than the previous rate. Researchers have also pushed the QKD record on land to over 500 km using a new technology called dual-field QKD (TF-QKD).

The team will then further expand the network in China and with its international partners in Austria, Italy, Russia and Canada. They also aim to develop small-scale and cost-effective QKD satellites and ground receivers, as well as medium and high Earth orbit satellites to achieve all-time ten thousand kilometer level QKD. The research findings have been published in the journal Nature. This article has been copied from the website https://codigooculto.com [4](You can read more at: https://codigooculto.com/ciencia/china-desarrolla-primera-red-comunicacion-cuantica-integrada-mundo/?fbclid=IwAR3PUmvOQNDk2nMHdhujP_qBj4WVzMeeEwjYsYc_r3sJhoF9x [5]).

---

4.   https://codigooculto.com

5.   https://codigooculto.com/ciencia/china-desarrolla-primera-red-comunicacion-cuantica-integrada-mundo/?fbclid=IwAR3PUmvOQNDk2nMHdhujP_qBj4WVzMeeEwjYsYc_r3sJhoF9xfZGcqIU4jw

VI. ELECTROMAGNETIC FIELDS

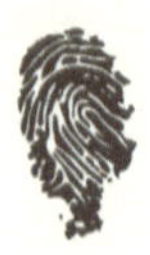

When the pandemic started it took me by surprise. I thought I knew everything, or almost everything, about the modus operandi that the elite would use for their development of the NWO. When that was in the Canary Islands and I was surprised that they put us in quarantine. It was quite an odyssey to go to the beach or the mountains, and going to the supermarket was like a movie. I began to sense within a few days that this was some false flag event. We began to send information to each other among acquaintances and discover what was happening. Then I got a video of a British electricity grid official filming a plate they were installing on 5G antennas, which was technically prohibited. The plate had a code that said 'COVID-19'. This aroused my curiosity greatly and pushed me to find out what this issue of 5G antennas was, with which until now I was not familiar with it. I saw news where people were burning antennas in France and England and they were blamed for the problem, but I didn't understand what relationship a supposed virus and an antenna could have. This is where my new research work began, which led me to publish this book a year later.

In this chapter we are going to address the most important part of the book. You must understand that matter is made up of energy, and energy is vibration. Sound is vibration. Waves are vibration. Thoughts, believe it or not, are vibration. Consciousness is vibration. Everything in the universe vibrates, there is absolutely nothing static, even though at first glance there appear to be things that do not move. In the same way, we are vibration. The vibration comes from intelligent energy, this from intelligent infinity, and this from Infinite Consciousness, which is the Universal Mind. This universe was created with multiple dimensions and planes of reality, and all of them are vibrational fields. The highest states of reality are called "spiritual", since they transcend the states of matter. The soul, however, is spirit, it is a portion of consciousness individualized and focused in a spiritual envelope. To experience the various states of reality he receives "vehicles", called in Sanskrit, "avatar". That avatar has 7 envelopes, or vestes (dresses), according to each dimension of the 7 of this base universe. They form a single being, or body of being, which is maintained and conscious by the mind of the individual in a vibrational field whose energy is known as 'aura'. This field is called the "biomagnetic field" and is about 9 meters in diameter, with its axis in the heart.

The science of vibration and waves has been well known for a long time, although it has been very little popularized. Magnetic use technologies have been implemented, but few with wave or sound technology. Before the era of Atlantis, there were already civilizations on our planet, such as Lumania, that had vehicles that moved by wave repulsion, without touching the ground. The waves were used in various interventions, especially by the plejaren (the Pleiadians), as is the case of the event where they divided the Red Sea (or Yam Suf (sea of reeds)) or the Yarden river (Jordan) so that the Israelites they passed dry. They also infused it in said town to use it against the inhabitants of the city of Yerijo (Jericho). The Hebrews did not know it, but that technique they were told to use was based on wave technology: going around the walls 7 times making noise. The vibration of the noise generated by the advance and shouts of more than a million people caused the structure to collapse. Nicola Tesla had also studied the implementation of these technologies, such as the "destructive ray", information that was later confiscated by the FBI after his death. With this knowledge, the Americans advanced in this science to equal the Soviets, who were already making it functional. The result was the installation of various military bases in various parts of the world with antennas capable of sending waves to the ionosphere so that they bounced wherever they wanted, causing earthquakes, hurricanes, rains or droughts.

I have already talked about this matter of geophysical weapons (HAARP) in chapter 1 (section D) of my book 'Recognizing the Time of the End' (2011), but on this occasion I will refer to other areas of said information and I will expand in other complementary areas, since they revolve around the same issue. The Soviets would have been using waves fired from HAARP-type antenna bases against the California coast to create a permanent state of psychological disorder. Each wave fulfills a specific function in the brain and its processes. Possibly this was the reason why the incident at the Chernobyl nuclear plant took place on April 26, 1986: the US attacked them to stop using this technology against them. Just two kilometers from the reactor was the city of Chernobyl II, where, precisely, the oldest HAARP structure built was located, and which supposedly stopped working. Could this be the machine that the USSR used to bombard California with low frequency waves? Ten years ago I made several posts on the then ProjectMagen blog about how the precursor of the television intended to create a machine that projected spectra through a screen. That occult man died without seeing his dream fulfilled, which was completed shortly after by another inventor. The idea of that man – I don't remember if his name was Robert Cook – consisted of the understanding that there are other planes of reality and they all intersect by waves. This principle is understood by quantum physics, and is part of the basis of string theory.

In addition to this, television emits 3 to 30 Hz, which, when hitting the person, infuses them into a kind of "trance" of the subconscious, predisposing them to be more easily docile to receive information than images and sounds. They try to project it. In this way, it is more efficient for any product seller to promote their material via television than through any other system, if they want to achieve a deep consumer impact on their client. The use of waves is also applied to music. This had a strong impact on me in 2010, when I was watching Abdullah Hashem's series, 'The Antichrist-Dajjal will be a Metamorphic Reptilian'. In his work he showed how the music industry used subliminal sound messages to program adolescents. Later I learned of testimonies from former Satanists and former witches who confessed that "the darkness" used music as a channel to possess young people. In one case, one of them told how he had been invited to a HeavyMetal concert, and while the band was playing he literally saw shadows coming to him and entering his body. Like the technique proposed by "Cook", waves played a crucial role in the transmission of entities from one plane of reality to another. But it is not my intention at this moment to talk to you about spiritualism or satanism, I only intend to expand a little on the matter of waves, sound, frequencies and vibrations. The story that "we are only matter" is an ambiguity that falls under its own weight: we are vibration. We are energy. That's why you put on a thermal sensor and it gives a temperature, you put on an electrical sensor and it shows a charge. What's more, you can be electrocuted, while a piece of wood does not produce conductivity.

And this doesn't stop here. Wave technology is so advanced that it is the cornerstone of the famous Blue Beam project, which I have talked about on so many occasions (see: 'Remote Vision I', chapters 16 to 20; Armageddon E-5, chapter 5, pp. 265-270; 'Recognizing the Time of the End', pp. 20-32). It is my assumption – understanding the elite's obsession with numerology – that Phase 1 of the Blue Beam will be perfected to fit the number '1'. After the Antichrist overture at the 2012 London Olympics, the next Olympics were postponed to the summer of 2021, and from that moment on, phase 2 could begin, or the idea could be introduced publicly. However, the Olympic Games are those types of large international events where the Illuminati excels at putting subliminal messages of their macabre intentions, like when they showed hospitalized people and a large hooded specter. What does this mean? The same as what Disney does: negative primacy. Disney is one of the elite's most important mass mind control structures, aimed at the mental transformation of children. The concept of phases 2, 3 and 4 of the Blue Beam are, in fact, elaborated with fantasy and "childhood" in the film 'Oz, the Magnificent', from 2013. There, if you know how to see between the lines (in each subliminal message and Illuminati symbology and vocabulary of witches) you observe the same thing I'm talking about. It only analyzes that the staging of "pyrotechnic fires" is used by the Illuminati to refer to the holographic, psychic and atmospheric sound deceptions that will be carried out to deceive humanity, and "if it were possible even the chosen ones" (Mark 13:22).

To develop phases 2, 3 and 4, the existence of quite advanced technologies is essential, most of which are not public knowledge, and the common citizen could think that they are mere "science fiction". These types of necessary advances have been the great developments that derived from electricity and radio (Hertzian waves) to reach unimaginable things, except for cinema. Thanks to the Schumann resonance, the waves travel within the ionosphere and their rebound propagates the waves, allowing telecommunications. Despite this, this technology is not enough to achieve the great objective or 'The Night of the Thousand Stars'. I will abbreviate it as 'TNTS'. As I mentioned in the first chapter, since the 1950s, the technology of the US and Russia has been far ahead in time. Only in Area 51 is technology used that is more than 60 years ahead of what we should be knowing at this moment as a civilization in the field of science. To achieve phases 2, 3 and 4 of the Blue Beam and achieve the great success of the TNTS, work has been done in various strategic areas:

1. Dispersion of metals in the troposphere by means of unmarked aircraft to ionize the atmosphere, deposit these chemicals in the crop soil and also be inhaled by the population. Many of these sprayed like aerosols that are breathed, and in the following days cases began of people collapsing hospitals due to respiratory failure (of course, later blamed on a pandemic).

2. Introduction of heavy metals, such as aluminum and mercury, into the bloodstream of the population through vaccines.

3. Introduction of nano devices through new vaccines.

4. Introduction of lithium, fluoride, lime and other minerals into tap water (pipes) and food to calcify the pituitary gland.

5. Blood poisoning through chemicals in food (additives, stabilizers, colorants, sweeteners, acidulants, pasteurizers, preservatives, transgenics, etc.).

6. Introduction of chimera viruses through vaccines.

7. Promotion of toxic and carcinogenic foods and junk food to weaken the immune system.

8. Implementation of low-frequency wave repeaters on orbital satellites with the capacity to transmit messages in any language, and holographic triangulation systems for projections in space.

9. Development of film holograms.

10. Radio frequency technology, wi-fi/bluetooth, and other very low, low, medium and high frequency wireless waves.

11. Mind control technology using images, words, sounds, phrases and social design concepts.

12. Hertz waves used to slow down critical reasoning processes, emitted by televisions.

13. Low and very low frequency antenna installations that launch waves into the ionosphere.

14. Use of agrochemicals that are absorbed by the roots and fruits and pass into the human body. And the fashion in 2020 of spraying highly dangerous components on city streets, dial to sterilize and disinfect.

15. Tracking systems through mobile phones, tablets and computers.

16. Installation of surveillance cameras in Smart-TVs, and "pan-dimensional plasma" conductive chips to facilitate the projection of spectra.

17. Development of automated drones and their combination with holographic coating fields.

18. Development of drones, cameras and satellites for surveillance, tracking and monitoring, heat and motion sensors.

19. Quantum computers interconnected with surveillance, security and information collection networks.

20. Development of artificial intelligence that collects information, directs security systems and monitors and controls all databases and surveillance in a centralized system.
21. Dimensional portals created for the opening of channels between parallel planes.
22. Technology and networks of biometric and sociometric control, tracking, surveillance and monitoring systems.
23. Installation of high-frequency antenna networks for bombardment of microtesla and vibrational resonance waves.
24. Artificially causing earthquakes at intersections of the Ley Lines to alter the "earth grid" - which prevents demons that have been locked under the Earth from being released -.
25. Introduction of pathogens and nano devices through implantable identification chips.
26. And finally release of nano devices in city water pipes.

I never tire of talking about The Night of a Thousand Stars over and over again, because more new elements always appear that add content to this scenario, and because it is a "masterpiece" of the Illuminati. The TNTS is an arduous work that has been launched with the sole purpose of making the appearance of the Antichrist a resounding success. The initial idea was intended to be carried out in 1983, but it was not achieved (the technology to achieve it did not yet exist), so it was attempted between 1995 and 1996, but not much progress had been made either, especially by NASA. It is the assumption of some that Ronald Reagan's claims about "war on aliens" at the UN in 1983 were a hint at this project. This suggests that the original NASA/UN document dates back long before 1994, when the Canadian researcher who released it – Sergie Monast – began appearing on television reporting on the aforementioned. Some allege that NASA is a cover, that the Secret Space Project investigates the colonization of space, while NASA actually fulfills the functions of fully implementing the installation of holographic projection satellites, camouflage drones, transatmospheric ballistic missiles and other exercises, while CERN and the LHC – among other "hadron colliders" – prepare the dimensional portals for exercise 3, and final, of phase 4 of the project.

Someone could argue that despite the links between these aspects, it is the word of Sergie Monast alone. The truth is that after Monast's statements a couple of former CIA agents acknowledged in an interview that this technology really existed and the project was under development. Years later, information was leaked from the CIA that recognized the authenticity of the plan. This suggests that the document that Monast obtained from NASA/UN could be much earlier, and would coincide with the known information that the UN was in fact created in 1945 with the sole purpose of pushing the world towards a world government that would end in the hands of the Antichrist. The antecedents of this go much further back and even reach back to 1871, when the Master Mason Albert Pike wrote to his friend, the Master Mason Giuseppe Mazzini about how the Illuminati was going to provoke three world wars in the coming years to achieve the goal of ending humanity and subject it to the feet of the Antichrist (these letters were preserved in the British Museum until 1977, when they were removed). Here you can see the original transcription of the text in English: https://ia801900.us.archive.org/16/items/albert-pike-letter-to-mazzini/Albert%20Pike%20Letter%20to%20Mazzini.pdf [1]. We are talking about a plan that had been studied for a long time, and there is testimony from former Satanists who confirm this, even referring to the members of British Freemasonry who pushed Darwin's theory of Evolution, which is an essential part of phase 1 of the Blue Beam Project, that is, this has been brewing for more than 200 years in the minds of the high degrees of Freemasonry.

This potential weapon was discussed in a memo from Marshall Chadwell, Deputy Director of Scientific Intelligence, to General Walter Bedell Smith, CIA Director of Central Intelligence, which was sent in October 1952, when the CIA was deeply involved in the investigation of the UFO phenomenon and flying saucers following an explosion of sightings. The memo was sent at the height of the Cold War and considered whether the number of UFO sightings could be predicted or controlled or, more ominously, even "used from a psychological warfare point of view, either offensively or defensively." ". He said studies showed that public concern, not just in the US but generally, with the phenomenon, was so strong that many people may be preconditioned to accept the unbelievable as truth. The memo added that news of possible extraterrestrial activity had the potential to cause hysteria and mass panic. Since 1947, the Air Technical Intelligence Center had received 1,500 official reports of sightings, plus more from the public and the press. In July 1952 there were 250 reports and, of all sightings, 20% remained unexplained. With so many sightings happening, there was a danger of false alarms of real military invasions of the Soviet Union, or worse, of real attacks being misinterpreted as "ghost" UFOs, the secret (now public) memo said.

---

1.   https://ia801900.us.archive.org/16/items/albert-pike-letter-to-mazzini/
Albert%20Pike%20Letter%20to%20Mazzini.pdf

The report added: "Immediate steps should be taken to improve both visual and electronic ghost identification so that, in the event of an attack, instantaneous and positive identification of enemy aircraft or missiles can be made. A study should be instituted to determine what use, if any, U.S. psychological warfare planners could make of these phenomena." Cold War paranoia was evident in the memo, which spoke of fears of a Soviet plot to use the UFO scare against the American public. The memo added that it would need to establish "what defenses, if any, should be planned in anticipation of Soviet plans to use them." Mr. Chadwell continued: "Other intelligence issues requiring determination include possible Soviet intentions and capabilities to use these phenomena to the detriment of US security interests." The memo also called for an investigation into how much the Soviet Union knew about UFOs and the reason behind why aliens or flying saucers were never mentioned in the Russian media. Chadwell signed his memorandum and added: "I consider this problem to be of such importance that it should be brought to the attention of the National Security Council so that a coordinated community-wide effort toward its solution can be initiated."

One of the theories aired since then was that the US was planning to initiate a "false flag" incident using hologram technology to stage a fake alien invasion as a pretext to introduce Martial Law or other dictatorial controls over the people. Hence conspiratorial proposals were also born around the government's High Frequency Active Auroral Research Program (HAAR). It was a United States military scientific project that has generated even more conspiracies than the Large Hadron Collider (LHC). It was established by the United States Air Force to study Earth's ionosphere, a highly charged and active part of the upper atmosphere. But many researchers and truth seekers always claimed that it was a cover for secret tests whose purposes are to control the weather or even to investigate "captured UFO technology" or create a false flag hologram, such as Project Blue Beam. The air force ended the project in 2014, but presumably the program is still continuing, since we are, without a doubt, working together where EVERYTHING leads to exactly the SAME THING: a global government run by the Antichrist. You can see more about this at this link: https://www.ufointernationalproject.com/frequently-asked-questions/uss-secret-plan-fake-alien-invasion-project-blue-beam-become-real/ [2].

The former Naval Intelligence officer, Milton William Cooper, points out in his work 'Behold a Pale Horse' (1991) that secret societies had been planning an "artificial threat" from "outside space" since at least 1917 to unite humanity in a single world government. They have shown this in cinematography, because alien films are the preparation for this agenda. Just look at 'Independence Day', not just the first one, but how obvious and clear they make it in the second movie. The young reporter Rick Clay, who anticipated this at the 2012 London Olympics, was murdered, Sergie Monast was also murdered in 1996, and Bill Cooper was first threatened when he wanted to document more information about this, and was finally murdered in 2001. We talk of one of the best elaborated and prepared conspiracies in history. Cooper linked the great fraud of the alien invasion with an additional pretext to restart the world's economy and include a new system in the New World Government. Following a chronological line, the Illuminati elite wants to push for a Third World War, of a thermonuclear nature, but divert

---

2.   https://www.ufointernationalproject.com/frequently-asked-questions/uss-secret-plan-fake-alien-invasion-project-blue-beam-become-real/

attention from it into a supposed alien invasion. Then the Antichrist would encourage the world to unite against enemies and establish a unified government that unites all logistical, military, infrastructure and war forces to save humanity from extinction, in the face of an imminent extraterrestrial invasion.

In 'Oz, the Magnificent' (2013), Disney leaves the symbology of this montage well exposed. Prophets such as Elijah (Elijah) or Yeshua (Jesus), and Paul of Tarsus himself, had warned that the appearance of the Antichrist would come with a great montage, worthy of Hollywood, with a 3D film projection in full atmosphere and with vivid sounds. Drones camouflaged as UFOs would shoot at planes, and vice versa. Motherships would be seen above Earth - as in the series 'V, Invasion' - but they would be holographic projections, not real ships. These Hebrews had warned in ancient texts that the Antichrist would carry out all kinds of artificial frauds and deceptions, making people believe that he had powers and pushing the world to see a completely fictitious spectacle of combat. Yeshua, Elijah and Pablo said that he would give orders to the stars to obey him, and of course, if he directs the assembly of the space holograms he will make the world see projections that supposedly make it appear that the stars are even moving from their positions in the opposite direction, as if leaving the sun when it should be at night, or the Moon where it was not its position. In addition to this, using their scarce language at that time, they describe the fictitious fight: <<there will be portents in the heavens>>. Well, as I said, I already address this in detail in my previous works, so I wanted to emphasize some details that I had not previously mentioned.

In 'I Pet Goat II' and 'Oz, the Magnificent' we find a coincidence that is repeated in other cases, such as Steve Jackson's Illuminati letters from 1995, about the Night of a Thousand

Stars, and that is that the symbol or code used To refer to that event, he is a "magician" with his hat and black suit, doing "tricks" with "pyrotechnics." Both the voices that people believe they hear, as well as the appearances of this new "god", such as the kidnapping of unsuspecting Christians, the alien invasion or the plague of demons are due to the technological advance that we have reached. It all comes from the colossal advance in applied science and knowledge. That is why I have expanded on this field before going into greater detail about the reasons for the various technologies that have been promoted, since these are an essential key to the triangulation of the systems that will be used to produce the great holographic deception, the great movie ever designed. We have: 1) Holograms, 2) Waves and 3) Portals. What is necessary for the soup that the Antichrist will offer as the last move, and his masterpiece, to take humanity into his pocket. No one will know if what they see on television is a 3D reproduction of a man performing miracles, because Hollywood can now invent anything you see through the "great eye" (television) that sees everything. You will be able to see that man flying on the news, walking on water, bringing the dead back to life... and people will not know that everything is done in a production room with color schemes, a harness and 3D animation design, and at public events he They will see things done that will simply be projected with holograms, while the populace believes that it is something real, that this being is a god and has superpowers.

Now, let's look at an example of patents for magnetic and wave technologies that were already known what effects they could cause, especially on people. And it must be linked to the above, taking into account that another added factor of Hollywood is the ideology of "magic" and "illusionism" (which are two different things, although culturally by mistake they define them as the same thing). Physiological effects have been observed in a human subject in response to stimulation of the skin with weak electromagnetic fields that are pulsed with certain frequencies close to ½ Hz or 2.4 Hz, so as to excite a sensory resonance. Many computer monitors and TV tubes, when displaying pulsed images, emit pulsed electromagnetic fields of sufficient amplitudes to cause such excitation. Therefore, it is possible to manipulate a subject's nervous system by tapping images displayed on a nearby computer monitor or television. For the latter, the image pulse can be embedded in the program material, or it can be overlaid by modulating a video stream, either as an RF (radio frequency) signal or as a video signal. The image displayed on a computer monitor can be effectively clicked using a simple computer program.

The invention relates to the stimulation of the human nervous system by means of an electromagnetic field applied externally to the body. A neurological effect of external electric fields has been mentioned by Wiener (1958) in a discussion of the grouping of brain waves through nonlinear interactions. The electric field was arranged to provide "direct electrical conduction of the brain." Wiener describes the field as being created by a 10 Hz alternating voltage of 400 V applied in a room between the ceiling and the floor. Brennan (1992) describes in US Patent No. 5,169,380, an apparatus for alleviating disturbances in the circadian rhythms of a mammal, in which an alternating electric field is applied across the subject's head using two electrodes placed a short distance from the skin. A device that involves both a field electrode and a contact electrode is the "Graham Potentiator," mentioned by Hutchison (1991). This relaxation device uses movement, light and sound, as well as an alternating electric field applied primarily to the head. The contact electrode is a metal bar in ohmic contact with the subject's bare feet, and the field electrode is a hemispherical metal helmet placed several inches from the subject's head.

In these three methods of electrical stimulation, the external electric field is predominantly applied to the head, so that electrical currents are induced in the brain in the physical manner governed by electrodynamics. These currents can be largely avoided by applying the field not to the head, but to areas of skin away from the head. Certain skin receptors can then be stimulated, which would provide an input signal to the brain along the natural afferent nerve pathways. It has been found that, in fact, physiological effects can be induced in this way by very weak electric fields, if pulsed with a frequency close to ½ Hz. The effects observed include ptosis of the eyelids, relaxation, drowsiness, sensation of pressure at a point centered on the lower edge of the eyebrow, dark purple and greenish-yellow moving patterns are seen with closed eyes, a toned smile, a feeling of tension in the stomach, sudden loose stools, and sexual arousal, depending on the precise frequency used and the area of skin to which the field is applied. The strong frequency dependence suggests the involvement of a resonance mechanism.

When mobile phones appeared, debates began about their health effects. In case people had tumors in the part of the brain closest to where they had the phone located all the time. Research in this regard combines biology and physics, two usually separate fields, and they have not been made clear due to corporate implications. Despite the Precautionary Principle, it would be masterful to see such a miracle as a global call for awareness about the dangers of mobile devices, Bluetooth, Wi-Fi and repeater antennas. On the other hand, society itself, addicted to new technologies and telecommunications, does not seem to be very willing to give up these "pleasures." It is known that plants produce calmodulin when exposed to radio frequencies such as microwaves. In the case of humans, these waves first affect the blood-brain barrier (highly selective permeability that separates circulating blood from the extracellular brain fluid in the central nervous system), making it permeable, and leading to a leak of alumina (a protein that is found in a large proportion in blood plasma, being the main protein in blood, and one of the most abundant in humans), in addition to destroying neurons and causing cancer. The laboratories that study this are divided, because, of course, some respond to the complacency of the companies that finance them (and that would be harmed by the results) and/or to negligence in the experiments due to being under pressure. Every new advance in telecommunications, from radio and radar, has been accompanied by an immediate wave of EHS (Electromagnetic Hypersensitivity) reactions that, depending on the person, have various effects. The people themselves who pass near cable towers or antennas, or live where they are located, have always complained about the physical discomfort it causes them. Now imagine the increase in Hertz waves as the range and power of the new installations expand.

It has been discovered that resonance can be excited not only by externally applied pulsed electric fields, as described in US Patents 5,782,874, 5,899,922, 6,081,744 and 6,167,304, but also by pulsed magnetic fields, as described in US Patent Nos. 5,935,054 and 6,238,333, by means of weak pulses of heat applied to the skin, as described in US Patent Nos. 5,800,481 and 6,091,994, and by subliminal acoustic pulses, as described in US Patent No. 6,017,302. Since resonance is excited through sensory pathways, it is called sensory resonance. In addition to the resonance close to ½ Hz, a sensory resonance close to 2.4 Hz has been found. The latter is characterized by the deceleration of certain cortical processes, as described in patents '481, '922, '302,

'744, '944 and '304. Excitation of sensory resonances through weak heat pulses applied to the skin provides a clue as to what is happening neurologically. Temperature-sensitive skin receptors are known to activate spontaneously. These nerves fire somewhat randomly around an average rate that depends on skin temperature. Therefore, weak heat pulses delivered to the skin periodically will cause a slight frequency modulation (fm) in the spike patterns generated by the nerves. Since stimulation through other sensory modalities results in similar physiological effects, frequency modulation of spontaneous afferent neural spiking patterns is thought to occur there as well.

It is instructive to apply this notion to stimulation using weak electric field pulses delivered to the skin. Externally generated fields induce pulses of electrical current in the underlying tissue, but the current density is too small to fire an otherwise inactive nerve. However, in experiments with the adaptation of crayfish stretch receptors, Terzuolo and Bullock (1956) have observed that very small electric fields may be sufficient to modulate the activation of already active nerves. Such modulation can occur in the stimulation of the electric field under discussion. Further understanding can be gained by considering the electrical charges that accumulate in the skin as a result of induced tissue currents. Ignoring thermodynamics, one would expect the accumulated polarization charges to be strictly limited to the outer surface of the skin. But the charge density is caused by a slight excess of positive or negative ions, and thermal movement distributes the ions through a thin layer. This implies that the externally applied electric field actually penetrates a short distance into the tissue, rather than stopping abruptly at the external surface of the skin. In this way, a considerable fraction of the applied field can be applied to some cutaneous nerve endings, so that a slight modulation of the type observed by Terzuolo and Bullock can occur.

In short, computer monitors and TV monitors can be made to emit weak, low-frequency electromagnetic fields simply by pulsing the intensity of the displayed images. Experiments have shown that the ½ Hz sensory resonance can be excited in this way in a subject near the monitor. The 2.4 Hz sensory resonance can also be excited in this way. Therefore, a television monitor or computer monitor can be used to manipulate the nervous system of people nearby. Implementations of the invention are tailored to the video stream source that drives the monitor, whether it is a computer program, a TV broadcast, a video tape, or a digital video disc (DVD). For a computer monitor, image pulses can be produced by a suitable computer program. The pulse rate can be controlled via keyboard input, so that the subject can tune to an individual sensory resonance frequency. The pulse width can also be controlled in this way. A program written in Visual Basic (R) is particularly suitable for use on computers running the Windows 95 (R) or Windows 98 (R) operating system. The structure of said program is described. The production of periodic pulses requires a precise synchronization procedure. This procedure is built on the GetTimeCount function available in the Application Program Interface (API) of the Windows operating system, together with an extrapolation procedure that improves the timing accuracy.

Pulse variability can be introduced through software, for the purpose of thwarting habituation of the nervous system to field stimulation, or when the precise resonant frequency is not known. The variability may be a pseudorandom variation within a narrow interval, or it may take the form of a sweep of frequency or amplitude over time. Pulse variability may be under the subject's control. The program that causes a monitor to display a pulsating image can be run on a remote computer that is connected to the user's computer by a link; the latter may belong in part to a network, which may be the Internet. For a TV monitor, the image pulse can be inherent to the video stream as it flows from the video source, or the stream can be modulated so that it superimposes the pulse. In the first case, a live television broadcast can be arranged so that the feature is embedded by simply lightly tapping the lighting of the scene being broadcast. Of course, this method can also be used to make movies and burn video tapes and DVDs.

Video tapes can be edited to overlay beats using modulation hardware. A simple modulator is discussed in which the composite video luminance signal is pulsed without affecting the chroma signal. The same effect can be introduced at the consumer end, by modulating the video stream produced by the video source. A DVD can be edited using software, introducing pulse-like variations to the digital RGB signals. Image intensity pulses can be superimposed on the analog component video output of a DVD player by modulating the luminance signal component. Before entering the television, a television signal can be modulated to cause pulses in image intensity by means of a variable delay line that is connected to a pulse generator. Certain monitors can emit electromagnetic field pulses that excite a sensory resonance in a nearby subject, through image pulses that are as weak as they are subliminal. This is unfortunate, as it opens a path for malicious application of the invention, whereby people are unknowingly exposed to the manipulation of their nervous systems for someone else's purposes. This application would be unethical and is of course not recommended. It is mentioned here in order to alert the public to the possibility of covert abuse that can occur while online or while watching television, a video or a DVD.

Half-Hertz sensory resonance experiments have been performed with the subject positioned at least a normal viewing distance from a 15″ computer monitor that was driven by a computer program written in Visual Basic (R), version 6.0 (VB6). The program produces a pulsed image with uniform luminance and hue across the entire screen, except for some small control buttons and text boxes. In VB6, screen pixel colors are determined by the integers R, G, and B, which range from 0 to 255, and set the pixel color contributions of the basic colors red, green, and blue. For a CRT type monitor, the pixel intensities for the primary colors may depend on the RGB values in a non-linear manner that will be discussed. In the VB6 program, the RGB values are modulated by small pulses RR, ΔG, ΔB, with a frequency that can be chosen by the subject or swept in a predetermined manner. In the sensory resonance experiments mentioned above, the ratios $\Delta R/R$, $\Delta G/G$ and $\Delta B/B$ were always less than 0.02, so the imaging pulses are quite weak. For certain frequencies near ½ Hz, the subject experienced physiological effects known to accompany excitation from the ½ Hz sensory resonance as mentioned in the background section. Furthermore, the measured field pulse amplitudes fall within the effective intensity window for the ½ Hz resonance, as explored in previous experiments and discussed in the '874, '744, '922, and '304 patents. Other Experiments have shown that one can also break out of the 2.4 Hz sensory resonance through screen emissions from monitors displaying pulsed images.

These results confirm that, in fact, a subject's nervous system can be manipulated through electromagnetic field pulses emitted by a nearby CRT or LCD monitor displaying images with pulsed intensity. The various implementations of the invention adapt to different video stream sources, such as video tape, DVD, a computer program, or a TV broadcast over free space or cable. In all of these implementations, the subject is exposed to the pulsed electromagnetic field generated by the monitor as a result of pulsing image intensity. Certain cutaneous nerves of the subject exhibit spontaneous spikes in patterns that, although quite random, contain sensory information at least in the form of average frequency. Some of these nerves have receptors that respond to field stimulation by changing their average spike frequency, so that the spike patterns of these nerves acquire a frequency modulation, which is transmitted to the brain. Modulation can be particularly effective if it has a frequency at or near a sensory resonance frequency. Such frequencies are expected to be in the range of 0.1 to 15 Hz. You can review all the content of the source here: https://patents.google.com/patent/US6506148B2/en [3].

In 1985 CNN had talked about 'EMF Weapons being used for Mind Control' (electromagnetic fields include 5G, Bluetooth, cell phone radiation, WiFi). This was recalled in an EraOfLight post from 2020. It has been reported that some US embassy workers in China and Cuba were attacked with microwave weapons and suffered brain injuries from their experiences. Research has found that exposure to ALL sources of microwave radiation, including 5G, Bluetooth, cell phone radiation, and WiFi, can disrupt the blood-brain barrier, cause leakage and kill brain cells, AS WELL AS cause all sorts of undesirable effects. Symptoms and health problems and increase the risk of cancer. In 1985, CNN special reports hosted by Chuck DeCaro feature the early use of radio frequency devices in the military and test their use for remote control of human behavior. The scientists interviewed, including Dr. Robert Becker and Dr. Ross Adey, show how electromagnetic fields and radio frequencies were tested as weapons of war against both

---

3.   https://patents.google.com/patent/US6506148B2/en

machines and humans, as well as against terrorism during the Cold War.

At the time, Russia was at the forefront of this technology with a device since the 1960s called the LIDA machine in psychiatric patients, to alter moods and behaviors by emitting pulsed EMF, heat, sound and flashing lights as a way of mind control. "Certain types of weak electromagnetic signals work exactly like drugs," a government scientist told CNN. Similar work by Dr. José Delgado achieved behavioral mind control through radio frequencies directed at the brains of animals and humans. Digging deeper into the segment reveals EMF and RF testing to induce hallucinations, manipulate judgment, alter brain function and intellect. Report presented by Elizabeth Rauscher, William van Bise and Chuck DeCaro.

"Last month, newspapers across the country carried an AP story about the Soviet "Lida" machine being tested at the Veterans Hospital in Loma Linda, CA. Lida uses low-frequency radiation to calm experimental subjects. Dr. Ross Adey is quoted as saying: "It seems that instead of taking Valium when you want to relax, it would be possible to achieve a similar result, probably in a safer way" with radio waves... "If you are thinking about investing in the companies marketing electrical devices for regenerating bones, check out "Electrifying Growth" by Richard Regis in Barren's May 16. Regis describes the various players (electrobiology, telectronics, biomagnetics, electromedical products, among others) competing in what has become a high-stakes competitive market and the patent wars being waged between them..." - Microwave News, June 1983. Coincidentally, the Russian Ministry of Health recently recommended parents reduce their children's exposure to WiFi. Source: https://eraoflight.com/2020/04/12/cnn-in-1985-emf-

weapons-being-used-for-mind-control-emfs-include-5g-
bluetooth-cell-phone-radiation- wifi/ [4].

Below I share a report from the StateOfTheNation website, dated April 1, 2020, related to radio frequencies, microwaves and millimeter waves by an electrical engineer, whistleblower and whistleblower, which exposes the health dangers of 5G. The person presenting this presentation currently works with Radio Frequency/Microwave/Millimeter Wave Engineer credentials (for over 25 years). 5G is the fifth generation of cellular communications. 1G was rolled out in the 1980s and they were those old school phones, the ones that only very rich people owned. Those phones were about 6" x 6" x 12", give or take. Many of the people who used these phones a lot had a region in their brain the size of a walnut that had literally been cooked. 2G came after that. 3G is the old school flip phone from the early 2000s. Then came 4G and 4G LTE. 5G is the next generation of cellular communications that is being deployed around the world. 4G LTE offers 10s of Megabits per second (Mbps) while 5G offers 100s of Mbps and goes towards Gigabits per second (Gbps). What does this give you? Now you can stream high resolution videos over your cellular network.

There are multiple variants of 5G deployed around the world. 5G in China has data encoded on a 28 GHz microwave carrier. 5G in Europe is supposed to operate on a 28 GHz carrier. Verizon wants to be like the rest of the world and operate at 28 GHz. The FCC recently auctioned 37 GHz, 39 GHz and 47 GHz for use in 5G applications. AT&T wants to operate at 39 GHz. T-Mobile has launched its version of 5G on a 400 MHz carrier. You're probably confused by all this and there is solid engineering logic behind it all. Let's start with a simple

---

4.   https://eraoflight.com/2020/04/12/cnn-in-1985-emf-weapons-being-used-for-
mind-control-emfs-include-5g-bluetooth-cell-phone-radiation-wifi/

calculation, wavelength and what wavelength is common for some RF frequencies, microwaves and millimeter waves: λ (wavelength) = v/f (v = speed of light in vacuum = 3 x 108 meters; f = frequency). Example 1: Determine the wavelength at 400 MHz. λ = v/f = 3 x 108 m/s/400 x 106 Hz = 0.75 meters = 29.5 inches. Example 2: Determine the wavelength at 850 MHz (cellular). λ = v/f = 3 x 108 m/s/850 x 106 Hz = 0.353 meters = 13.9 inches. Example 3: Determine the wavelength at 1.5 GHz (Global Positioning System or GPS). λ = v/f = 3 x 108 m/s/1.5 x 109 Hz = 0.2 meters = 7.87 inches. Example 4: Determine the wavelength at 2 GHz (Very close to many 4G LTE bands). λ = v/f = 3 x 108 m/s/2.0 x 109 Hz = 0.15 meters = 5.9 inches.

Example 5: Determine the wavelength at 2.45 GHz (WiFi, first resonant frequency of a water molecule/operating frequency of a microwave oven). λ = v/f = 3 x 108 m/s/2.45 x 109 Hz = 0.122 meters = 4.8 inches. Example 6: Determine the wavelength at 5 GHz (WiFi upper band). λ = v/f = 3 x 108 m/s/5 x 109 Hz = 0.06 meters = 2.36 inches. Example 7: Determine the wavelength at 14 GHz (approximate satellite TV and Internet). λ = v/f = 3 x 108 m/s/14 x 109 Hz = 0.021 meters = 0.843 inches. Example 8: Determine the wavelength at 28 GHz (5G in China, Europe, Verizon). λ = v/f = 3 x 108 m/s/28 x 109 Hz = 10.7 thousand meters = 0.421 inches. Example 9: Determine the wavelength at 39 GHz (AT&T 5G). λ = v/f = 3 x 108 m/s/39 x 109 Hz = 7.7 thousand meters = 0.303 inches. Example 10: Determine the wavelength at 60 GHz (WiFi, unlicensed frequency band). λ = v/f = 3 x 108 m/s/60 x 109 Hz = 5 millimeters = 0.303 inches. Example 11: Determine the wavelength at 90 GHz (crowd control machine that makes skin feel like it is on fire). λ = v/f = 3 x 108 m/s/90 x 109 Hz = 3.3 thousand meters = 0.13 inches. What is the wavelength? It is the length of the electromagnetic wave. From examples 1 to

11, we can see that as we increase the frequency, the wavelength becomes smaller. In general, the longer the wavelength, the deeper it will penetrate your body. The shorter the wavelength, the less it will penetrate...

90 GHz penetrates to a depth that makes your skin feel like it's on fire. T-Mobile's 400 MHz 5G has a long wavelength that will penetrate very deep into your body. Everything else is somewhere in between. Human blood is very good at converting radiofrequency, microwaves and millimeter waves into heat. This is the basic premise on which many medical devices work. These waves will undoubtedly induce currents in the nerves, since they are ultimately conductors. We can only speculate what the outcome may be, but the possibilities are almost endless. Anxiety, insomnia, depression, ADHD are all neurological... Disrupting nerve signals and replacing them with radio frequency waves can also cause things like irritable bowel syndrome and all these "new diseases" that have emerged in recent years. 10 or 20 years. Let's summarize what we've learned so far: 1) Lower frequencies have longer wavelengths that penetrate deeply; 2) Higher frequencies have shorter wavelengths that do not penetrate deeply. Before we get into the details of 5G and the coronavirus, let's first talk about how you can protect yourself from these radio frequency, microwave, and millimeter waves. Do not attempt to use metal except in limited applications and circumstances. You can inadvertently set up a cavity resonance using metal and generate very strong fields and make things worse.

There is also a 7.83 Hz field that exists everywhere in the universe. If you isolate a person from this field using a thick steel Faraday cage, they will die in about 3 to 4 weeks. Please do not try this at home and if you do, you have been warned... If you must completely insulate yourself, a house with mounds of earth or a house built into the side of a mountain is much safer. It is much better to convert waves into heat. Carbon-impregnated foam is known to be one of the best and most cost-effective ways to convert radio frequency, microwave and millimeter waves into heat. Once converted into heat, there is no longer a wave. Use carbon-laden foam if you can. More is better, but eventually you run into practical limitations. Make sure you don't build perfect squares and rectangles, to avoid cavity resonances. Alternatively, drywall, wood, fiberglass insulation, books, furniture, mattresses, regular glass, and all sorts of common things will convert radio frequency, microwave, and millimeter waves into heat. Remember, lower frequencies penetrate deeper and need more thickness of protection than higher frequencies. 5G running at 28 GHz is stopped dead by drywall, especially at a humidity level of 55% to 60%. T-Mobile 400 MHz 5G penetrates deeply through your home and everything in it.

That's why, "it travels farther and delivers the stronger signal." If 5G 28 GHz does not penetrate deep into the body, how can they get 5G to activate the coronavirus that is in their lungs...? 5G spreads in the mouth and nose, down the throat and into the lungs. It will also spread through the ear canals and excite your inner ear, the nerves and that entire region of your brain that is very close to your inner ear... In example 8, we determined that the wavelength of a data carrier of 28 GHz microwave is 10.7 millimeters or 0.421 inches. This small wavelength will propagate through the openings of the mouth and nose into the lungs, where there will be small microwave fields and currents. A lot of heat will also be generated in this process, because blood easily converts microwave fields into heat. Let's analyze this and prove that yes, this really happens using state-of-the-art microwave field analysis software. I'm sure you're freaking out now and saying, "Oh my God, how can I stop this from happening to me?" So before we start the technical deep dive, let's discuss a simple solution on how to stop this. This is the only instance in which we advocate the use of metal. You can get one of those practical and stylish dust masks that everyone uses and cover it with some type of metallic fabric. Copper compression socks can be used for this purpose. A single layer of copper compression sock material covering your mouth, nose and ears will greatly reduce the 28 GHz field and offer plenty of protection.

Don't wrap the cloth around the back of your head. Creating a metallized cylinder offers the opportunity to create cavity resonances, and your head will be in the middle of the resonator. This is not good and we want to avoid it. Use just enough to be effective and no more. Brick walls, foliage, bushes, forest, drywall, and carbon-impregnated foam are known to stop 28 GHz microwave fields in their tracks. Use everything to your advantage. The main thing is that if you know where the 28 GHz antennas are, you want to keep something between you and as much isolation as possible. The 28 GHz fields don't penetrate car glass very well and you are safe driving one. Make sure the windows are closed and you'll be fine. Let's start with the outside of the body and then we will move to the mouth, nose, throat and lungs. Many of the 5G deployments are using Phased Antenna Technology. This means that one can concentrate a lot of power in a very small area and direct it to follow one person. You can also "track" multiple people at the same time. There are 2 sources of microwave energy in this situation, A) the cell tower transmitter, B) your smartphone. The Institute of Electrical and Electronics Engineering (IEEE) Standard C95.1-2005 states that a maximum power density of 10 milliwatts/square centimeter is the maximum power density to which one should be exposed.

This is for 9 minutes for every 24 hours. Now think about your cell phone. It contains a 500 milliwatt transmitter and we can assume that it emits out of an area of approximately 1 cm x 3 cm, which means that the power density is 166.67 mW/cm2. When your smartphone is against your head, the power density is 16 times higher than that recommended by the IEEE...!!! Even if we assume that the power is divided equally between 5 sides of your smartphone, it is still 166.67 mW/cm2/5 = 33 mW/cm2, which is 3 times higher than recommended by the IEEE. The IEEE limit is the maximum exposure limit for a total of 9 minutes in a 24-hour period! If half of this is transmitted to your brain, which it is, it is still about 15 mW/cm2 or 1.5 times the IEEE limit! We haven't done any real math, just rough calculations and we can see that using smartphones doesn't seem that safe as it goes against the recommendations of the world's most knowledgeable radio frequency, microwave and millimeter wave communications body. The outside of your body lights up with all types of radio frequency and microwave signals from CDs to daylight. We know this because we can look at the FCC's Frequency Allocation Plan and see that there are no unused frequencies below 20 GHz. No one has ever asked: What is the cumulative effect of being illuminated 24/7? weekdays? Answer: Who knows...! In the United States, it is SAFE until it is proven unsafe.

Not only are we literally being heated by radio frequency and microwave energy sources, but we are also being fed GMOs (genetically modified organisms) in our food. Is our government really taking care of us? Who on this blessed green earth are they representing? Answer: TO THE MONEY...! After a few laps, we are now ready to start observing how a 28 GHz microwave signal propagates in the mouth and throat, towards the lungs. In our next article we are going to use a high quality 3D electromagnetic field solver to analyze this and present the results. We will start with a simple case and move on to more complex problems. The first case will be a simple 1" long cylinder of seawater (saline) that has 0.3" internal diameter and 0.4" external diameter to approximate the ear canal. We can then define the cylinder as blood, and see how much signal reaches the bottom of the ear canal, as well as how much is converted to heat along the way... source: https://www.bibliotecapleyades.net/scalar_tech/ esp_scalartech_cellphonesmicrowave160.htm [5].

In a study of the correlation between coronavirus cases and the presence of 5G networks by Bartomeu Payeras i Cifre from March-April 2020, he presents a work that leaves a lot to think about. Fortunately, the official statistical material that is published daily is a basic and valuable tool that we have made use of. It should be noted that in these publications, in general the methodology used to count cases of coronavirus infections does not offer real data. In Spain and many other countries, it has not been calculated, as there are not enough tests for such analyses. But this does not alter the result of this work, since it is based on the comparative, not absolute, method of contagion. For this reason, to avoid a statistical error, we will choose to compare the density value of confirmed coronavirus cases (expressed in number of cases/1000 inhabitants) instead of absolute values. Since the counting criteria by the health authorities within the same state or city is the same, the comparison of the values published for different cities or regions will be equally reliable for statistics. Comparisons between different countries of confirmed cases, excluding the so-called asymptomatic cases, will be equally reliable. The possible exception of a non-transparent

---

5.   https://www.bibliotecapleyades.net/scalar_tech/

esp_scalartech_cellphonesmicrowave160.htm

country that could manipulate the publication of its data is beyond our reach. The method used was to compare the index (number of cases/1000 h) between countries with or without 5G technology.

Between regions of the same country with or without 5G technology. Between cities in the same state with or without 5G technology. Between different neighborhoods of the same city with the 5G network map of said city. Comparing states with common borders with and without 5G technology. Comparing the case of one state within another, such as the case of San Marino. The data for each scheme has been taken on the same day. A biologist from the University of Barcelona, specialized in microbiology, has published research papers. He worked and researched at the Hubber pharmaceutical laboratories in Barcelona with smallpox bacteria and viruses. He created and worked in the Department of Marine Microbiology at the Oceanographic Laboratory of Palma de Mallorca, and carried out clinical analyzes at the Center d'Anàlisis Clínics in Palma, they also carried out studies on genetic engineering: Episomal exchange between Paracolobacter and Citrobacter C-3 with bacteriophage. They also studied biogram, a method to evaluate the activity of vitamin B12, and even studied marine bacterial contamination in the Port of Maón. He is also a professor of mathematics, physics and chemistry and biology at IEM. He discovered the Dalí Code with which he encrypted his messages in his paintings. Their graphic results and data published below: The 9 countries with the most infections on the planet, indices of 5 countries with the most infections in Europe, indices of 4 nearby countries on the same latitude (Portugal, Spain, Italy, Greece), indices of Italy , San Marino, Croatia, especially from Italy graph of infections and 5G network, Spain with 5G coverage and indices, also Barcelona, Madrid, New York, the "border effect" between Mexico and the USA, also 5G networks and indices in Canada, USA and Mexico, also Africa, the Persian Gulf, the 5G Network and US military bases and finally China and its neighboring countries.

4G coverage is general and therefore does not serve in this case to compare areas of "coronavirus" incidence. But the 5G map is the one that most closely matches map A. Which shows that the 5G factor is decisive. The African country with the most cases of coronavirus is the Republic of South Africa. The only one that has 5G. In the case of China, to know whether or not the result obtained is that of a random phenomenon, the statistical analysis of the results of an experience must be completed with the calculation of the probability that the event will occur. The probability calculation is obtained by dividing the number of favorable cases by the number of possible cases. If the result shows that it is not a random phenomenon, we must assume that it is causal, which is sufficient reason to analyze the causes. To eliminate any upward error we will always opt for the most conservative numerical option. Let's then calculate the probability of three of the examples analyzed above. Probability that the 9 countries with the most infections on the planet are countries with 5G networks. There are 194 countries on the planet. As of March 6, 2020, according to GSMA, there are 24 countries with 5G technology (1).

Pr = 24/194 x 23/193 x 22/192 (nine times in total) =

= 0.1237 x 0.1191 x 0.1145 x 0.1099 x 0.1052 x 0.1005 x 0.0957 x 0.0909 x 0.0860 =

= 1.47 x 10 (raised -9). The probability is 1 in 680,000,000

If we include Japan, which also has 5G and with an index similar to South Korea:

The probability is 1 in 8,500,000,000

Probability that the 5 countries with the most infections in Europe have 5G networks. In Europe there are 49 countries of which today it is difficult to know which ones are currently deploying 5G, since there are 5 that have declared a moratorium and many others do not have operational networks although the companies publish as if they already were when only They have signed agreements. We will calculate it downwards, as a conservative option, we will assume that about 15 countries have the 5G system operational.

$Pr = 15/49 \times 14/48 \times 13/47 \times 12/46 \times 11/45 = 0.00157$. The probability is 1 in 637

The case of San Marino. The case of San Marino is highly significant since being located within the Italian territory, with a similar culture, economy, and social level, it has much higher infection rates. The only difference is the exposure time of its citizens to 5G radiation, because it was the first state in the world to implement this technology on September 4, 2018, while in Italy it was June 5, 2019. This opens the doors of the debate on the probable influence of 5G on the increase in the infection rate: $Pr = 1/194 \times 1/194$. The probability is 1 in 37,636.

It is obvious that these figures are eloquent enough to not make it necessary to add the calculation of the other cases. The results on page 8 of the City of Barcelona indicate that sociological factors do not have a significant influence on the case rate, but we do see a clear relationship with the 5G coverage map, which added to the 4G coverage gives us a correlation between mobile coverage and proportion of coronavirus cases. If we have more data, this study should be expanded to other cities. Conclusion:

1st. The results obtained clearly demonstrate a clear and close relationship between the rate of "coronavirus" cases and the location of 5G antennas.

2nd. This study does not analyze the beneficial or harmful effects caused by 5G electromagnetic radiation on humans. But it does point in the direction of a possible cause-effect in the current pandemic.

3rd. It is significant, original and exclusive to this pandemic, which presents a "border effect", with marked differences between contiguous states with or without 5G implementation. It is especially significant that the countries bordering China have very low infection rates. Also look between Mexico and the USA or between Portugal and Spain, etc.

4th. The case of San Marino is especially important. The first state in the world to implement 5G, therefore, the state where its citizens have been exposed to said radiation the longest, and suspiciously, the first state in the world in infection rate. The probability of this happening is 1 in 37,636.

5th. In the cities studied: Madrid, Barcelona and New York, the aforementioned correlation is also observed. In the study of the City of Barcelona (page 8) it is seen that the socioeconomic factor has the most influence.

6th. It is very significant that on the African continent, with few health resources, but without 5G, the rate is very low, except for some antennas in the Republic of South Africa; which coincidentally has the highest numbers of infections in Africa.

7th. The indices are diluted. The indices of some regions are influenced by cities with 5G, but the index of these cities is diluted in those of the region to which they belong. Therefore, it is more significant, as is the case of Spain, to compare single-provincial Autonomous Communities, rather than those that are made up of 3 or more of the old provinces. Thus we see that some communities with 5G such as La Rioja, Madrid, Navarra, present rates between 4 and 8 times higher than others without 5G. The same thing happens in other cities in the world where the 5G network does not cover the entire territory of the state or region.

8th. These data and results have the value of being taken "in vivo", not based on prospective or laboratory studies. Never in history have we had so much epidemiological information on a disease in humans to be able to carry out scientific studies.

A formula to be able to answer the question of cause-effect would be to be able to disconnect, at least as a preventive measure, the 5G networks, and see the results of the evolution of coronavirus cases. It would also be to study the index in a state that has declared a 5G moratorium once the pandemic began and study if the statistics change. For everything said and calculated here, I consider it urgent to take into consideration the data and conclusions of this study. Given the current serious circumstances of the pandemic, it is the responsibility of the media and the political and health authorities to take urgent measures. The fact of knowing about this study and not acting could be considered at the very least negligence or even prevarication. Already in a study by Steven Weller, Bachelor of Science at Monash University conducted a study on EHS (Electromagnetic Hypersensitivity) published on November 27, 2013. It was presented in an information session on EHS for health professionals, research scientists, civil servants governments and interested members of the public. Below I will present the complete work, with which, given its coverage and scope, after it I will conclude this chapter of the book. Steven Weller:

I felt compelled to write this personal case study because through my own personal experiences I discovered that there is a serious lack of understanding of what Electromagnetic Hypersensitivity (EHS), also commonly known as Electrosensitivity (ES), is and its cause. For some people, EHS can be completely disabling and, in some extreme situations, can lead to hospitalization due to aggravation of a pre-existing medical condition, development of tachyarrhythmias, which can sometimes result in loss of consciousness, and other acute situations. Effects on the neurological system. The main problem that people suffering from EHS face is that they are in a precarious position where there is a complete absence of government support. The WHO states that EHS is "not a medical diagnosis", so the medical profession ignores the patient's symptoms and often misdiagnoses them. This can lead to unnecessary and ineffective medications being prescribed. Only Sweden recognizes EHS as a functional impairment, while the Austrian Medical Association has provided guidelines on the diagnosis and treatment of EHS-related diseases. My hope in writing this case study is to dispel the misconceptions that some members of the scientific community, government agencies, and the general public have about this functional impairment.

I also hope that by detailing my own personal experience with EHS, I can help those who may be suffering from similar symptoms recognize the cause and help them understand how they can manage their condition and, to some extent, protect themselves. Conflict of interest statement: I would like to declare that I have no conflict of interest. I have no financial or political gain from writing this personal case study and declaring my sensitivity to EMR. By making such a statement regarding my sensitivity, there is a real possibility that I am putting my career in IT at risk. I have come to the conclusion that my health and the health of my children are much more valuable to me than the convenience of a cell phone or wireless Internet access. What is electromagnetic hypersensitivity (EHS)? EHS, as functional impairment, has been known to the scientific community for many years. In the 1970s it was known as microwave disease or radio wave disease, the same symptoms as EHS, just with a different name. The Powerwatch.org.uk website lists a total of 130 studies related to the topic of EHS and has categorized them as follows: 69 studies with positive findings, 27 studies with null findings and 24 studies that provided important information but did not were positive nor a null finding.

"People who live within 100 meters of a wireless facility of any kind tend to report symptoms such as dizziness, nausea, memory loss, inability to concentrate, irritability, increased blood pressure, peculiar pressure behind the eyeballs, joint pains that move through the body, pain in the bottom of the feet, high-pitched noises in the ears, an itchy systemic rash, and even internal bleeding, all symptoms of radio wave illness. Clinics report an immediate increase in respiratory illnesses: bronchitis, flu, pneumonia and asthma during the first weeks of commissioning of the PCS base station and hospitals are flooded." Source: http://www.laleva.cc/ environment/ taskforce_eng.html [6]. Microwave syndrome: a preliminary study in Spain. Epidemiological study: "Insomnia, cancer, leukemia in children and brain tumors are the most frequently described clinical entities (Dolk et al., 1997; Hocking et al., 1996; Maskarinec et al., 1994; Minder and Pfluger, 2001; Selvinet al., 1992). Furthermore, the clinical consequences of exposure to microwave radiation such as radar have been evaluated from military and occupational studies (Balode, 1996; Garaj-Vrhovac, 1999; Goldsmith, 1997; Johnson-Liakouris, 1998; Robinette et al, 1980). A specific symptomatology, related to radar exposure at low levels of RF, has been termed "microwave illness" or "RF syndrome" (Johnson-Liakouris, 1998). With few exceptions, functional disturbances of the central nervous system have

---

6.   http://www.laleva.cc/environment/taskforce_eng.html

typically been described as a kind of radio wave disease, neurasthenic or asthenic syndrome.

Symptoms and signs include headache, fatigue, irritability, loss of appetite, drowsiness, concentration or memory difficulties, depression and emotional instability, actually reversible if RF exposure is stopped. There is a large and coherent body of evidence of biological mechanisms that support the conclusion of a plausible, logical and causal relationship between RF exposure and neurological disease." Source: https://www.emf-portal.org/en /article/13498 [7]. What are the key points? The main problem facing people suffering from EHS today in Australia is that there is a complete lack of government support. In addition, there are a number of other concerns which I have listed below which are by no means the complete story on this topic:

1. The general public, as well as the medical profession in general, do not seem to understand what EHS is and what causes it. Doctors do not have the tools or methodology (training) to identify or treat those who suffer. Although my doctor indicated that he had read some material on EHS, he suggested that I was probably suffering from a migraine (similar symptoms, a band of pressure around the head) and that I should take ibuprofen (an anti-inflammatory/pain reliever) which in my case is ineffective in treating the symptoms and certainly does not address the cause. More concerning is the possibility of misdiagnosis and prescription of unnecessary medications that could result in further health complications due to the unwanted side effects that some medications may have as a result of prolonged use.

2. There appears to be no consensus within the scientific community on RF safety. Some scientists and scientific bodies suggest that there is no evidence of harm, while others, such as

---

7.   https://www.emf-portal.org/en/article/13498

the WHO and IARC, have classified all microwave transmitters as potential carcinogens.

3. Very little research is being done on EHS to validate it as a real condition or to confirm the cause.

4. While scientists debate whether EHS is a psychological and/or physiological disease and whether sufficient evidence can be established to link it with EMR, patients are left in limbo without any adequate protection, support or recognition of their health problems. It is not clear why a "diagnosis of exclusion" approach cannot be adopted to verify that EHS is a health problem.

5. The burden of proof for the existence of EHS as an impediment, like proof of RF security in general, appears to be unreasonably high. RF-emitting devices are not handled in a manner consistent with the handling of other substances that may affect health, including drugs, medications and prostheses and medical devices, where manufacturers have to demonstrate the absence of risk to the health of the population and maintain post-marketing. Surveillance for years after a drug or device is first marketed.

6. The current testing methodology for checking sensitivity using challenge testing, which I will go into more detail about in this study, has some potentially serious flaws that I will go into more detail about in this study.

7. "Positive studies, studies that show the effects of EMF, are being analyzed in depth for possible errors that lead to the observation of the effects. "Negative studies are more commonly accepted at face value and their quality is not being questioned because they provide evidence 'as expected.'"

My experience with EHS. I am 44 years old and have been using computers my entire adult life. I am an IT professional with a bachelor's degree in Biochemistry and Microbiology. I have always considered myself an early adopter of technology and discovered by accident that I was sensitive to certain frequencies of Electromagnetic Radiation (EMR). My discovery also occurred long before I learned through my subsequent research that there was a label for my condition, also known as EHS or Electromagnetic Hypersensitivity. My first memory of being sensitive to radio frequencies was in late 2001, when wireless networks were just starting to become popular. I had no preconceptions or fears about the technology nor did I know that RF could be potentially harmful. I looked forward to the freedom it would bring me. No more cables cluttering the desk, free to do my work on my laptop at the kitchen table while having breakfast. Being an IT expert, I had decided to purchase the most powerful wireless Wi-Fi router available at the time, capable of transmitting 108 Mbs per second and having an effective range of 100m+, which was twice as fast and twice the range of the cheaper more common. Wireless routers at that time.

The first time I used my wireless router I started to feel pressure in my head, pressure in my chest, tingling sensations in my hands and face within a few minutes of use. I also noticed (and my wife did too) that my temperament changed to being more agitated and short-tempered when using my Wi-Fi enabled router. After turning off my wireless router, I was left with a headache that persisted for several hours. At first, I didn't think about it and didn't immediately associate it with my use of wireless technology. It was only on subsequent use that I felt the same symptoms. If it persisted for a longer time, I would find that in addition to the symptoms mentioned above, I would feel a burning sensation in my intestinal region and the pressure in my chest would sometimes cause my heart to beat irregularly (arrhythmia) followed by stronger than normal heartbeats. (like my heart was trying to jump out of my chest). I soon realized that a consistent pattern was developing with using my wireless router and the symptoms I was experiencing. It was not a nocebo effect: it was real, constant and most unpleasant. It was at this point that I made a conscious decision not to use a wireless network to connect to the Internet. Definition of nocebo effect: First of all, the word nocebo (from the Latin "I will do harm") is a harmless substance that creates harmful effects in the patient who takes it. The nocebo effect is the negative reaction experienced by a patient who receives a nocebo. These reactions are the result of the subject's expectations about how the substance will affect them. Although they originate exclusively from psychological sources, nocebo effects can be psychological or physiological. Source: Wikipedia.

In 2007, I bought a Sony PlayStation 3. I didn't use the built-in wireless networking feature because it had a wired LAN I could connect to. However, the PS3 controller is a Bluetooth wireless device that runs at 2.4 GHz, just like my router but with significantly lower power density (the PS3 controller is a class 2 Bluetooth device, so it only will generate a maximum of 2.5 mW). I found that I didn't have the same sensations I felt with the router (not completely absent, but barely noticeable and easily tolerable). Realizing that I could possibly use low-power wireless devices without major problems, I decided to buy a Nintendo Wii for my children for Christmas several years later, but after using the Wii a couple of times I had to get rid of it as I will now explain. The Wii controllers also use Bluetooth 2.4GHz (online documentation suggests they operate at a maximum output of 3.83mW) which is the same frequency as the PS3, however the all-too-familiar EHS symptoms reappeared and were not pleasant. The difference in transmit power levels could be a potential cause and cannot be completely ruled out, but I would say it is very unlikely. Instead, there is a notable difference in the amount of data that is transmitted. My PS3 controller will only send information occasionally, such as when a button is pressed, which is much more infrequent than a Wii controller which is practically always transmitting, as it needs to send telemetry data to indicate the position and movement of the controller to through space and time.

The amount of information being transmitted seems to be a key in my sensitivity because I have a very similar problem regarding 3G USB modems compared to 3G cell phones. A person can be 3-5m away talking on a mobile phone and I don't feel anything significant compared to someone using a laptop at the same distance that is connected to a 3G internet USB stick that downloads video in real time which can be quite intense. The amount of data packed into the signal appears to be a differentiating factor. Of course, this doesn't mean I'm not sensitive to cell phones; I certainly am. I can only use a mobile phone near my head for 30 seconds or so before switching the phone to my other ear due to a lot of discomfort I feel. Nowadays I hardly use my cell phone and only keep it for emergencies. I switch it to flight mode most of the time, but if I need to use it, I operate it hands-free. Before the launch of smart meters on my street, but after I discovered that I am sensitive to certain RF frequencies, I took precautionary measures in my home by ensuring that I only used wired connections for Internet connectivity and that all devices with wireless capability had said features set to disabled I was able to function normally and had no major issues with sleep or health. I did not suffer any more headaches or palpitations. I could tell he was in good health. However, in late August/early September 2011, Powercor launched wireless smart meters on my street. I resisted the installation of a smart meter.

However, not having a smart meter installed in my property did not help me as I was severely affected by my neighbors' 2 smart meters that were installed next to my room 3m away. It was shortly after installation that I discovered that I was waking up at specific times each night, sometimes feeling as if someone had taken a long, sharp needle and quickly stuck it in my head. Once I woke up, I found it very difficult to go back to sleep. Times fell in a fairly consistent range in the early morning hours. Every morning I woke up with a severe headache that lasted all day and made it quite difficult to concentrate and complete simple tasks. On several occasions I woke up with my heart beating irregularly. I was feeling the same symptoms I had previously experienced with my wireless router. 2012 was a very difficult year for me because for 6 months I had to travel interstate every Sunday night to work on an IT project for an interstate client. I would stay in hotels that have DECT (digital cordless phones) that transmit constantly, even when not in use, in addition to being radiated by the hotel's wireless Internet. The office I worked in was located under a cell tower and also had wireless access points so staff with wireless laptops could access the corporate network.

I would be flying with a national airline that began allowing its business class passengers to use wireless-enabled iPads. When I got home, I was in a terrible state that was exacerbated by emissions from smart meters. To make matters worse, I had become sensitive to things that normally didn't bother me. Being around transformers (phone charges, laptop power modules, light dimmers) left me feeling the same symptoms I felt when exposed to wireless RF. Being close to my hot plate and extractor hood also affected me. I became allergic to my deodorant which I had been using for 10 years without problems and it suggests that the RF was interfering with my immune system. I had constant headaches, felt extremely lethargic, and completely lost motivation to do anything with the family. I would wake up feeling just as tired when I got out of bed in the morning as I did before I went to bed. I even discovered that I had become a rudimentary mobile phone base station detector. I could feel a cell phone tower long before I saw it. I can no longer drive through suburbs where smart meters have just been installed without developing a severe headache that can last for days. I have been to my local GP many times and he cannot explain what is wrong with me. Blood tests and ECG tests return to normal.

Of course, an ECG will only show heartbeat irregularities in my case if I am exposed to high levels of EMR (but still within the basic restrictions of the ARAPNSA RF standard), which was absent from the doctor's office at the time. Painkillers were prescribed, but they offered very little relief. I was referred to a neurologist who indicated he had never heard of EHS, he said he didn't fully understand wireless technology so he couldn't give me an informed opinion. He suggested that I have an EEG and an MRI to verify that I do not have brain disorders or tumors. Of course, the results were negative. It's important to understand that when I say I have a headache, it's not a normal headache where sudden movements cause sharp pain, like when you're hungover or dehydrated. Instead, it's a constant pressure and dull ache in my head. My face feels exhausted as if I have been working a 24 hour shift and can sometimes be accompanied by an itchy sensation on my skin (head and face) when I am in the presence of microwave RF frequencies. EHS is not restricted to certain age groups. I was 32 years old when I decided I was sensitive to wireless technology. My condition has progressively worsened as the amount of man-made RF in our environment has increased. I know without a doubt that wireless RF is causing these problems because when I go to remote areas where the EMR is very low, I feel fine after several days.

A recent trip to southern NSW, away from large population centers for a few weeks, showed me that my health problems were related to EMR. It is important to understand that it takes time for the effects to wear off in some people, meaning there is no instant relief. I recently painted my house with RF protective paint and installed RF blocking curtains and my sensitivity has been greatly reduced. Now I can sleep better, be around transformers and electrical plates without feeling sick, but the use of mobile phones and wireless networks is still a problem for me and something I avoid as much as I can. Despite taking precautionary measures in my own home at great cost, I am deeply concerned by the lack of support, care and understanding from power companies and the various government departments I have contacted on this issue. . In fact, I've become a prisoner in my own home because venturing out into the neighborhood for long periods of time leaves me exhausted and feeling sick for days. I am forced to sleep in the back of the house because the master bedroom on the first floor is still receiving RF penetration through the unshielded floor. Effectively, I am denied the front parts of my house if I do not want my health to deteriorate substantially. What other patients have said:

Case 1: "I feel extremely isolated and marginalized by the community in which I live. Both my husband and mother think that I am simply making up the symptoms or that they are psychosomatic in nature. "The condition seems very difficult to understand for people who do not hear the doorbell, have headaches or insomnia, and even when people have these symptoms."

Case 2: "It was nothing like the occasional headache I have experienced in the past, where the slightest movement produced a throbbing sensation. "This headache consisted of pressure all over my skull with a tingling sensation on my scalp... My zest for life faded."

Case 3: "I have been experiencing intense ringing in my ears and burning/burning sensations on the sides of my head since I moved into our neighborhood."

Case 4: "Fatigue, depression, excessive sleeping, stress, sometimes anger, pain, difficulty concentrating, inability to concentrate, housework is also difficult to do".

There are countless example cases on the Internet around the world. Stop Smart Meters Australia has maintained a health record and documented over 160 cases as of November 2013. How do scientists try to verify if a person is EHS? Most scientists will perform what is called a challenge test. The challenge test is performed using a radio transmitting device that usually operates at a specific frequency, i.e. 914 MHz to simulate a mobile phone. These tests are usually carried out double blind. What this means is that the scientist performing the test and the person being tested do not know whether the box is transmitting or not. Typically the box will have a readout with some numerical codes that the tester can record and use later to determine whether the transmitter was active or not and then correlate this with the "feelings" of the subject. The limitations of challenge testing are numerous and include:

1. Probably the most important fact that people need to realize is that provocation testing is not a biologically based test, but rather requires the subject to respond with how they feel, which of course is very subjective and therefore Therefore, it cannot realistically be considered an objective test.

2. Some challenge tests require the subject to give

feedback on the severity of symptoms and rate it in comparison to previous exposures (challenge tests are usually performed as a series of stepwise sequential exposure tests); Again, this is very subjective and not objective as most people cannot remember exactly how something felt hours or days later. If we could remember what pain feels like, along with the intensity, I would seriously doubt that women would choose to become pregnant voluntarily and opt for a natural birth more than once! Pain is a private emotional experience. Pain intensity cannot be measured directly; Responses to supposedly painful stimuli can be measured, but not the experience itself.

3. They are set to a specific frequency of operation to which the subject may not actually be sensitive. Reviewers claim that the device simulates a mobile phone, but this is debatable as it does not communicate with one or more cell towers nor is it clear what type of data is being sent (simulation of a voice call - low data speed vs data/video transmission - high data rate or just a carrier signal), the modulation pattern used to send the data or whether the data transmission is even simulated. My experience at EHS has shown that the amount of information conveyed in a short window of time is a key factor in my feelings of ill health.

4. Tests often do not simulate the environment that the person claims is affecting them. We are surrounded by EMF from a variety of sources every day. When I was suffering from RF emissions from my router, I was also using a computer that was also emitting RF (from the wireless card and to a lesser extent from the CPU due to its internal clock speed), I was also sitting in front of a

19" CRT monitor. , there were also a number of power transformers present in the room. Using these devices without wireless enabled did not cause any problems for me. However, the EMR effects of multiple devices are additive.

5. The testing procedure is often poorly defined due in part to those performing the test not fully understanding the subject's EHS condition, i.e., delayed reaction and delayed recovery times are not always considered. EHS is not like flipping a light switch that results in an instant reaction, although there are some sufferers who can feel the emissions shortly after they are turned on. There may be considerable delay times between the start of signal transmission and the appearance of symptoms. The same goes for recovery time, which can take anywhere from hours to several days. One can see where a situation may arise where a subject has not fully recovered from an active cue and is then tested with a false cue and asked how it feels. Guess what? They will give an answer stating that they are still suffering, which will lead them to the conclusion that EHS is not real or at least not related to EMR. Some provocation testing protocols attempt to take this into account by having the subject attempt to evaluate intensity with respect to past experiences that are of dubious value (see point 2 above).

6. Each subject is unique (body mass, current illnesses, medications, allergies, age, immune system sensitivity, genetic predisposition, etc.), so a standard set of tests with set exposure times and time intervals between exposures may not be sufficient or appropriate.

7. There is a definite psychological component that will

influence test results and reinforce the belief that EHS is a nocebo (psychosomatic) effect. An analogy would be to perform a test on a mouse by connecting electrodes to it and delivering shocks every time a light is turned on. After a while, the mouse will be conditioned so that by simply turning on the light, the mouse will react the same as if it were actually feeling the effects of an electric shock. The same goes for humans. Use a phone a lot and get serious headaches and then present the user with a phone-like device and tell him that you are testing his sensitivity to mobile frequencies without him knowing if the transmitter is active or not and you can bet there is a good possibility that they will develop some form of reaction. This reaction is natural and the result of conditioning, as we try to avoid situations where we feel uncomfortable/painful by applying behavior learned through experience as a result of previous painful episodes. See "Nocebo Effect or Real Deal" detailed later in this study. An experiment similar to that described above in mice was recently reported on the BBC and can be viewed by clicking on the link provided: http://www.bbc.co.uk/news/science-environment-23447600 [8].

8. For those suffering from EHS, provocation testing is a form of torture. It creates unnecessary anxiety which in itself can lead to the appearance of similar symptoms that can interfere with the test and lead to a confusing result.

9. Depending on where the test is performed, results may be contaminated by other sources of EMR which may

---

8. http://www.bbc.co.uk/news/science-environment-23447600

include nearby computers or wireless routers, DECT phones, cell towers, EMR from transformers, fluorescent lights, etc. is emitting RF, but while it is on, it is certainly creating EM fields that can interfere with the test, especially when testing with a simulated signal.

10. When conducting group studies, people who have to withdraw prematurely from the trial because of the disabling effects they are experiencing are often not included in the study results. Current methodology for testing sensitivity is inconsistent and often relies on poorly defined testing protocols. This is due in part to the fact that there appears to be a poor general understanding of people's electrical sensitivity by the scientific community and the fact that most tests do not have a biological basis, i.e. Provocation, which we know is very subjective, can be manipulated to show inconclusive results. Although challenge testing is typically performed as a double-blind study, that is, the scientist and study participant do not know whether the device is transmitting or in sham mode, the testing protocol can be set up in such a way that a challenge occurs. insufficient recovery time. allowed before performing the next test. Subjects can, through learned behavior, also affect outcomes, particularly in the case where the testing protocol requires the subject to compare feelings from a current exposure test to previous exposures. For EHS testing to be meaningful and realistic, scientists should seek to establish biological tests that are used in conjunction with a provocation device that can measure heart rate variability and heart palpitations (as recently demonstrated by Dr. Magda Havas in 2010 and

reconfirmed in a repeat experiment: http://www.ncbi.nlm.nih.gov/pubmed/23675629 [9]), brain responses, brain scans, immune response, sleep studies, blood chemistry, etc.

Dr. Dominique Belpomme, Professor of Oncology at the Descartes University of Paris, is conducting research on electrohypersensitivity with the Association for Research and Treatments against Cancer (ARTAC) in Paris. The ARTAC group has been following several hundred patients with EHS for the past four years and has documented that these patients have clear and consistent changes in oxidative metabolism, and also in blood flow to the limbic system (as measured by Doppler studies). Dr. Belpomme believes that these changes in the limbic system directly correlate with many of the cognitive changes (memory problems, difficulty concentrating, etc.) that these patients experience. The ARTAC group hopes to publish a series of papers on their findings over the next year (Dart, 2012). I look forward to the results of their research when they are published, which will demonstrate and confirm that EHS is real and not a nocebo effect as some scientists would have us believe. The big question I have is whether we need to find biological markers before we accept that this is real. There is enough evidence to make a diagnosis on the pattern of symptoms alone; this is what I think happens in Sweden. While scientists fight over testing methodology and industry demands testing, people suffer.

It is also interesting to note that an email I received from an Australian scientist who offered to test me with a challenge testing device for EHS stated the following: "I would ask you to sign a consent form, as the test is likely to generate symptoms that would be uncomfortable for you. To me, this is a tacit

---

9. http://www.ncbi.nlm.nih.gov/pubmed/23675629

acknowledgment that EHS is probably real. Nocebo effect or the real deal. Scientists readily know that we learn to withdraw or alter our behavior in response to a conditioned stimulus. Definition of conditioned stimulus: "A previously neutral stimulus that, after repeated association with an unconditioned stimulus, elicits the response effected by the unconditioned stimulus itself." In the context of EHS, an analogy I would suggest is that an inactive mobile phone, router or provocation testing device (physical object) be considered as the neutral stimulus and the RF it emits when turned on as the unconditioned stimulus that causes pain or results in some form of health impact. Therefore, it is very plausible that EHS suffers, through learned behavior, associated visual and auditory elements (hearing nearby people talking on a mobile phone or the phone ringing) capable of emitting RF such as a mobile phone, iPad, mast. mobile phone base station and other antennas with their condition and making their bodies react accordingly.

Such behavior reinforces the belief of some scientists that EHS is a nocebo effect. What scientists need to understand is that the original mechanism that triggered this learned behavior in most cases is real and is not a psychologically induced condition. People only need to look at my particular case history to see evidence of this, which is as follows:

1. I work in IT and embrace technological advances and was looking forward to the freedom that wireless technology offers.

2. I had no preconceived ideas and was completely uninformed of the possible health impacts when I first used Wi-Fi.

3. The physiological reaction I experience in the presence of Wi-Fi is real and reasonably consistent with each exposure. I say "reasonably consistent" because depending on my state of health (did I have a cold? Did I get a good night's sleep? I'm

still recovering from a previous exposure, etc.), the duration and intensity of the exposure will see the type and duration of symptoms that vary within a common set that I have experienced previously. One hour of exposure does not always induce heart palpitations. But they have only occurred when I am exposed to wireless (pulsed) RF.

4. Symptoms disappear when I go to remote locations away from wireless transmitters, suggesting that an underlying health problem is not the cause.

5. RF shielding alleviated my symptoms, suggesting that other environmental concerns or stress are not a significant factor.

I mentioned "most cases" above because I don't doubt that there may be cases where some people who are of a neurotic disposition, may have read an article suggesting harm, become obsessed and anxious to the point where they experience an event. real nocebo. These cases are the exception and not the norm. [I will now talk about] smart meters and EHS. Unfortunately, some authorities assume that because SM radiation emissions are short-lived and apparently lower in energy density than other wireless devices typically found in and around people's homes, they are safe. What many people don't know is how many times these meters actually communicate. We are told that the smart meter transmits SMS as messages 4 to 6 times a day (depends on your service provider), which may be true for your home's personal data, but what is not said is that for mesh networks, the average duty cycle also includes transmissions to maintain the network, time synchronization, and network message management (i.e., transmitting data from other houses). This can lead to between 10,000 transmissions to 190,000 transmissions or more per day. Nobody sends that many SMS messages on their mobile phone. Many of these devices are located on a wall or in wall cavities where people spend a significant amount of time (i.e., bedroom or living room walls).

It has been shown in a recent Victorian medical report titled "SELF-REPORTING OF SYMPTOM DEVELOPMENT FROM EXPOSURE TO RADIO FREQUENCY FIELDS FROM WIRELESS SMART METERS IN VICTORIA, AUSTRALIA - A SERIES OF CASES" that smart meters appear to be causing people who They were previously not sensitive to RF frequencies to become EHS. Additionally, people who previously self-diagnosed as having EHS found their condition worsened dramatically. This medical report has been written by a doctor using data obtained from a health record maintained independently by Stop Smart Meters Australia. More than 150 people have registered their health complaints. The case study only looks at those who were fully identifiable and agreed to have their de-identified data made public in a health report amounting to a total of 92 individuals. As I described in my introduction, I am self-diagnosed as EHS having identified my sensitivity over 10 years ago. In terms of the medical report findings mentioned above, I fit into the second category in that my condition (despite previously being able to manage it quite successfully) has worsened after mesh-networked wireless smart meters were installed in my neighborhood. Below I list the specific EHS symptoms of my smart meter:

1. Constant headaches: pressure in my head.

2. Insomnia: I find it very difficult to get a good night of uninterrupted sleep.

3. Lethargy and concentration difficulties.

4. Sharp pains like a hot spike that go through my head and occasionally in the intestinal region.

5. Burning pain in the intestinal region.

6. Pain in the joints, especially in the elbows, fingers and sometimes knees.

7. Irritability and feelings of anxiety - I find that I am more prone to angry outbursts when exposed to RF from the smart meter. My wife can certainly attest to that!

8. Heartbeat irregularities and occasionally palpitations when near a smart meter for a long period of time.

I am sensitive to very low power densities. What also seems to affect me is the amount of data being sent in a very short time interval. Perhaps this is an area that deserves further investigation to see if this could be a potential cause of the health effects claimed to result from exposure to certain pulsed radio frequencies with high data transmission rates. The problem I face now is that I have effectively become a prisoner in my own home. Leaving my house into an environment that has steadily increased EMR makes me feel exhausted, sore, and trapped. Moving interstate where there are currently no smart meters is an option, but if new cell tower rollouts continue, high-speed wireless networks as part of the NBN rollout and other states follow Victoria's lead in mandating rollout of Metros devices I will eventually run out of places to go and become an EMR haven as I move to increasingly remote locations. Career options will diminish and my job is already under threat as I struggle to continue working in the IT industry, where wireless networks and smart wireless devices are becoming the norm.

I am facing the dilemma of how I can support my family. What kind of life will they have and what kind of opportunities are they missing out on as we move to isolated places to escape this human threat to my health? What steps can you take to protect yourself? The most important actions that can be taken to protect yourself from exposure to ubiquitous human-caused RF emissions are as follows:

1) Turn off all wireless devices in the home – avoiding them is the best protective measure. It is important to understand that the effects of wireless technology are additive when exposed to multiple frequencies and the damage caused accumulates over a lifetime. The ARPANSA RF standards say "In situations of simultaneous exposure to fields of different frequencies and depending on the nature of the exposure and the distribution of RF absorption within the body, the combined effects of exposure to frequency exposure sources multiple can be additive". (rps3 page 18). If you must use wireless devices, at least turn them off before you go to bed at night.

2) Replace digital cordless phones (DECT) with corded phones. Most DECT base units transmit all the time, regardless of whether you are on a call or not. Again, if your cordless phone is valuable to you, make sure it is not in your room.

3) Put your iPad in airplane mode when you don't need Internet access. Also, do not rest it on your lap when using wireless technology, as "epidemiological studies of men evaluated for infertility were consistent in demonstrating decreased sperm motility associated with cell phone use. Most of the in vitro (laboratory) studies, which involved exposing human semen samples to controlled RF exposure from cell phones, generally noted a decrease in sperm motility, among other adverse effects. Similar findings were seen in animal studies of a specific type of rat. "We suggest that oxidative stress or antioxidant depletion are plausible mechanisms for these non-thermal effects of RF exposure."

4) Distance is your friend as the wireless signal strength drops following the inverse square rule i.e. Strength = 1 / Distance. Put as much distance between you and transmitters, including smart meters. This may mean moving your bed to

another room if the smart meter is located on the wall in your room.

5) Rooms can be protected with special carbon-based paint and windows can be covered with RF shielding curtains. More information is provided below.

6) Install bed canopies made with the same RF shielding materials as the curtains mentioned above.

7) Strengthen your body by exercising regularly and eating good healthy foods high in natural antioxidants. This will put less stress on your body, giving it a chance to deal with potentially harmful man-made RF emissions. Although RF energy is not sufficient to damage DNA directly, independent researchers have shown that it causes damage through indirect pathways. "A large body of research has shown that microwave radiofrequency causes increased production of free radicals and reactive oxidant species in living tissues, and that this increased oxidative stress damages DNA. This damage can and does occur at power levels well below the levels that could produce damage by thermal mechanisms." Special note: DNA damage can potentially lead to cancer.

8) Try to maintain regular sleep habits by not varying your bedtime too much if possible. Make sure all EMF sources (including radio frequency) are not near the head of the bed. This would include clock radios, small appliance transformers, mobile phones and cordless phones. And remember to turn off electric blankets before getting into bed to go to sleep, if you use them. Do not place the bed immediately behind or near where the power meter is installed.

9) Although the medical profession generally does not know what EHS is or how to treat it, a visit to the doctor is essential to confirm that other possible serious causes of your symptoms are excluded with appropriate medical testing.

In my case, I don't have wireless devices in my house. My master bedroom was located at the front of the house on the first floor. My neighbor had 2 smart meters installed in his garage, which is 3m from my room. I moved my bed to the back of the house on the ground floor. My home office is also located at the front of the house and was unusable as an 8 hour shift would cause me to suffer major headaches, concentration problems and extreme lethargy. To reclaim these rooms, I decided to paint the front rooms with charcoal paint. A single layer reduces signal intensity by 10,000 times. 2 Coats reduces the signal 100,000 times. By coupling carbon paint with RF protective curtains, it is possible to reduce RF penetration into a room to negligible levels. Carbon paint works by reflecting most of the signal. However, protective paint must be applied with caution because it is conductive and therefore must be properly grounded. Another issue is that due to the reflective qualities of carbon paint, it is important that you do not use wireless devices in these rooms, otherwise most of the RF cannot escape and will bounce back and therefore increase your exposure.

After taking these protective measures, I can use my office again, but I am reluctant to move into my master bedroom as the RF emissions from the smart meter can infiltrate my room through the unshielded floor (I live in a 2 - History House). Shielding is expensive and for some it does not always improve the situation. When I am in rooms that are completely shielded I seem to feel different and not necessarily better than an unshielded room that has very low RF. Rooms that have shielding and devices that have transformers (amplifiers, dimmers, etc.) still seem to affect me. I'm not sure if the conductive properties of the charcoal paint are causing the spread of other electromagnetic fields that I may be sensitive to and therefore affect me. An example is that I had a UPS (uninterruptible power supply, battery backup that recharges with AC power) in my computer room that seemed to affect me only after I painted the room with charcoal paint. Turning off the UPS caused my EHS symptoms to dissipate. I never had this problem before painting the wall or before smart meters were installed in the neighborhood. Therefore, it is important to understand that there can be side effects with protective paint. If I were given the choice again whether to use protective paint, I would still do it, because without it my quality of life would have suffered drastically. Heart palpitations and endless headaches are not something I would want to endure every day of my life.

The problem I face now is that I have effectively become a prisoner in my own home. Venturing into this now toxic environment leaves me feeling exhausted, sore, and trapped. Moving from one state to another where there are currently no smart meters is an option, but if new cell tower rollouts continue, high-speed wireless networks as part of the NBN rollout and other states follow Victoria's lead. require smart meters from the public and will eventually run out of places to go and become an EMR haven as I move to more and more remote locations. Career options will diminish and my job is already under threat as I struggle to continue working in the IT industry, where wireless networks and smart wireless devices are becoming the norm. I am facing the dilemma of how I can support my family. What kind of life will they have and what kind of opportunities are they missing out on as we move to isolated places to escape this man-made madness?

What I think needs to happen... Firstly, governments must recognize that the environment, health and safety is real and can be a serious health problem, as Sweden does. Additionally, medical professionals need to be educated about what EHS is, how to diagnose it, and how to treat it. It is necessary to establish educational programs in universities that cover this topic. The public must also be educated and informed about the risks of using wireless devices clearly without bias or unwanted influence from those who market these devices. The media often portrays those who are suffering in a poor light, leading to hurtful comments and ridicule from uneducated members of the public, this must change. Scientists often weigh in on the argument suggesting that EHS is a psychosomatic illness based on what I believe are flawed scientific studies that use challenge testing as a basis for their claims. More research may be required, but those who are suffering should not be held hostage by bickering scientists and politicians as they argue the validity of EHS and testing techniques. The symptomatology and causal factors of EHS are known and have been known for years.

I urgently ask ARPANSA to take this issue seriously and investigate the claims made by people on their complaints register as well as the health register they had created for Stop Smart Meters Australia. A recommendation should be made to the government and the National Health and Medical Research Council (NHMRC) to fund research on EHS as well as to conduct a post-deployment surveillance study of smart meters with a focus on health. It is also recommended that the ACMA follow its industry code and the Radio Communications Act, which includes the implementation of a precautionary principle, especially now that the IARC published its monograph this year justifying why RF is categorized as possible Group 2B carcinogen. You should ensure that wireless access points and cell towers are not located near or in schools, libraries or hospitals. All schools should be required to adopt a free wireless policy and use wired internal/intranet connections until it can be proven beyond doubt that Wi-Fi is secure. We should not risk the health of our children at any cost. The government should provide more funding to independent research scientists to further investigate the possible biological effects RF may have, particularly when Australia's top ARPANSA scientists suggest there are gaps in their knowledge, particularly in the area of non-toxic interactions. thermal.

Are they real or are they artifacts of the testing process? Let us make an effort to find out, since the future health of our nation depends on it. Before the installation of mobile phone base stations or the deployment of smart meters in a suburb, a surveillance study that measures the current health status of households should be carried out to create a baseline reference point and avoid potential problems of recall bias. Further surveillance studies should be conducted after the installation of the radio transmitters at established intervals to determine if there have been notable changes in public health. Telcos should be required to rationalize the deployment of mobile base stations so that resources are shared between service providers when capacity is unsubscribed, especially as our suburbs are surrounded by base stations without due consideration. to the announcement by IARC and WHO. Public health must take a higher priority than technological conveniences, especially when there is no evidence of safety and many people complain of insomnia, headaches, neurological disorders and other disabling symptoms. <<Strange times are these in which we live when the old and the young are taught falsehoods in school. And the person who dares to tell the truth is called both a lunatic and a fool.>> (Plato 427 BC). [I will put the sources and additional content links at the end of the book to make reading it more comfortable and educational.]

As if that were not enough, 5G antennas are not only spread across the surface of the Earth. Elon Musk's SpaceX project proposes the orbit of 20,000 satellites to "provide" internet to all of humanity. How do you provide internet from a satellite? Or do you use cables or do you use waves? As with telephony, to reach any part of the globe you must extend network cabling and/or position communication satellites. Do you know why the microwave we have in the kitchen is so effective? Because it bombards microwave waves from various angles. These waves excite the products because they hit the atoms, accelerating them. Due to this they break up the water molecules. And it must be considered that there should be no metal parts, so that it does not produce sparks, as in MRI machines. Have you ever imagined what it would be like to be inside a turned on microwave? Well, that remains to be seen, and more and more intensely. Now imagine that these waves come from above (by satellites), from the sides (by 5G antennas) and that they bounce around in the atmosphere (by HAARP antennas), and we are in the middle, full of our bodies with heavy metals (introduced by water, breathing, food and vaccines) and surrounded by wave and chip electronic devices (smart phones, smart watches, smart TVs, computers, tablets...). They can explode our devices, destroy our heads, hypnotize us, psychologically upset us, make us sick, fry us...

It sounds like fiction, but the technology is there, it is an immutable fact, and whoever has the power of the switch has the power to do all this. We just need to leave that button in the hands of artificial intelligence and we will see what it means to act fully without humanity or moral conscience. Bartomeu Payeras, a biologist specializing in microbiology, also studied the relationship between COVID-19 cases and the deployment of 5G networks, and his study can be reviewed here: https://drive.google.com/file/d/ 12PCGswdo5POgwOtnMGG0hswtXIAeoQKv/view ?usp=sharing [10], and at: https://www.bitchute.com/video/

aNhvfySVScpu/ [11]. But in this regard all is not lost. The human body generates a biomagnetic field of 6-9 meters by Ampere's law. According to the same electrical and magnetic principles, the soil makes an earth-air connection. Therefore, footwear, usually rubber-based, avoids this connection, causing the body to absorb all the waves, while, if you are barefoot, the waves pass over the body. The same thing happens when we are among trees, which isolate electromagnetic waves. The less you are exposed to wireless devices, such as Wi-Fi, Bluetooth, smartphones or high-frequency antennas, the better your physical and mental health. The same applies to radio waves, television, conventional telephones (landline, cable, home) and electronic equipment (such as tablets, computers, etc.).

---

10.   https://drive.google.com/file/d/

   12PCGswdo5POgwOtnMGG0hswtXIAeoQKv/view?usp=sharing

11.   https://www.bitchute.com/video/aNhvfySVScpu/

VII. CORPORATECRACY

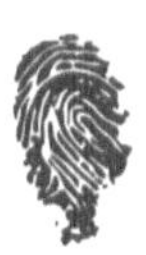

If you run a company, do you look for annual financial or moral benefits? Does love pay bills? Does kindness grow corporations? Do nobility expand companies? Good intentions, no matter how nice they are, are of no use in terms of industrial benefits. Every year companies compete to achieve greater profits. In the corporate pyramid are the pharmaceutical companies. Above them is only the banking structure, and below them, the governments. It is the pharmaceutical companies that finance and manipulate politics and the news, and therefore determine the decisions of the WHO. Every year, for a century, they promote the story of new potegenic buds, to sell their drugs, pills, treatments and injections. Despite paying million-dollar fines for their scams, people continue to believe in them, because they believe in the medical system and television. They do not understand that television is a tool of mind control, used to mold and design the system of social thought. The medical system earns commissions for drugs they prescribe, since recommending fresh fruit and vegetables, sun, beaches and fresh air do not generate profits for multinationals.

Pharmaceutical laboratories work hand in hand with military scientists on many occasions, and for governments, in the creation of chimeras. These are not created to be transmitted through the air, because an uncontrolled Ebola would kill the very scientist who created it. The chimeras are inoculated intravenously, and this is carried out through annual vaccination campaigns. The medical-pharmaceutical sign tells you, "Do you have a headache? Take this pill." That pill is a placebo that stimulates the disappearance of the headache, but leaves another component in your body. Over the years, a pill for your blood pressure controls it, but it damages your heart; later, a pill for your heart controls it, but it annoys your pancreas and stomach, and so on. They look for lifelong drug addicts, because it is a secure business with fixed profits. This is a kind of planned obsolescence, where you go to check something and they fix it while they remove two other parts so you have to return, or they sell you a printer that may last a decade, but contains a chip that causes it to fail after a while. 3 years so that you are forced to buy a new one. Selling solutions is not strategic, creating permanent clients is.

If you create a pathogen, include the antidote, then you are the Bill Gates of health, creating virus-susceptible programs and attacking them with viruses to sell them the antivirus. But the most macabre thing about this is that in reality the virus is not the problem but the excuse. A virus, as cellular waste, is nothing, nor can it do anything. What can do it is the fear propaganda of the media, which weakens the body due to cellular stress. The suggested person then goes to the doctor and is prescribed cocktails that are deadly to his body and take him to a truly terrible state. They are drugs, even if they are called legal. And they are the main cause of most deaths worldwide each year. Add to that the aerosols dispersed by airplanes, which release heavy metals, anthrax and various other toxins that people end up breathing, fumigations in fields or even in cities and nursing homes, and to top it off, the propagation of high-frequency waves that create a bacterial collapse of the organic microbiota. You already have your pandemic, and it was never a virus.

When talking about corporate monopoly, many people think that the affairs of companies are not necessarily a problem for social life, or if they are, they are actually based on internal corruption and governments simply investigate them a lot. What really happens is that for about a hundred years the power of companies has surpassed the power of government entities. Just as banking power had previously subjugated the state, multinational corporations slowly began to be above the law, to the point of seeing that not even politicians who wanted to stand up to this corporatocracy were able to get anywhere. I have already spoken many times about the infamous Rockefellers, how they monopolized the oil lobby, put themselves at the top of banking, pushed the pharmaceutical system, bought education books, pushed and have financed the most prestigious universities and research centers and even They have given land to political establishments, as is the case of the UN. The Rockefellers pushed a campaign all these decades to eliminate from the US.

Most people consider that what is happening in the world right now is under the control of experts and well-intentioned professionals. Well, the CDC is a vaccine company, Google has agreements with vaccine companies, Microsoft patents vaccines, doctors receive commissions for vaccinations, politicians traffic in the price of vaccines, the WHO is financed by Gates - who is a financier of vaccines -, the news programs are financed by companies - mostly pharmaceutical companies, vaccine manufacturers -, Facebook fact-checkers - who will have censored something from you at some point - belong to a Gates lobby... they all benefit from the sale of vaccines . They all have close business ties and strong vested interests with pharmaceutical companies and their laboratories. Doesn't the UN know this? What if I told you that World War II was the first step towards this Agenda 2030 plan? WWII promoted the Union of Nations for the interests of the Rockefellers and the

Rothschilds. They brought Harry S. Truman to power to create the UN, and the Rockefellers themselves gave up the land where the United Nations general building is now in Manhattan – also being the owners of the WHO -, just as the Rothschilds did with the Knesset (the Parliament of Israel). The Rockefellers are the main promoters of the pharmaceutical monopoly. They created it.

Traditional medicine and replace it with their new business, taking oil to create drugs, and getting the FDA (the Drug and Drug Administration) to accept it. This was achieved slowly, through bribes, blackmail, "accidental" deaths, threats and other strategies very typical of these families. Coca-Cola did the same to avoid being rejected for the compounds found in its drinks, so Rockefeller would have no problem monopolizing the market with its drugs. In the last 10 years, thousands of eminences of traditional and homeopathic health, as well as biologists, chemists, bacteriologists and scientists, have been found dead. Few have followed up on this "phenomenon", but it is clear from what is happening now why this is. Let's just look at the death of Kary Mullis, who was not old, but died a couple of months before this pandemic began. Kary was the creator of the PCR test, and who since the AIDS scam did not stop saying that his test only detected bacteria, not viruses, and was not an absolutist test, but a complementary one, and had to be corroborated with other confirmatory tests. What would Kary have said about the absurd use of his test to diagnose a disease, much less determine a pandemic?

Doctors constantly warn that they are censored and threatened, telling them that they will lose their jobs and could go to jail if they talk about what really happens in hospitals. This pressure increased after hundreds of professionals from all fields of medicine uploaded their opinions about what was happening on the networks. Since then they have been strictly prohibited from speaking publicly, apart from the fact that the Bill Gates lobby has created a social media censorship network, together with its friends at Google, to eliminate any opposition to the hoax of such vaccines, the assembly of the such a pandemic and to veto all opinions on alternative medicines. Because? Gates is a friend of the Rockefellers, and his main business these last two decades has been vaccines. Zuckerberg, owner and CEO of Facebook, is he allied with these clowns? In July 2020, he openly said that the safety of vaccines should be reviewed, despite the fact that Facebook kept censoring opinions on the matter. Zuckerberg has been on trial for Facebook's vaccine censorship. This is somewhat contradictory. Facebook that "punishes" weeks and up to a month for making certain types of comments.

This comes, they maintain, from the Fact Checkers, who ridiculously belong to Bill Gates' lobby. It is precisely Gates who does not want the good reputation of the poison and technologies in which he has invested so much time and money to be defamed. But this does not stop there, there is more… the parent company of YouTube – which by the way deleted my account of almost 10 years when talking about this book that you are now reading – is Google, which invests directly in AstraZeneca injections/ Oxford. This explains this dilemma much more. Google, working from Silicon Valley, has automated "health" systems to be telematic with artificial intelligence, so that it is not that there is a supposedly "independent" "data verifier" that reviews information, but that the algorithms merely detect keywords that criticize the lobby, and they automatically block you. And that's not all, Google partnered with the US military on transhumanism programs, where DARPA also operates. That is why pseudo-vaccines have nano DNA tracking and modification technology.

<u>WHO IS THE PFIZER COMPANY?</u>

Let's look at who the good guys are who want to puncture their "antidote". One of the famous companies that "manufactures" this "vaccine" "against" the bug, Pfizer, has a reputation that precedes it (see: https://www.mp-22.com [1], https://lbry.tv /@elinvestigador:0/ Historia—%C3%A9tica—de-la- [2]Farmace%C3%BAtica-Pfizer-que-comercializa-las-Vacunas-Covid19.-:6 [3], https://www.justice.gov /opa/pr/just...gest-health-care-fraud-settlement-its-history [4]and https://www.bitchute.com/video/ zVHaSlw2PWrT/ [5]). The former vice president of Pfizer revealed how they bribe Governments, Medical Institutions, Universities and scientists. He has received fines for various dark actions.

- Name of parent company: Pfizer
- Total penalty since 2000: USD $4,747,652,947
- Number of records: 80
- Full list: https://violationtracker.goodjobsfirst.org/parent/pfizer

There are 5 groups of main crimes (defined groups) and their total penalty, according to the number of records, and the corresponding fine: for health-related crimes $3,373,675,000; for crimes related to government contracting, $1,161,001,892; for security-related violations, $104,004,655; for violations related to competition, $98,166,568; for crimes related to the

---

1.   https://www.mp-22.com

2.   https://lbry.tv/@elinvestigador:0/Historia--%C3%A9tica--de-la-Farmace%C3%BAtica-Pfizer-que-comercializa-las-Vacunas-Covid19.-:6

3.   https://lbry.tv/@elinvestigador:0/Historia--%C3%A9tica--de-la-Farmace%C3%BAtica-Pfizer-que-comercializa-las-Vacunas-Covid19.-:6

4.   https://www.justice.gov/opa/pr/just...gest-health-care-fraud-settlement-its-history

5.   https://www.bitchute.com/video/zVHaSlw2PWrT/

environment, $5,324,642. Regarding the 5 main types of main crimes and the total penalty according to the number of registrations: for off-label or unapproved promotion of medical products, $3,373,675,000; by False Claims and related law, $1,161,001,892; for violation of safety of medications or medical equipment, $103,840,000; for Foreign Corrupt Practices Act, $60,216,568; for illegal commissions and bribes, $34,700,000. And well, the list goes on, but if you want to go deeper I recommend looking at the tables. Pfizer became the world's largest pharmaceutical company largely by purchasing its competitors. It has also grown through aggressive marketing, a practice it pioneered in the 1950s by purchasing unprecedented advertising in medical journals.

In 2009, the company had to pay a record $2.3 billion to settle federal charges that one of its subsidiaries had illegally marketed a painkiller called Bextra. Along with questionable marketing, Pfizer has for decades been at the center of controversies over its pricing, including a price-fixing case that began in 1958. In the mid-1980s, advocacy organizations such as the Public Citizen Health Research Group They charged that Feldene, a widely prescribed arthritis drug from Pfizer, created a high risk of gastrointestinal bleeding among the elderly, but the federal government, despite reports of dozens of deaths, refused to place restrictions on the medication. A June 1986 article in The Progressive about Feldene was titled "Death by Prescription." The Food and Drug Administration expressed further concern over reports of dozens of deaths related to heart valves by Pfizer's Shiley division. In 1986, when the death toll reached 125, Pfizer ended production of all valve models. However, at the time they were implanted in thousands of people, who were concerned that the devices could fracture and fail at any time.

In 1991, an FDA task force accused Shiley of withholding information about safety issues from regulators to gain initial approval for its valves and that the company continued to keep the FDA in the dark. A November 7, 1991, investigation in the Wall Street Journal claimed that Shiley had been deliberately falsifying manufacturing records related to valve fractures. In the face of this growing scandal, Pfizer announced that it would spend up to $205 million to resolve the tens of thousands of valve lawsuits that had been filed against it. Still, Pfizer resisted an FDA order to notify patients about new findings that there was an increased risk of fatal fractures in those who had the valve installed before age 50. In 1994, the company agreed to pay $10 million to resolve this issue. The Justice Department accuses them of having lied to regulators when seeking approval for the valves; also agreed to pay $9 million to monitor valve patients at Veterans Administration hospitals or pay for device removal. In 2004, Pfizer announced that it had reached a $60 million settlement of a class-action lawsuit brought by users of Rezulin, a diabetes drug developed by Warner-Lambert, which had removed it from the market shortly before Pfizer acquired the company in 2000. The recall came after dozens of patients died from acute liver failure caused by the drug.

In 2004, in the wake of revelations about the dangerous side effects of Merck's painkiller Vioxx, Pfizer agreed to discontinue television advertising for a related drug called Celebrex. The following year, Pfizer admitted that a 1999 clinical trial found that elderly patients taking Celebrex had a very high risk of heart problems. In 2005, Pfizer pulled another pain reliever, Bextra, from the market after the FDA mandated a "black box" warning about the drug's cardiovascular and gastrointestinal risks. In 2008, Pfizer announced that it would provide $894 million to settle lawsuits that had been filed in connection with Bextra and

Celebrex. With the acquisition of Wyeth (formerly American Home Products) in October 2009, Pfizer faced a new set of legal problems. The summary of the legal proceedings in Wyeth's last annual financial report before the deal was announced ran for 14 pages. Most of the lawsuits discussed were product liability cases involving hormone therapy, childhood vaccines, the antidepressant Effexor, the contraceptive Norplant and, most importantly, the combination diet drug known as fen-phen, which had been removed from the market after reports that its use was linked to potentially fatal damage to heart valves. Those findings triggered a wave of tens of thousands of lawsuits against the company.

Pfizer has been at the center of controversy over its pricing for more than 50 years. In 1958 it was one of six pharmaceutical companies accused by the Federal Trade Commission of fixing prices on antibiotics. The company was also accused of making false statements to the United States Patent Office to obtain a patent on tetracycline. In 1961, the Department of Justice brought criminal antitrust charges against Pfizer, American Cyanamid, Bristol-Myers, and top executives of the three companies. Two years later, the FTC ruled that the six companies named in its 1958 complaint had conspired to fix tetracycline prices. The commission also found that "irregularities played a significant role" in the issuance of the tetracycline patent to Pfizer. In 1964, the FTC ordered the six companies to readjust their prices and told Pfizer to grant a tetracycline production license to any company that requested one. In 1967, a federal jury found Pfizer, American Cyanamid and Bristol-Myers guilty of conspiring to control the production and distribution of restraint of trade, conspiracy to monopolize and monopoly. Each of the companies received a maximum paltry fine of $150,000. In 1970, a federal appeals court ordered the case be returned to district court. Pfizer and other companies agreed to pay about $136 million to settle a class action case and other civil lawsuits that had been filed on behalf of consumers and state and local governments. Subsequent settlements raised the amount to more than $150 million.

Pfizer, along with the other big pharmaceutical companies, were the subject of a series of lawsuits brought by state attorneys general and other parties challenging the industry's pricing practices. In 1996, Pfizer was one of 15 large pharmaceutical companies that agreed to pay more than $408 million to settle a class-action lawsuit accusing them of conspiring to fix prices charged to independent pharmacies. In 1999, Pfizer pleaded guilty to criminal antitrust charges that its former Food Science Group unit participated in two international price-fixing conspiracies, one involving the food preservative sodium erythorbate and the other involving the food enhancer maltol flavor. Pfizer agreed to pay fines totaling $20 million. In 2000, amid widespread criticism about the high price of AIDS drugs, Pfizer offered to donate a two-year supply of its drug Diflucan worth $50 million to the South African government. However, in 2003, after acquiring Pharmacia Corp., Pfizer withdrew from the company's plan to license its AIDS drug Rescriptor for low-cost distribution in poor countries.

In 2002, Pfizer resisted cooperating with a General Accounting Office investigation of the industry's pricing practices but relented after president and CEO Henry McKinnell was served with a subpoena. Later that year, Pfizer agreed to pay $49 million to resolve charges that one of its subsidiaries defrauded the federal Medicaid program by overcharging for its cholesterol-lowering drug Lipitor. In 2003, as Congress was discussing legislation to legalize the importation of cheap prescription drugs from Canada, Pfizer tried to undermine the practice by telling major Canadian pharmacies that they would have to start ordering directly from Pfizer instead of through wholesalers. . This put Pfizer in the position of cutting off supply if it suspected pharmacies were selling to the US market. The following year, Pfizer announced that it would begin requiring wholesalers to report orders from individual pharmacies. In 2016, the Justice Department announced that Pfizer would pay $784 million to resolve allegations that Wyeth failed to pay rebates to Medicaid for two of its drugs. Later in 2016, the UK Competition and Markets Authority fined Pfizer the equivalent of $107 million for charging excessive and unfair prices for an epilepsy drug.

After World War II, Pfizer caused a scandal when it bypassed traditional drug distribution networks and began marketing its products (especially the antibiotic Terramycin) directly to hospitals and doctors, making unprecedented use of eye-catching advertisements in the Journal of the American Medical Association. A prominent article in the Saturday Review in 1957 exposed the company for tactics such as running advertisements for its antibiotics that featured the names of doctors who supposedly endorsed the product but turned out to be fictitious. In 1991, Pfizer paid a total of $70,000 to 10 states to settle charges related to misleading advertising of its Plax mouthwash. In 1996, the Food and Drug Administration ordered Pfizer to stop making unauthorized and misleading medical claims about its antidepressant Zoloft. In 2000, the FDA warned Pfizer and Pharmacia, co-marketers of the arthritis drug Celebrex, that the consumer advertisements they were running for the drug were false and misleading. Two years later, the FDA ordered Pfizer to stop publishing a series of magazine ads that the agency said misleadingly suggested that its cholesterol-lowering drug Lipitor was safer than competing products.

In 2003, Pfizer paid $6 million to settle with 19 states that had accused the company of using deceptive advertising to promote its drug Zithromax for children's ear infections. In 2004, Pfizer's Warner-Lambert subsidiary agreed to pay $430 million to resolve criminal and civil charges it paid doctors to prescribe its epilepsy drug Neurontin to patients with ailments for which the drug was not approved. Documents later came to light suggesting that Pfizer orchestrated delays in publishing scientific studies that undermined its claim of Neurontin's other uses. In 2010, a federal jury found that Pfizer committed racketeering fraud in its marketing of Neurontin; The judge in the case later ordered the company to pay $142 million in damages. In 2007, Pfizer's subsidy, Pharmacia & Upjohn, agreed to pay $34.7 million to resolve federal charges related to the illegal marketing of its human growth hormone Genotropin. In 2009, Pfizer agreed to pay $2.3 billion to resolve criminal and civil charges related to the improper marketing of Bextra and three other drugs. The amount was a record for a health care fraud settlement. John Kopchinski, a former Pfizer sales representative whose complaint helped launch the federal investigation, told the New York Times: "Pfizer's entire culture is sales-driven, and if I wasn't selling drugs illegally, I wasn't seen as a team player." John Kopchinski, a former Pfizer sales representative.

As part of the settlement, Pfizer had to enter into a Corporate Integrity Agreement with the Inspector General of the Department of Health and Human Services. In 2010, Pfizer disclosed that over a six-month period the previous year it had paid $20 million to about 4,500 doctors and other medical professionals to consult and speak on the company's behalf. This was the first time the company made its expenses of this type public. In 2011, Pfizer agreed to pay $14.5 million to settle federal charges that it illegally marketed its bladder drug Detrol. In 2011, the FDA told Pfizer that its "Online Resources" web page about Lipitor contained misleading statements. In July 2012, Pfizer agreed to remove claims related to breast and colon health from its Centrum multivitamin advertising as part of an agreement to resolve a lawsuit brought by the Center for Science in the Public Interest. In November 2012, Pfizer revealed that it had taken a charge against profits of $491 million in connection with an "agreement in principle" with the US Department of Justice to resolve charges related to improper marketing of the drug. for Rapamune kidney transplant by Wyeth. That deal was finalized in July 2013. Pfizer later reached a $35 million settlement over the Rapamune charges brought by more than 40 state attorneys general.

In 1976, Pfizer was one of many companies revealed to have made questionable payments to foreign government officials. The company said about $265,000 had been paid to officials in three countries, but did not identify them. In August 2012, the U.S. Securities and Exchange Commission announced that it had reached a $45 million settlement with Pfizer to resolve charges that its subsidiaries, especially Wyeth, had bribed doctors and other healthcare professionals. abroad to increase overseas sales. In 1971, the Environmental Protection Agency asked Pfizer to end its long-standing practice of dumping industrial waste from its Groton, Connecticut plant into Long Island Sound. The company was reported to be disposing of about 1 million gallons of waste each year by that method. In 1991, Pfizer agreed to pay $3.1 million to settle EPA charges that the company severely damaged the Delaware River by failing to install pollution control equipment at one of its plants in

Pennsylvania. In 1994, Pfizer agreed to pay $1.5 million as part of a consent decree with the EPA regarding its dumping at a toxic waste site in Rhode Island. In 1998, Pfizer agreed to pay a $625,000 civil penalty for environmental violations discovered at its research facility in Groton, Connecticut.

In 2002, New Jersey fined Pfizer $538,000 for failing to adequately monitor wastewater discharged from its Parsippany plant. In 2003, shortly after Pfizer acquired Pharmacia, the company (along with Solutia and Monsanto) agreed to pay about $700 million to settle a lawsuit over PCB dumping in Anniston, Alabama. In 2005, Pfizer agreed to pay $22,500 to resolve EPA claims that the company failed to adequately notify state and federal officials of a 2002 chemical release from its plant in Groton that seriously injured several employees and required an emergency response. important. Also in 2005, Pfizer agreed to pay $46,250 to settle charges that its Pharmacia & Upjohn operation had violated federal air pollution rules at its Kalamazoo, Michigan, plant. In 2008, Pfizer agreed to pay a $975,000 civil penalty to settle federal charges for violating the Clean Air Act at its former manufacturing plant in Groton, Connecticut, from 2002 to 2005. New Jersey environmental groups have criticized it for A cleanup plan devised by Pfizer and the EPA for the American Cyanamid Superfund site in Bridgewater, which is considered one of the worst toxic waste sites in the country, is inadequate. Pfizer inherited responsibility for the cleanup through its 2009 purchase of Wyeth.

Pfizer also reportedly engaged in questionable practices abroad. In 2000, the Washington Post published a major exposé accusing Pfizer of testing a dangerous new antibiotic called Trovan on children in Nigeria without receiving proper consent from their parents. The experiment occurred during a 1996 meningitis epidemic in the country. In 2001, Pfizer was sued in US federal court by thirty Nigerian families, who accused the company of using their children as human guinea pigs. In 2006, a panel of Nigerian medical experts concluded that Pfizer had violated international law. In 2009, the company agreed to pay $75 million to resolve some of the lawsuits that had been filed in Nigerian courts. The US case was settled in 2011 for an undisclosed amount. Classified US State Department cables made public in 2010 by Wikileaks indicated that Pfizer had hired investigators to unearth Nigeria's former attorney general as a way to gain influence in one of the remaining cases. Pfizer had to apologize for the revelation in the cables that it had falsely claimed that the group Doctors Without Borders was also administering Trovan during the Nigerian meningitis epidemic.

In January 2012, a group of Pfizer employees in Puerto Rico filed a lawsuit against the company in federal court, charging that it failed to properly manage its pension plan and caused losses totaling hundreds of millions of dollars over the past decade. . In 2010, a federal jury awarded $1.37 million to a former Pfizer scientist who claimed she was sickened by a genetically engineered virus in a company lab and was later fired for raising safety concerns. Pfizer is one of the numerous pharmaceutical companies that for many years took advantage of a provision of the Internal Revenue Code (Section 936) that granted special tax credits for its operations in Puerto Rico and was widely criticized as a form of corporate welfare. A 1992 report by the U.S. General Accounting Office found that Pfizer enjoyed $156,400 in tax savings for each of its 500 employees on the island. The amount was said to be 636 percent of the company's compensation costs. There was a move during the Clinton administration to eliminate Section 936, but Pfizer and other pharmaceutical companies managed to phase out the termination over a decade. During that period, pharmaceutical companies began registering their operations in Puerto Rico as foreign entities, allowing them to escape taxes entirely as long as they did not send profits back to the mainland United States.

The companies then pressured Congress to enact a repatriation tax exemption that would allow them to bring all of their foreign profits back home and pay them an artificially low tax rate, supposedly to stimulate domestic job creation. When that holiday went into effect for 2005, Pfizer repatriated more foreign profits than any other company — $37 billion — and enjoyed an $11 billion tax break while cutting rather than adding to its American workforce. In 2014, Pfizer launched an effort to take over AstraZeneca that was designed not only to swallow up a competitor but also to reduce its tax bill by locating the combined operation's headquarters in Britain. When AstraZeneca resisted the controversial move, Pfizer abandoned the bid. Then, in November 2015, Pfizer announced a similar deal, worth $160 billion, to merge with Allergan and move the combined company's headquarters to Ireland. The plan was abandoned when the Obama administration introduced new tax rules.

Connecticut. In 2001, Pfizer opened a new $270 million research facility in New London with the help of a $60 million grant package from state and local officials. The city also used its power of eminent domain to assemble the site used by the company, angering local residents and sparking a court challenge that reached all the way to the U.S. Supreme Court. In that case, Kelo v. New London judges upheld the city's right to take private property for economic development projects. In 2009, however, Pfizer announced that it would close its New London operation and relocate 1,400 jobs to its campus in nearby Groton, Connecticut. In 2001, the company committed to an $800 million expansion of its Ann Arbor research laboratories after receiving a state and local tax subsidy package worth more than $70 million. However, five years later, the company announced it would abandon the facility and eliminate more than 2,000 jobs. The company also said it would eliminate 250 jobs in Kalamazoo, where in 2003 it received a 20-year subsidy package worth up to $635 million.

NY. In 2003, New York city and state officials offered Pfizer up to $47 million in hopes that the company would create 2,000 new jobs at its Manhattan headquarters and other New York City locations while retaining more than 5,000 positions. By 2010, Pfizer had instead eliminated a large number of jobs in the city, in part due to the closure of its former manufacturing plant in Brooklyn. In December of that year, Pfizer agreed to pay the city a $24.7 million fine, double the tax subsidies it had received. Source: By Philip Mattera, https://cienciaysaludnatural.com/historia-criminal-de-pfizer/ [6].

Why is there such a rush and obsession? Because of Trump, the globalists have accelerated many things that were supposed to go at their own pace since the end of 2016. Trump hindered their plans, as the Kennedy family has been doing, however, they do whatever it takes to get them out of the way. The elite wants to poison humanity no matter what, because they don't want so many people nor do they want them thinking. They want a few to perform certain functions and feed the draconians, and for the rest to have all the resources for that Illuminati leadership. Think, why could tests like PCR secretly vaccinate the "vaccine resistant"? Yes, to the "divergents", who take the test for various reasons of pressure, but would necessarily get vaccinated. In November 2020, Johns Hopkins University (JHU) published a study suggesting that Wuhan coronavirus test swabs may carry "tiny star-shaped microdevices," capable of delivering vaccines to

---

6.   https://cienciaysaludnatural.com/historia-criminal-de-pfizer/

people without their knowledge or knowledge. consent. Because more than half of the US is "vaccine reluctant," meaning most people want nothing to do with "Chinese virus" shots, "science" has apparently developed a hidden injection technology to secretly vaccinate people through the nasal or anal PCR test sticks that are stuck in their orifices.

One post noted: JHU's Patrick Smith wrote in an article about the study that these tiny star-shaped microdevices were "inspired by a parasitic worm that sinks its sharp teeth into the intestines of its host." Sounds fun, right? "David Gracias, a professor at the Whiting School of Engineering, and gastroenterologist Florin M. Selaru, director of the Johns Hopkins Inflammatory Bowel Disease Center, led a team of biomedical researchers and engineers who designed and tested shape-changing microdevices that mimic the how parasitic hookworms attach to an organism's intestines," Smith wrote. Known as "theragrippers," these microdevices made of metal and "shape-changing thin film" are coated with heat-sensitive paraffin wax that is delivered to the body undetected. Each of these chips is no larger than a grain of dust. Once inside the body, the star-shaped devices react to heat by closing and sticking to the intestinal wall with small spikes. The centers of these now closed stars are capable of delivering any medicine implanted inside them, in this case substances from the microscopic vaccine against the Wuhan coronavirus (COVID-19).

"The claim is that powder-sized 'theragrippers' can be deployed on the tips of PCR test rods and delivered to the innocent 'victim,'" writes John O'Sullivan for Principia Scientific International. "This may be totally immoral - and probably illegal - but it is certainly feasible..." "Thousands of these sinister miniature theragrippers can be deployed in the gastrointestinal tract through a simple innocent swab administered as part of the COVID-19 test already carried out by millions of people around the world. You simply wouldn't feel anything," he adds. You can watch a video about this technology at this link: https://www.brighteon.com/6bbf3d1b-d9b6-4047-9772-dd277bfe3324 [7]. Does Fauci know about the vaccines hidden in the swabs? PCR test? If the PCR test swabs contain this hidden technology, which seems possible, then people who believe they are simply being "tested" for Chinese germs could also be vaccinated without authorization. This is music to the ears. from Anthony Fauci, who recently complained that vaccinating large numbers of people against WuFlu would be difficult due to "vaccine hesitancy."

Using the word "hesitation" implies that people are simply not sure whether they should get vaccinated, when in reality most people are sure about not getting vaccinated at all. A Gallup poll conducted late last year found that about half of Americans will not get vaccinated. "Colored people" were very sure at the time that they would not receive the vaccine, although the number of "vaccine hesitants" of all races has only increased since then. Put pressure on your legislators to answer the question of whether people get vaccinated secretly or not. Right now, it is crucial for ordinary people to contact their legislators to demand answers. Since "Congress belongs to the pharmaceutical industry," to quote a top FDA medical adviser, you're likely to get a runaround, but it's always worth a try. President Donald Trump also warned that the pharmaceutical industry was contributing "enormous sums of money to politicians" who then do their bidding. There was even an article published in Helpdesk Report about "vaccination hesitancy" and the strategies that Big Pharma and corrupt lawmakers can

---

7.   https://www.brighteon.com/6bbf3d1b-d9b6-4047-9772-dd277bfe3324

use to overcome it. One of these strategies consists of hiding the microscopic vaccines in the PCR test rods.

Keep in mind that the pharmaceutical industry spends much more money than any other industry trying to influence politicians. Some of them are almost certainly on board programs like this that essentially trick people into getting vaccinated who would otherwise say no to the vaccine. "This is particularly worrying because if for some reason you have to go to the hospital like I did, they give you a test," wrote a concerned Principia Scientific International commenter. "Just the other day, this same thought suddenly crossed my mind," wrote another. "Whether it's true or not, it doesn't matter, but I'm glad I decided under no circumstances, regardless of the consequences (no family, so nothing to lose), that I would take a vaccine test. I'd rather die slowly of hunger. No It's a joke. Sources for this article include: VaccineImpact.com, NaturalNews.com, Principia-Scientific.com, naturalnews/Ciencia y Paciencia, and https://religionlavozlibre.blogspot.com/2021/02/los-pcr-could-vaccinate-in-secret-los.html?m=1 [8]. Dr. Mike Yeadon, former scientific director and former vice president of Pfizer Global, assures that in the United Kingdom the pandemic is over. He denounces the false positives due to mass testing with the PCR technique and the uselessness of confinements. He warns that there is something "with a very bad smell" around the possible mandatory nature of the vaccine: http://www.laprensa.com.ar/495563-Coronavirus-el-fraude-of-the-second-wave.note.aspx [9].

---

8.   https://religionlavozlibre.blogspot.com/2021/02/los-pcr-podrian-vacunar-en-secreto-los.html?m=1

9.   http://www.laprensa.com.ar/495563-Coronavirus-el-fraude-de-la-segunda-ola.note.aspx

In just two months, since the start of mass vaccination in 2021, the wave of deaths and people with adverse side effects such as paralysis flooded the media. Doctors are prohibited from speaking publicly about this. The so-called cytokine storms, blood clots, the Delta variant, etc., were the same: side effects of pseudo-vaccines. By the end of summer 2021, 33 million adverse effects had been reported worldwide, with 11 million deaths. Clearly, the newsmen were prohibited from reporting these events. Conventional deaths are called "covid deaths," and deaths from injections are called "natural deaths." Following this line, in one year more people could die from these injections than all the deaths in World War II. Just watching the video at conferences of a 160 kilodalton protein, Cas9, cutting the DNA chains, in injected people, made it clear that it was true that they were destroying human DNA. As the months go by, more people know about the deception, but more individuals have given in to the persecution and pressure to get vaccinated, with the fact that without the vaccination certificate it will soon be impossible to be part of the system, and ultimately, no one You will be able to eat, pay services or rent, and even receive a salary, as was prophesied in the book of Revelation almost 2,000 years ago.

Obviously, less is reported than it is so that there is no opposite reaction of the masses to vaccination. I could write an entire chapter on this alone, but I leave that task to the reader, as an exercise in their own research and verification. I'll give you some nudges, though: From the CDC, 3,150 people vaccinated in ONE DAY are "unable to perform normal daily activities, unable to work" after vaccination. This is a massive 2.7% of people who [10]can no longer work after receiving the Pfizer vaccine: https://www.cdc.gov/vaccines/acip/meetings/

---

10.   https://www.cdc.gov/vaccines/acip/meetings/downloads/slides-2020-12/

slides-12-19/05-COVID-CLARK.pdf

downloads/slides-2020-12/slides-12-19/
[11]05-COVID-CLARK.pdf [12]; Portuguese health worker, 41, dies two days after receiving Pfizer covid vaccine when her father says he 'wants answers': https://trib.al/eEWi66p [13]; Mexican doctor hospitalized after receiving COVID-19 vaccine: https://www.reuters.com/article/health-coronavirus-mexico-vaccines-idUSKBN2970H3 [14]; Gregory Michael, 56, an obstetrician who had his practice at Mount Sinai Medical Center in Miami Beach, died due to a strong reaction to the COVID vaccine: https://www.local10.com/news/local/2021/01 /07/did-miami-beach-doctor-56-die-from-receiving-covid-19-vaccine/ [15]and https://www.dailymail.co.uk/news/article-9119431/Miami-doctor-58- dies-three-weeks-receiving-Pfizer-Covid-19-vaccine.html [16].

Hundreds of Israelis become infected with Covid-19 after receiving Pfizer/BioNTech vaccine: https://www.rt.com/news/511332-israel-vaccination-coronavirus-pfizer/ [17]; 75-year-old Israeli dies 2 hours after receiving Covid-19 vaccine: https://www.israelnationalnews.com/News/News.aspx/293865 [18]; Death of a Swiss man after Pfizer vaccine:

11.   https://www.cdc.gov/vaccines/acip/meetings/downloads/slides-2020-12/slides-12-19/05-COVID-CLARK.pdf

12.   https://www.cdc.gov/vaccines/acip/meetings/downloads/slides-2020-12/slides-12-19/05-COVID-CLARK.pdf

13.   https://trib.al/eEWi66p

14.   https://www.reuters.com/article/health-coronavirus-mexico-vaccines-idUSKBN2970H3

15.   https://www.local10.com/news/local/2021/01/07/did-miami-beach-doctor-56-die-from-receiving-covid-19-vaccine/

16.   https://www.dailymail.co.uk/news/article-9119431/Miami-doctor-58-dies-three-weeks-receiving-Pfizer-Covid-19-vaccine.html

17.   https://www.rt.com/news/511332-israel-vaccination-coronavirus-pfizer/

https://www.reuters.com/article/us-health-coronavirus-swiss-death-idUSKBN29413Y [19]; 88-year-old woman collapses and dies several hours after being vaccinated: https://www.israelnationalnews.com/News/News.aspx/293952 [20]; thousands of people negatively affected after getting Covid-19 vaccine: https://m.theepochtimes.com/thousands-negatively-affected-after-getting-covid-19-vaccine_3625914.html [21]; Hospital worker with no previous allergies in intensive care with severe reaction after Pfizer Covid vaccine: https://metro.co.uk/2020/12/16/hospital-worker-in-intensive-care-after-suffering-severe -allergic-reaction-to-covid-vaccine-13763695/ [22]; four volunteers develop FACIAL PARALYSIS after taking Pfizer Covid-19 jab, prompting FDA to recommend "case surveillance": https://www.rt.com/usa/509081-pfizer-vaccine-fda- bells-palsy-covid/ [23]; The investigation was launched when 2 people die in a Norwegian nursing home days after receiving Pfizer's Covid-19 vaccine: https://www.rt.com/news/511623-norway-covid19-vaccine-deaths/ [24].

Hundreds of people sent to emergency room after getting COVID-19 vaccines: https://m.theepochtimes.com/hundreds-sent-to-emergency-room-after-getting-covid-19-

---

18.	https://www.israelnationalnews.com/News/News.aspx/293865

19.	https://www.reuters.com/article/us-health-coronavirus-swiss-death-idUSKBN29413Y

20.	https://www.israelnationalnews.com/News/News.aspx/293952

21.	https://m.theepochtimes.com/thousands-negatively-affected-after-getting-covid-19-vaccine_3625914.html

22.	https://metro.co.uk/2020/12/16/hospital-worker-in-intensive-care-after-suffering-severe-allergic-reaction-to-covid-vaccine-13763695/

23.	https://www.rt.com/usa/509081-pfizer-vaccine-fda-bells-palsy-covid/

24.	https://www.rt.com/news/511623-norway-covid19-vaccine-deaths/

vaccines_3644148.html [25]; US officials report more severe allergic reactions to COVID-19 vaccines: https://www.google.com/amp/s/mobile.reuters.com/article/amp/idUSKBN29B2GS [26]; NHS said not to give the Covid vaccine to those with a history of allergic reactions: https://www.google.com/amp/s/amp.theguardian.com/world/2020/dec/09/pfizer-covid-vaccine-nhs-extreme-allergy-sufferers-regulators-reaction [27]; COVID-19, single dose vaccine leads to 'increased risk' of new coronavirus variants, South African experts warn: https://news.sky.com/story/amp/covid-19-single-vaccine-dose-leads-to-greater-risk-from-new-coronavirus-variants-south-african-experts-warn-12180837 [28]; The CDC reveals that at least 21 Americans have suffered life-threatening allergic reactions to the Pfizer COVID vaccine: www.dailymail.co.uk/health/article-9119029/amp/At-21-Americans-life-threatening-anaphylaxis-receiving -Pfizers-vaccine-CDC-reveals.html [29]; Woman experiences side effects of COVID-19 vaccine: www.everythinglubbock.com/news/local-news/woman-experiences-side-effects-of-covid-19-vaccine/amp/ [30]; COVID vaccine side effects are more common after

---

25.   https://m.theepochtimes.com/hundreds-sent-to-emergency-room-after-getting-covid-19-vaccines_3644148.html

26.   https://www.google.com/amp/s/mobile.reuters.com/article/amp/idUSKBN29B2GS

27.   https://www.google.com/amp/s/amp.theguardian.com/world/2020/dec/09/pfizer-covid-vaccine-nhs-extreme-allergy-sufferers-regulators-reaction

28.   https://news.sky.com/story/amp/covid-19-single-vaccine-dose-leads-to-greater-risk-from-new-coronavirus-variants-south-african-experts-warn-12180837

29.   http://www.dailymail.co.uk/health/article-9119029/amp/At-21-Americans-life-threatening-anaphylaxis-receiving-Pfizers-vaccine-CDC-reveals.html

30.   http://www.everythinglubbock.com/news/local-news/woman-experiences-side-effects-of-covid-19-vaccine/amp/

the second dose: www.boston.cbslocal.com/2021/01/05/covid-vaccine-s [31].

According to a doctor with a specialty in virology, <<the Pfizer vaccine has a pig rhinovirus vector. It is an RNA gene (RNA) that synthesizes its unit 1, unit 2 and RBD (Receptor-Binding Domain) for the 'S' protein. That vaccine is a gene... in fact, it is not a vaccine, it is actually a gene, genetic therapy.>> It is a gene that, upon entering your cell, orders your body what to do, and causes it to be generated by The receptors do a certain job, <<by the B lymphocytes and by the entire cascade of enzymatic reactions, the generation of antibodies, so that when you become infected with coronavirus you already have the antibodies and do not get sick. Now, does the vaccine eliminate the coronavirus? Yes, but that's not the problem. The problem is the following: every exogenous, synthetic, foreign, non-natural gene inserted by this injection will go through a process called retrotranscription. Your body is going to convert it into DNA, and polymerases are a family that is going to help insert that foreign gene into genetic memory. Those are all the proteins that unwind, and that DNA, through a system similar to that of nucleases, cuts a piece and inserts the DNA, and the histone is wound again. In other words, they made you a transgenic, genetically modified organism. What is the danger of it? The danger is that when it comes to hitting, they hit badly, and they cause autoimmune diseases...>> Among them, <<you lose mobility, you can't breathe and you can even die. Mutations, etc.>> Vaccines are supposed to be attenuated viruses and bacteria, but this is not that, this is a gene, and yes, they attach to your DNA. That's what I dedicate myself to.>> You could see your body's responses 10 years from now, when you suffer from paralysis.

---

31.   http://www.boston.cbslocal.com/2021/01/05/covid-vaccine-s

The genetic engineer, Luis Marcelo Martínez, maintained in another interview – this time with a program from Paraguay – that these pseudo-vaccines will contain nanochips, based on data that is documented in the scientific literature. It is the use of insertional mutagenesis, nano technology to sterilize the population and change human behavior. Atypical bilateral pneumonia is an example of the inconsistency of calling the coronavirus a respiratory disease, since it is assumed that respiratory viruses first attach to the lung closest to the heart, since it arrives with the first puff, not simultaneously. It is said that it started in China, but it doesn't have to be due to a virus, but rather that there they inhale synthesized garbage in the air, dust from broken monitors, they pulverize the garbage and release it into the air, that gives you pneumonitis. He adds that 5G technology, based on scalar waves, can generate massive inflammation, multi-organ failure, cytokine storm, thrombotic phenomenon, and they call that 'covid-19'. They assume that pneumonia and pneumonitis must be caused by a virus, but that is not a scientifically proven fact. Doctors must keep an open mind and open themselves to various possibilities, to the multifactoriality and multicausality of the 'health-disease' process. How many causes can there be? In cities, chemical agents are sprayed, particles are sprayed on the streets, and people breathe it. People essentially get sick from fear, from a nocebo effect. People die from wrong procedures, from intubating people, causing their natural exercise of lung, liver and kidney function to fail. An interview participant adds that UNESCO's article 16 of dietetics talks about the protection of future generations, which is being violated, in addition to all international treaties.

Another professional and scientific expert called this a "terrible program of activation of pathogens, viruses, bacteria, parasites, fungi, algae, archaea and more undifferentiated pathogens, which normally exist, commonly, in the microflora of the cavities of the the bodily spaces that make up each of our bodies, called the respiratory, digestive, intestinal system, etc. From the skin to our most internal organs we have microorganisms, which live in symbiosis, in normal behavior, habitual mutualism, and that in a continuous balance does not have to be causing us any alteration. But if these microorganisms are activated, through a very intelligent, strategic system, designed to be able to, in a moment, just raise, by raising the knob, increase the voltage of the microtesla, so to speak, the electromagnetic frequency of the environment, which emit signals so strong that they can, invisibly, and inadvertently, activate many microorganisms, and turn them into aggressive elements to our cellular "economy." For that reason it is not a virus, it is all the microorganisms that can be activated depending on the person, depending on the pathogen that is activated, it will cause digestive, respiratory, neurological, urinary, hormonal, cardiocirculatory disorders, and that is what is entering hospitals.>>

He added that <<a patient is not coming in with a viral condition, because if that were the case there is not even an antiviral that is being used in a hospital for what they so often call covid, if no antiviral is used. We are using everything, but less antivirals in hospitals, that is, we are not against a virus, we are with a complicated mutisystemic patient. Complicated by something that is causing your entire body to go into chaos, not respiratoryly, of course. That is the consequent, final part, but prior to that we are experiencing very common signs and symptoms. Of those who are listening to me, who can feel insomnia, continuous pain in the head, shoulders and back, continuous dizziness, typical ringing in the ears, feelings of

anxiety and anguish, panic attacks, and in an unjustified way? Who has tachycardia, increased pulse unexpectedly? How many have gastric disorders, gastritis, which surely puts the focus on the pylori? No. They are diverse symptoms because the microorganisms that are activated by the electromagnetic frequency of the environment, which rises from more than 100 microtesla to 700 microtesla, are going to blame starting this weekend, the last day of October 2020, this season of celebrations, they are going to blame these days, the "negligence" of the people who go out into the streets or the places where they are going to socialize, they are going to blame the holiday, but that is not it. Because starting on Friday they began to increase the voltage-volume of the frequencies that are maximum allowed up to 80 microtesla, no more than 100. Well, we have 600, 400, microtesla levels of electromagnetic frequency in the environment, and people begin to burst like crab in a pot.>>

<<Alkalize yourselves, drink liquids that cause alkalization. Vegetables, legumes, vegetables, sea water. Yes, all that helps. You can also use chlorine dioxide, CDS, MMS - even if they have a lot of criticism - that helps the microorganisms calm down their state of aggression again. It helps oxygenate tissues, particles that have two parts of oxygen. Perfect, they do it very well. For the patient who is already complicated, and demands to be managed in a specific way, according to the metabolic picture that this imbalance presents>> <<We are not waiting for a vaccine, you have to cure yourself. The best vaccine is the one you produce in your antibodies. Humanity has to enter a point where it produces its own antibody, and that antibody in a state of fear or panic cannot be produced. Herd immunity, collective immunity, is what can overcome a pathogen activation pattern, but as long as we are alkaline, as long as we drain to the ground, positive charges. Look for nature, rivers, seas, beaches, forests, mountains,

fields, trees. That is the place where all this positive charge that causes acid or morbid metabolism that activates pathogens is practically precipitated to the ground. And it activates them in such a way that it activates a particular sign or symptom in each person.>>

I recommend you investigate LUCIFERASA. Nice name. Although she has been clearly ridiculed in the mass media, Carrie Madej has appealed to conscience after having learned what the new vaccines brought, and where DARPA (the US department for the development of sophisticated military technologies) is involved. .): A call to the world, I looked at the advantages and disadvantages and it terrifies me. I want you to know about this, you need to be very well informed, because this new vaccine is not like your normal flu vaccine. This is something very different, this is something very new, this is something completely experimental for the human race. And it's not just about being a different vaccine, but the technologies that are being introduced by this vaccine can change the way we live. Who we are and what we are. And very fast. I think that, you know, some people that you may know, these names, Elon Musk, who is the founder of SpaceX. And Tesla Automotive, as well as Ray Kurzweil, who is one of the important people at Google, these people are self-proclaimed transhumanists, they believe that we should go to Humans 2.0 and they are great proponents of this.

There are many other people that maybe you would know their names, they are also involved in this, you should look up. I think the easiest way to explain this is to go to one of those who are most advanced for the vaccine, and go into the story a little and tell them how they want to make the vaccine, and I think that will be revealing. So, for example Moderna is one of those at the forefront of the vaccine for Covid-19, you should know that Moderna was founded by a person from Harvard, Derek Rossi. And this researcher was actually very successful in taking modified RNA and being able to reprogram a stem cell in the body and change the function of the stem cell, he actually made it genetically modified, you understand? So, you can, I proved that you can genetically modify something using modified RNA, so they founded Moderna on this concept. He's like the "new kid on the block," you know? It hasn't been around for long, in fact, they haven't even made any vaccines for humans before, they haven't made any medicine for humans before, this will be the first thing they do. You should know that Moderna was in the news recently, because they are really accelerating... it's like the other companies, they are accelerating the vaccine... [End of video transcript].

"Shock at the revelation of an enzyme called Luciferase that makes Bill Gates' implantable Quantum Dot microneedle vaccine delivery system work," is the title of an article by Geoffrey Grider, dated May 3, 2020. in 'Now The End Begins'. The publication in question claims: An enzyme called LUCIFERASE is what makes Bill Gates' implantable vaccine work, the 'VACCINE ID'. Bill Gates is building something we call 'Human Implantable Quantum Dot Microneedle Vaccine Delivery System', and it's made up of several things. I want to draw your attention to one component, the quantum dot microneedles that will deliver the vaccines, and a very, very unique biochemical that makes it all work. If you are standing while reading this, you may want to sit down. Today we bring you the 'near-infrared bioluminescence luciferase enzyme', which is the chemical that will make the quantum dot vaccine readable through a special application for mobile devices. That's right, the enzyme that will power Bill Gates' human-implantable Quantum Dot microneedle vaccine delivery system is called

Luciferase—that's what makes the vaccine readable long after the victim has been injected.

Bill Gates is building something we call the human-implantable quantum dot microneedle vaccine delivery system, and it needs an enzyme called Luciferase to make it work. Remove the word 'human' and it becomes 666. With each passing day, it becomes clearer to those of us who are Bible believers that we are living in a unique time period. So unique, in fact, that we could be witnessing the reign of Antichrist and the Mark of the Beast system coming together before our very eyes. Please note that I use the word "might" out of an abundance of caution when writing articles like these, but when I'm alone with my thoughts, I'm completely convinced that's exactly where we are. 100%. The wise man will understand. Have you heard of Luciferase? Over the past few weeks we've shown you a massive Bill Gates project that's all-encompassing and almost unbelievable. That expression is an Old English term that means something that is so incredible that you almost can't believe it. The Nazi concentration camps in the Holocaust are a great example of that. When the films came out of what happened there, it was so astonishing that it was difficult to comprehend that something like that could happen. But it happened that it happened. And what is happening right now, the Antichrist system, is equally difficult to understand, but here we are.

Bill Gates is building something we call the Human Implantable Quantum Dot Microneedle Vaccine Delivery System, and at its center we have the COVID-19 vaccine that he wants to give to every human on Earth, there will be quantum dot microneedles, a brand ID2020 digital identification device and a human implantable device for buying and selling cryptocurrencies with a patent number of 0 **6** 0 **6** 0 **6**. The digital ID will come in the form of something called an Immunity

Passport. All of these things, and all funded by one man, Bill Gates, together represent at least one striking precursor to the global Mark of the Beast system. That's at least an estimate, taken to its logical extreme, it could very well be the actual Mark of the Beast system. Source September 2020: https://stillnessinthestorm.com/2020/09/must-read-an-enzyme-called-luciferase-is-what-makes-bill-gates-implantable-vaccine-work-vaccine-id/ [32]. Microsoft cryptocurrency monitoring system patent registration is WO2020060606A1: https://patentscope.wipo.int/search/en/detail.jsf?docId=WO2020060606 [33]. But the "great Gates" has also been interested for more than a decade in the VMAT2 gene (vesicular monoamine transporter 2), which is said to be located on human chromosome 10 as a protein encoded by the SLC18A2 gene. VMAT2 is an integral membrane protein that transports monoamines, particularly neurotransmitters such as dopamine, norepinephrine, serotonin, and histamine, from the cellular cytosol to synaptic vesicles. It sends nigrostriatal and mesolimbic dopamine-releasing neurons, VMAT2 function is also necessary for the vesicular release of the neurotransmitter GABA.

On April 13, 2005, Bill Gates gave a conference to the DoD (US Department of Defense) at the Pentagon (http://stateofthenation.co/?p=13275 [34]), talking about this gene and the importance of removing it. According to Gates, this gene is what promotes "religious fanaticism", although this statement is contrary even to the descriptions found on Wikipedia regarding VMAT2, where it is presented as the source

---

32.   https://stillnessinthestorm.com/2020/09/must-read-an-enzyme-called-luciferase-is-what-makes-bill-gates-implantable-vaccine-work-vaccine-id/

33.   https://patentscope.wipo.int/search/en/detail.jsf?docId=WO2020060606

34.   http://stateofthenation.co/?p=13275

of "spirituality" (https: / /en.wikipedia.org/wiki/ Vesicular_monoamine_transporter_2 [35]). In fact, on another analogous page, Wikipedia has a space for its alternative name: 'God Gene' (https://en.wikipedia.org/wiki/God_gene [36]). The false prophet Gates said that they had the "vaccine" to "cure" this "evil", called 'FunVax'. The operational version of it was ready in 2009 and was used in Iraq (https://www.youtube.com/ watch?v=xptxL6xzhRc&feature=youtu.be [37]). Gates claims that they would have used influenza (flu) viruses and rhinoviruses to release in large numbers of people.

To continue to the next section of this book, I share this with you: The mandatory vaccination law No. 27491, enacted in January 2019 in Spain, says: Art. 13. Certification of compliance with the National Vaccination Calendar must be required in the procedures for: a) Entry and exit of the school year, both mandatory and optional, formal or informal; b) Carrying out medical health examinations that are carried out within the framework of law 24,557 on occupational risks; c) Processing or renewal of DNI [National Identity Document], passport, residence, prenuptial certificate and driver's license; d) Processing of family allowances in accordance with Law 24,714 and non-remunerative monetary allowances, whatever their name, stipulated by current regulations. The dissemination prior to the implementation of this article, its execution and the deadlines thereof, will be specified in the regulations, in such a way as to favor the population's access to vaccination at all stages of life without preventing the realization of these procedures. Art. 14., Failure to comply with the obligations provided for in articles 7, 8, 10 and 13 of this law will generate actions by the

---

35.   https://en.wikipedia.org/wiki/Vesicular_monoamine_transporter_2

36.   https://en.wikipedia.org/wiki/God_gene

37.   https://www.youtube.com/watch?v=xptxL6xzhRc&feature=youtu.be

corresponding jurisdictional health authority, aimed at carrying out vaccination, which will range from notification to vaccination. compulsive

VIII. MANIPULATION – MANUFACTURED CONSENSUS

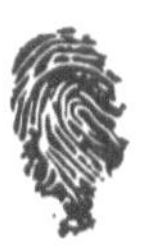

It has been said that there are documents that prove that the World Bank exported "covid-19" forecasting devices already 2 years before the pandemic. The 'COVID-19 Strategic Preparedness and Response Programme', labeled 'FOR OFFICIAL USE ONLY', dating back to 2017-2018, referred to all records of instrumental transport and test apparatus for prognosis of "covid-19" to different countries around the world, mainly China and several countries in Europe. The countries where this was exported, in order of dollar cost amount, were in 2017: Switzerland, Germany, the European Union, the United States, Ireland and the Netherlands. In 2018, the destination territories were: the European Union, Germany, France, the United Kingdom, the Netherlands, Switzerland, the United States, Japan, Singapore, China and Hong Kong. The labels of the products had the reference, 'Covid-19 Diagnostic Test Instruments and Apparatus'. These tests had the code from 2017: 300215. Those from 2018 had the code 902780. French soldiers had already made this known at the beginning of 2020, explaining that in Wuhan there was a combination of 5G waves and virus cocktails. They theorized that this exercise combined with vaccines would be aimed at changing human biology to control the population.

Alfred L. Webre, former advisor to former US President Jimmy Carter, is part of an international court of 30 judges from 3 continents that demands answers on what have been proposed as international emergency measures, because they violate rights constitutional. On November 29, 2020, they filed a lawsuit that ruled to strictly prohibit all covid vaccines worldwide, because they are programmed to use RNA to reprogram the DNA of humanity in order to lead it towards transhumanism (https://rumble.com/ved89x   -international-tribunal-against-global-vaccination.html [1]). Now, personally I think that the fact that certain people do not have the proper arguments for a debate or to defend themselves does not mean that their principles are wrong. It is logical that anyone thinks that a "truth" must come from a professional in their field, and hearing from someone without a university degree in said field, or without scientific degrees, is not taken seriously. That is why it is so important that in these next chapters we evoke those who know more about the aforementioned. I don't think that everything the news says is a lie, but most of it is, and the other part is manipulated. It is not that all scientists and doctors lie, but that we are only talking about two or three, who are bought. And above all, I personally do believe that there is a bat virus, but it is not killing the world, and it is not the reason for the current problem. The "batman virus" is just a scapegoat. What would be behind this are the questions whose answers are very important and broad. Here are some examples of what you should be understanding:

1st - adapt society to accept the deprivation of their basic rights to health and movement.

2nd - teach society to abdicate their rights assuming that the "government" knows what is best for them, better than themselves, even ignoring common sense or their own intuition. Thus, to even receive financial aid or food vouchers they force

---

1.   https://rumble.com/ved89x-tribunal-internacional-contra-la-vacunacin-global.html

you to fill out extensive forms, and depending on the country they go much further, asking you about your hours of sleep, your bank transactions, your children, your employment, your marital status, they tell you. where you can buy and where you can't, what you can spend that money on and what you can't, they prohibit you from traveling if you are receiving aid, etc. And this is getting worse.

3rd - the progressive succession of propaganda of deprivation of civil rights.

4th - the progressive succession of conditioning propaganda towards a dangerous world, full of viruses and lethal enemies for which the only savior are magical injections. Any other alternative is strongly criticized and discredited.

5th - adapt people to being overcrowded and cloistered in their homes to be easily controlled, monitored and censused by the government. In this way, television fans are even more programmed.

6th - create social apathy and increasingly break social and family ties. The pro-masks against the anti-masks, the pro-vaccines against the anti-vaccines, those who believe the state's versions and those who do not, those who believe in the existence of the bug and those who do not, those who repeat the propaganda television against those who investigate on their own, those who defend social distancing against those who reject it, and so on.

7th - make people betray each other and see each other as enemies, losing trust in each other. The vaccinated fear the vaccinated and those who do not wear muzzles, and from looking at them ugly, many begin to criticize them and even insult them... this is only the beginning.

8th - expand a "safety distance" that actually makes it easier for surveillance drones, high-frequency waves and satellites to geolocalize and bombard frequencies to keep people in a state of lethargy, non-use of their judgment and control of movement (know where they are and what they are doing at all times), and prevent them from conspiring against the government or raising seditions. Furthermore, they avoid crowds because at their zenith each person creates (consciousness) a biomagnetic field, and the unification of people produces a strong electromagnetic change – or "spirit" – as a unified consciousness.

9th - weaken the immune system, both by not breathing pure oxygen and by damaging the skin with gels that prevent natural contact with bacteria with which we have always been in communion. For years they have been poisoning the population with food, water and air, not only to benefit the industry, but because it calcifies the pineal gland, which is our connection to our mental potential.

10th - keep society in a state of alarm to lower their state of vibration, which makes them more likely to get sick and accept the following propaganda of social control, so that they do not protest and docilely accept martial law when it is imposed, as if it were a salvation for the state. That is why they are encouraged to wear a muzzle, since it is a symbol of censorship and a reminder of danger.

11th - reduce the elderly population - before the global euthanasia law - to prevent governments from losing millions of dollars in pensions and health aid.

12th - know who is in favor of the truth, to discredit them and remove them from the equation, and on the contrary support and finance those who support government propaganda.

13th - impose new civil control laws, starting with the control of what is published on social networks.

The first phase of manipulation is the alteration of facts and figures, and the incorrect use of words. A typical example is when they tell you that someone dies "of" covid, instead of saying that they die "with" covid. Of course, it's like if you have the flu and you're driving your car, but you get into an accident and die, and the death certificate says that you died from the flu. Maybe a sneeze would have made you lose control for a moment and caused the accident, but how do we approach things here? Did the flu kill you? To begin with, the virus was not really isolated from public information, so it is not known what we are talking about when assuming that someone has "covid" (much less if autopsies are not performed). PCR tests do not detect covid. Starting with this elementary factor, the entire debate falls under its own weight. The story of PCR and other fraudulent tests has been the efficient tool to create a pandemic, but a pandemic of false positives, and thus categorize healthy people as sick, so that the entire population would be under the control of draconian regulations, without exception. . It is used in airports – the big business of PCR, where they earn from €40 to €120 per test – because prohibiting travel would be a violation of human rights, a crime that has crept into jobs, where the majority suffer the pressure to If you don't get a puncture, you can't continue working, even though this is a crime.

The German virologist Christian Drosten presented PCR as a way to detect viruses, even though Mullis himself said that this only defines bacteria. If this Sars-Cov-2 was never isolated, nor purified, nor sequenced, nor is there any photograph of it, what is the test based on? Or, what is a vaccine based on? Drosten has played crazy time and time again when questioned about this, just as Robert Gallo did when saying that HIV caused AIDS, saying that he photographed the virus, but never presented real evidence. Today it is the same, where the evidence of Sars-Cov-2 is computer images, and the supposed sequence of the virus is nothing more than a reconstruction manufactured with numbers on a computer. These types of pawns, like Fauci, are the ones the WHO needs, because the pharmaceutical industries seem to pay them a fortune to benefit their interests and help the emerging Super State. 80.22% of PCR tests give false positives, and an example of this is published on a government page that explains this from the beginning of the pandemic, and which took this reference from studies conducted in China at the beginning of the 2000s. statistical analyzes of cases that occurred in Wuhan: https://www.ncbi.nlm.nih.gov/pubmed/32133832?fbclid=IwAR26NyA6AxMz7oZDkSr29LAQUyvZYr5r8T[2].

The website https://pubchem.ncbi.nlm.nih.gov [3], which maintains all US studies on viruses, has, in the covid-19 section, a tab that leads to the area of tests manufactured for the same, that is, they had to be invented to detect this Sars-Cov-2. But the patent is not from now, but from 2015. In the Components section it has the Patents, which belong to none other than the Rothschilds. The patent, US-2020279585-A1, holds that: A method is provided for acquiring and transmitting biometric data (e.g., vital signs) of a user, where the data is analyzed to determine whether the user is suffering from a viral infection, such as COVID-19. The method includes the use of a pulse oximeter to acquire at least pulse rate and blood oxygen saturation percentage, which is transmitted wirelessly to a smartphone. To ensure that the data is accurate, an accelerometer inside the smartphone is used to measure the movement of the

---

2.   https://www.ncbi.nlm.nih.gov/pubmed/
32133832?fbclid=IwAR26NyA6AxMz7oZDkSr29LAQUyvZYr5r8TbuwuxRXRRKt
kHoXvU9YA2ZOwo

3.   https://pubchem.ncbi.nlm.nih.gov

smartphone and/or the user. Once accurate data is acquired, it is uploaded to the cloud (or host), where the data is used (alone or in conjunction with other vital signs) to determine whether the user is suffering from (or is likely to suffer from) a viral infection, like COVID-19. Depending on the specific requirements, the data, changes to it, and/or determination may be used to alert medical personnel and take appropriate action." Are you surprised?

Well, Bill Gates and George Soros have also bought Mologic, one of the companies that tests for such covid, as was learned on July 20, 2021. Two days later, the CDC announces that from December 2021 the RT-PCR test, and in its place another tool will work, yes, the test of these individuals, the so-called SARS-CoV-2 test, which is supposed to be approved by the FDA (American Food and Drug Administration). And now what do they want? A procedure that yields more false positives, that allows the numbers to be manipulated and, above all, that introduces more elements into the person that they want to inoculate. Just as Fauci became the scapegoat at the time, a scapegoat, so they will say that the PCR is not the correct test, and they will bring a worse one. Since there was no quantified virus isolation of 2019-nCoV available for CDC use at the time the test was developed and this study was conducted, assays designed for the detection of 2019-nCoV RNA were tested with characterized strains. of in vitro transcribed full-length RNA (Gene N; GenBank accession: MN908947.2) of known titer (RNA copies/μL) added to a diluent consisting of a suspension of human A549 cells and viral transport medium (VTM) to mimic a clinical sample. This was completed with computer numbers, completing a human-like sequence, which was supposedly a virus. In other words, the virus was never isolated, purified or sequenced, so neither PCR nor vaccines make any sense.

An official Argentine report says that in mid-July 2020 (after 4 months of strict confinement), there were 2,200 deaths supposedly from the disease called covid-19 (average age of the dead: 80 years, and others with previous serious illnesses), in a country of 45 million people. The matter doesn't work. This was seen everywhere. With such a low fatality rate it is absurd to talk about a pandemic, even an epidemic. On the one hand, the elderly were the main victims of this, why, then, was the rest of the population locked in their homes as if death were outside with its hood and scythe waiting to take anyone who went out for a walk? The only thing outside were the 5G antenna installers. And on the other hand, people with previous health problems died. What is the mystery? Statistically that applies to anything that can take the life of an elderly person over 80 years old and someone who is already in very poor health. Consequently, since the story did not work, from that date onwards, they began to inflate the figures, everywhere (and in recent years they have altered the meaning of pandemic so that it is applicable to media scandal uses). In the case of Argentina - which I have taken as a reference - by order of the Argentine Ministry of Health, reporting every illness (even a cold) as if it were the disease called covid-19, << any cold we have during this winter **is coronavirus** until proven otherwise>> (secretary of access to health, who gives the daily report, on July 8, 2020). Then-President Donald Trump retweeted a figure updated by the CDC (US Center for Disease Control), in mid-August 2020, of deaths from the disease called covid-19. Only 6% of the 153,504 reported deaths, that is, 9,210 were actually said to have died from the disease. The remaining 94% of the dead had 2-3 other serious illnesses, and most of them were very old; 90% in nursing homes.

The Union of Lawyers for the Argentine Truth achieved the first legal autopsy in Argentina of a person who died supposedly from the disease called covid-19. Do you want to know the result of that autopsy? He was negative for the disease called covid-19. In other cases, in Italy and Germany, autopsies showed death from blood clots and respiratory distress, not a virus. This phase of deception comes from the large financing behind it. In each country, between US$2,000 and US$7,000 are paid to hospital centers per person they report as having died from covid. They pay for people treated "with covid", that is, a system (PCR) is used on people that will clearly diagnose them as sick in 80% of cases, and then they treat them. They basically do experiments on healthy people. They also get paid to intubate people. Quite a business. And let's not talk about the commissions that health personnel receive for prescribing drugs, since pharmaceutical companies give them percentages for using their products. Corruption is already expected from politicians, but from the media and the medical system, it is surprising. But this is how the strategists of the Antichrist, the Rockefeller mafia and their henchmen, have achieved their plans: 1° bribes, buying off all the people in high places, or 2°, if they do not let themselves, they appear dead, or they have to resign. Considering the power of the Rockefeller empire, this is child's play for them: they have all the economic power on the planet.

An Austrian parliamentarian does a PCR test on a Coca-Cola and guess what, the result was positive. This went viral on December 11, 2020. All the parliamentarians in the Austrian Parliament were amazed when the liberal general secretary of the Freedom Party of Austria, Michael Schnedlitz, carried out a PCR test on a woman during his speech. Coca Cola and guess what, the result was positive. Addressing Austrian Health Minister Anschober and the rest of the government, Schnedlitz told them after taking the test that he "spends tens of millions in tax money on testing and testing, but that in principle, this is a pure and simple redistribution." massive amount of tax money in favor of the pharmaceutical industry." Furthermore, he accused the Austrian government of promoting "the policy of closures, bankruptcies, mass unemployment, an economic crisis and a social crisis. Furthermore, they have stolen our children's education by forcing our little ones to wear masks in schools. "Countless patients have stopped being treated in hospitals and, therefore, a health emergency has been artificially caused in our country." It seems that more and more people are waking up across Europe to what is happening. A virus is being used as an excuse to destroy nations by taking arbitrary, dictatorial and totally disproportionate measures that will end up destroying everything. Will we wake up one day in Spain? We are already beginning to doubt it: https://www.eldiestro.es/2020/12/un-parlamentario-austriaco-hace-un-test-pcr-a-una-coca-cola-y-adivinen-el-resultado-fue -of-positive/[4]

The Italian association Codacons has carried out PCR tests: 95% are false positives. They also denounce corruption in hospitals. Nine prosecutors are investigating serious fraud to obtain public funds, deliberate intimidation tactics, false protocols and murders: https://superocho.org/watch/rO9pYlnGbP64tca [5]. But not only the PCR is used as a devirtualization trick. A masterstroke is to use the definition of asymptomatic to imply that anyone can be sick even if they do not show symptoms. It is the same hoax of Barack Obama

---

4.   https://www.eldiestro.es/2020/12/un-parlamentario-austriaco-hace-un-test-pcr-a-una-coca-cola-y-adivinen-el-resultado-fue-de-positivo/

5.   https://superocho.org/watch/rO9pYlnGbP64tca

to detain any person, indefinitely, simply because of suspicion of some possible terrorist link. A healthy person who has no symptoms is like a sober person who, according to a decree, states that he really has alcohol in his blood but does not know it, and is labeled a drunk. You know that someone has something by the symptoms, but the trick here is population control.

Dr. Enrique Costa Vertcher: "The pandemic is a fraud, because the flu has miraculously disappeared and they count everything as Covid." Dr. Costa is an internist and graduated in Medicine and Surgery from the Faculty of Medicine of Valencia in 1979. He has been practicing as a family doctor for more than 40 years and does so from a holistic and comprehensive vision since he believes that Medicine is a unitary science. Catholic, married and father of a family. He is the author of several books: "AIDS. Trial of an innocent virus" (1993), "Children of a terminal god" (2001), which are out of print and will be reissued shortly. "Vaccines, a critical reflection" by Ediciones "i" (2014), "Iatrogenia, the medicine of the beast" Editorial Cauac (2019) These last two titles are currently on the market and can also be purchased on Amazon. Part of an interview, where he explains with arguments why in his opinion the pandemic is a great fraud:

<< You affirm that the pandemic is a story and that everything is a lie from the beginning to the end. What are your arguments based on and how did you reach that conclusion so contrary to the official information that we all know? >>

<<I am a doctor who, to begin with, is very distrustful of the veracity of the multiple diseases caused by new viruses that the press presents to us every few years (AIDS, influenza A, Ebola...) since all of them, for me and for some dissident doctors and scientists, they have been true "artifacts" that, yes, there is no doubt that they have contributed to the business of multinationals but to the detriment of the health and tranquility

of thousands of citizens. Well, when last January we were informed by the press that a "new" virus had appeared in Wu Han, I began to distrust and thought: "here we are again with this season's story that presents us with a new virus"; But my suspicion reached its peak when we were informed that this new virus, which appeared in the middle of winter, caused the same symptoms as the winter flu. It is important to know that the symptoms were the same as those of the flu: At first, a cold, cough, fever, breathing difficulties, loss of smell and taste appear... and, if it becomes complicated, severe pneumonia, acute bronchitis and profound and... death in elderly people or sick people weakened by previous chronic illnesses; We repeat, this new virus, curiously, caused the same thing as the flu. It is as if this "new" virus had hijacked and taken over the same symptomatic picture of the flu and, furthermore, its same winter period, because the flu occurs in winter since it is a disease caused by the aggression of the cold. Then I thought it was a trick or hoax to market another new virus-artifact hacking this year's winter flu syndrome.>>

<<The fact that this fraudulent substitution has occurred is that you can verify that this year's flu cases have disappeared and have all been replaced by cases of covid-19, which confirms my suspicions and, thus, if you look at the epidemiology center of the Carlos III Institute you will see that since January of this year the flu has disappeared (miraculously?) in Spain and, since then, all are cases of covid-19... It is the first year In the history of medicine in which there are no cases of flu in the middle of winter... how about it? But the covid-19 pandemic has been something more complex than the flu. The press and official media tell us that there have been many more thousands of deaths and you tell us that it has been like the flu every year. How do you explain it? This year's flu should have caused, more

or less, the death of a similar number of citizens as it usually does each year, but, in fact, this year it could have caused a few thousand more; But this increase does not mean that this year's flu has been more aggressive and, of course, it does not indicate that it has been a new, more aggressive virus but rather that it has a perfectly clear explanation that, in addition, is known to everyone, although not recognized, and it is due to circumstances and events that occurred, precisely, as a consequence of having been declared, officially and by the entire press, a non-existent or unreal pandemic; That is to say, having alarmed citizens in an exaggerated and terrifying way about the existence of a pandemic and the draconian measures that have been adopted have caused a state of panic as evident as it is overwhelming that, as a logical consequence, the number of deaths skyrocketed , especially among the elderly, who have turned out to be 95% of the deceased.>>

<<Every year, if you remember, you will remember that, in the winter, all the country's television stations report, on two or three occasions, that hospitals are overflowing with flu cases and patients accumulate in the hallways; It is something that happens every year when the cold waves come; However, as far as I know, it has been the first year that due to flu cases there have been public appearances by Ministers of Health, Defense, Chiefs of the Police and the Civil Guard... giving press conferences, while all the news programs were trying to terrorize the staff, from early morning until night; You will remember that last March and April it seemed as if we were in a state of war or facing an invasion of aliens instead of suffering from the seasonal flu each year.>> << So you admit an *increase in mortality from the flu this year. year due to the alarm motivated by the declaration of the pandemic* >>; <<if so...>> << *Can you explain how the declaration of a pandemic and the state of alarm could have*

influenced the increase in mortality among the population affected by flu or other diseases? >> <<Of course I admit this increase in mortality from this year's flu due to the causes mentioned and which I will now explain: What is called the "placebo" effect exists and is well known to medicine, which is about a beneficial effect on recovery from any illness; It is an effect that we could call psychosomatic of a beneficial nature that occurs when the patient is confident that he will be cured soon and occurs when he is convinced that his illness is simple and easy to cure, when he believes that his doctor knows the illness and knows how to cure it... that is, if the patient is optimistic and confident in his or her speedy recovery, that feeling and conviction acts as a beneficial effect to achieve healing; In fact, many times, this placebo effect is enough to achieve, on its own, a total cure.>>

<<But there is also, of course, the opposite case, the "nocebo" effect that is produced by a terrified mental state, a feeling of restlessness and a conviction that the illness you are suffering from is a serious and fatal illness, when you know that Its cause and treatment are unknown and, furthermore, it is a disease that is destroying many people and that doctors do not know how to address and cure it... When a patient with the flu or another illness experiences this negative mental state, of restlessness and stress and this conviction of doom and hopelessness... suffers from the nocebo effect which, of course, will make recovery difficult and, in many cases, is enough to lead to a fatal outcome; That is, it acts in the opposite direction to the placebo effect. If you have understood what the placebo and nocebo effect is...>>

<< *I ask you: How do you think the citizens who have had the flu this year and have been classified as infected with coronavirus have felt, after hearing to the Spanish press to say that we were being attacked by a new terrible and deadly virus, to see those press conferences of high command of the army and politics, to hear*

doctors warn of how serious and unprecedented the situation was and to be reminded, every night, the number of deaths that had occurred that day in the country? What effect do you think could have been caused on flu patients with this scenario... The placebo or the nocebo? >>

He adds that it is clear that the press and the government have created a huge nocebo effect that surely has not benefited any flu sufferer, but is there any other factor that has contributed to increasing the number of deaths attributed to covid-19? Of course yes and we could describe them with the following qualifying adjectives:

a) Hygienic factors: In order to protect the elderly population in nursing homes from infection, we all know that they have been mercilessly "arrested" inside their rooms without being able to leave or interact or meet with each other in common places for more than six months; They were served by scared people dressed as astronauts who told them that they were contagious and that they no longer touched them or approached them. They served them food from a distance as if they were plagued and, to make matters worse, they could not see their relatives, children. and grandchildren, during all that time being abandoned for months; I have witnessed the deep sadness that this situation has caused in two elderly people who were my patients and who have been able to tell me about it. This inhuman situation of rejection and abandonment has produced a nocebo effect, depression and a feeling of hopelessness such... that it has taken away many of our elderly.

b) Toxic or iatrogenic factors: As it was a "new" virus, a multitude of experimental medications with unknown effects have been tested on the patients, such as medication against AIDS or medication against malaria, in addition to antibiotics and antipyretics and sedatives by the ton.

c) Protocol euthanasia: In some autonomous communities, by political order of the health ministries, protocols have been ordered that induced sedation with opiates and barbiturates, as the only treatment, for those over eighty years of age despite the fact that all doctors We know or should know that a person with respiratory failure, especially if they are elderly, if they are sedated with opiates and/or barbiturates, death is induced due to respiratory arrest and, finally, in many elderly people, due to the fact that they are 80 years old. or more, they have been restricted, by protocol prescription, from entering hospitals so as not to take the place of the youngest in times of scarcity.

d) Fictitious or camouflage factors: Politicians, in order to justify their draconian and meaningless measures, have subsidized hospitals and autonomous communities based on the number of covid-19 cases they declared and, that very appetizing incentive, has caused many deaths from other diseases such as heart attacks, strokes, cancers... etc., to have been classified as deaths from coronavirus... in this way the subsidy increased in volume.

<<All these factors, perfectly proven and verifiable, have been and continue to be the cause of the increase in the lists of deaths from covid-19; which, together with the long list of false positives, has contributed and contributes to the maintenance, by the press and the government, of the general hallucination of terror of the coronavirus that has frightened the population and that, due to that collective fear or to this general paranoia, citizens have allowed themselves to be arrested at home without having symptoms of any kind, to be muzzled and to have their jobs suspended and plunged into misery and to be prohibited from visiting family and friends, That is, due to the general state of panic and fear of the false pandemic, citizens have renounced their basic human rights.>> << *So for you and for the doctors*

who maintain your point of view... all this movement of masks, hand washing with gel, restrictions on the free movement of people, the general stoppage of work and economic activity, the closure of temples and the alteration of the liturgy... in reality, Is it a consequence of having taken the annual and seasonal flu for a false pandemic of a "new" highly infectious, aggressive and deadly virus? >> <<No more nor less, that's how it is, although it seems incredible at this point in the film. And, furthermore, you and other citizens can verify it without needing to be doctors but, yes, using common sense or the most basic Aristotelian logic: If you enter, through the Internet, the epidemiology center of the Carlos Institute III or in the INE and look for the statistics of deaths and their causes in Spain in this year 2020, you will see that in March and April of this year there is a large increase in deaths due to supposed covid-19, this large increase translates into an enormous and outstanding statistical curve in the shape of a Gauss bell that goes from the second week of March to the first week of April.>>

<< What happened in that short period of time? What could have caused so many deaths in Spain? The explanation is this: If you remember or review the newspaper archive you will see two facts that were the cause of this increase in mortality: The first was the delayed arrival of winter in the month of March, which lowered temperatures and brought widespread rains throughout the country. country and the second factor that had a negative influence was that on March 14 the government implemented the "state of alarm" that forced millions of Spaniards to stand in long lines outdoors, in the cold and rain; As we have explained before, the flu is a disease caused by the aggression of cold and humidity and, that is why it normally appears in winter when cold waves arrive. This year winter arrived in March and coincided with the government order that

forced millions of Spaniards to suffer cold in the long lines that formed at the doors of supermarkets and other services and, due to those long stays outdoors going through cold and humidity, the flu and the deaths from it skyrocketed during the last three weeks of March and the first of April; but, after these weeks, they were reduced without doing anything, spontaneously and immediately, when the rains and the cold disappeared in the second week of April, that is, when the warmth arrived.>>

<<From the arrival of the heat, the sick and the deceased suddenly disappeared and the curious and contradictory cases of "asymptomatic" infected people appeared. This nice and novel medical concept called "asymptomatic patient" wants to describe a possible patient who, in an inexplicable or "miraculous" way, has no symptoms, even though he is infected by a "new" highly aggressive and deadly virus... But, what? Can you be infected by a highly aggressive and deadly virus and not have any symptoms or, in other words, be so confident? Is that logical? Well, even though it doesn't make any sense, everyone swallows that logical impossibility, including doctors, who are hearing about such a case for the first time. In fact, for a doctor with 40 years of practice, as is my case, that is an impossible novelty, it is an unknown and inexplicable medical "neologism"; But despite this, during the spring and summer, as people no longer got sick or, much less, died from the flu because it was no longer cold, the cases of "asymptomatic" infected people have multiplied to reach 1,700,000 Spaniards and the numbers are increasing, without stopping, as more PCR tests are carried out, which are tests that the WHO itself admits give a high percentage of false negatives and that, in addition, its own inventor and creator, the deceased Dr. Kary Mullis has spent more than 20 years saying that his PCR test is useless in diagnosing viral diseases.>>

<<I wonder how many millions of "asymptomatic" infected people will be needed for the politicians, journalists and doctors who maintain the hallucination to reach the logical and elementary conclusion that there is no pandemic and that the supposedly "infected" In reality, they have nothing and nothing is wrong with them and, therefore, are they asymptomatic? But, despite this evidence and against all logic, they stick to their guns and announce that a new wave is expected this winter; By the way, in this we do agree with them, but, yes, clarifying that we already predict that the wave that will come this winter will not be of "asymptomatic" infected but will be, like every winter, of common flu and that it will bring the same symptoms (colds, fever, cough, pneumonia...) and the same deaths as always. The new concept of "asymptomatic" infected is a mockery of the medical logic of all time and a media excuse to maintain the collective hallucination and panic of the existence of a pandemic that, in reality, does not exist and never has existed.> > You can see the same example here years ago, where Iñaki Gabilondo and Mercedes Mila talk about Influenza A. The Spanish journalist explains on Channel 4 about the psychosis of Influenza A organized and orchestrated by private interests and the Pharmaceutical Industry: https://lbry.tv/@elinvestigador:0/ que-tiempos-aquellos-en-los-que   -TVs-were-not-100-bought-by-international-lobbies:1[6]

I must remind the reader that most of the content has already been deleted from the Internet, so we barely found the extracts, and when we wanted to upload them to other platforms to rescue them, they were no longer there. Yes, for a year now (around February 2020) I have saved many links to reports, articles, documentaries, interviews, conferences and more, about

---

6.   https://lbry.tv/@elinvestigador:0/que-tiempos-aquellos-en-los-que-las-tv-no-estaban-100-compradas-por-lobbies-internacionales:1

the "covid" plot, but, unfortunately, information bias is no longer a thing. of Chinese or Cuban communism, but has entered the West. Facebook, Twitter, YouTube, Instagram, and others are leading among the platforms that cut off the heads of all those who want to report the truth. Likewise, Google, Wikipedia and the main news networks disguise information or discredit it. However, a few contents are still available, and we try to upload them to Rumbel, DailyMorion, VK or other networks, such as those that are already becoming popular to replace Whats App, such as Telegram or Signal. For example, this is an interview with former Russian counterintelligence agent Daniel Estulin, on this topic (from August 26, 2020), which as of the first week of February 2021 has not yet been deleted: https:// www .youtube.com/ watch?v=sKD5pR4AkgI&fbclid=IwAR0mxb-5MHWQKaWOj5Kbhm59J7u2dnm1iE18X23gAeiz3nuNyzXqJ_etlW [7].

Senator Dr. Scott Jensen of Minnesota says the AMA is encouraging American doctors to aggregate coronavirus death counts across the country. Scott Jensen is a doctor, physicist and Republican state senator, who reported that he received a 7-page document ordering death certificates to be filled out as caused by coronavirus in people who had not even been infected. Jensen also reported that hospitals are paid more if they list patients diagnosed with COVID-19, and three times more if they say the patient received a ventilator: https://thespectator.info/2020/ 04/09 /hospitals-get-paid-more-to-list-patients-as-covid-19-and-three-times-as-much-if-the-patient-goes-on-ventilator-video/?fbclid=IwAR082E8PlpCYINOvwzfHe4Zg7DJUDsYj0Qg2vFkY -Ylkh03eFfo8KUbTd4 [8]. Here where the senator reveals that

---

7.   https://www.youtube.com/watch?v=sKD5pR4AkgI&fbclid=IwAR0mxb-
5MHWQKaWOj5Kbhm59J7u2dnm1iE18X23gAeiz3nuNyzXqJ_etlWI

hospitals receive funds if they alter figures: https://thespectator.info/2020/04/09/hospitals-get-paid-more-to-list-patients-as-covid-19-and- three-times-as-much-if-the-patient-goes-on-ventilator-video/?fbclid=IwAR0IPaZPa8HI7ppWYrDjHovDz_RfdYzwqsjlb6Ek II, [9]and https://www.valleynewslive.com/content/news/MN-Sen-Dr- - [10]569489461.html?fbclid=IwAR024X_z29Tyl-6md-JKjpJlHPZakXnyhayLaFBI5gY44OYZbbcsRPI-Gh8 [11].

Regarding other content, before online censorship accelerated, I managed to transcribe some notes about California doctors, virologists, scientists and other health personnel who recorded themselves telling things that I will now put here, but paraphrasing. I start with an American virologist Judy Mikovits who worked with Antoni Fauci, but when she opposed him and revealed the truth about viruses and vaccines in court, they put her in jail for 5 years to silence her (you can see a little about this matter here : http://barcelona.indymedia.org/newswire/display/530720 [12]). If you don't suspect the false

---

8.   https://thespectator.info/2020/04/09/hospitals-get-paid-more-to-list-patients-as-covid-19-and-three-times-as-much-if-the-patient-goes-on-ventilator-video/?fbclid=IwAR082E8PlpCYINOvwzfHe4Zg7DJUDsYj0Qg2vFkY--Ylkh03eFfo8KUbTd4

9.   https://thespectator.info/2020/04/09/hospitals-get-paid-more-to-list-patients-as-covid-19-and-three-times-as-much-if-the-patient-goes-on-ventilator-video/?fbclid=IwAR0IPaZPa8HI7ppWYrDjHovDz_RfdYzwqsjlb6EkFHSQJQRqoUVf1Mnd-II

10.   https://www.valleynewslive.com/content/news/MN-Sen-Dr--569489461.html?fbclid=IwAR024X_z29Tyl-6md-JKjpJlHPZakXnyhayLaFBI5gY44OYZbbcsRPI-Gh8

11.   https://www.valleynewslive.com/content/news/MN-Sen-Dr--569489461.html?fbclid=IwAR024X_z29Tyl-6md-JKjpJlHPZakXnyhayLaFBI5gY44OYZbbcsRPI-Gh8

prophet Fauci, think how curious he is officially the "highest paid official" in the US (Forbes magazine revealed that he earned $417,608 in salary in 2019, which means he will earn about $2.5 million for his work between 2019 and 2024). Let's look at some of Mrs. Mikovits' statements in one of these videos that YouTube deleted, "You can be affected-infected without developing the disease, then you are immunized, and this can help other humans develop immunity" [...] "the idea that the virus went from bat soup to humans in Wuhan is absurd... it jumped from a cell culture in the laboratory" [...] "if you don't have the inflammatory marker, it doesn't matter how you get infected, you won't get sick... you are immune." [...] "What they say does not correspond to an infected virus but to an injected virus. Influence of the flu vaccine, absolutely. That means that when you get the flu vaccine it can trigger a new family of viruses."

He goes on to state, "this coronavirus is nothing more than a bad cold, and it is impossible for it to be passed from one person to another through the cough of a healthy person, it does not work that way, and it is more likely that it has been injected." [...] "Dogs and cats are carriers of coronavirus... this virus was not transmitted to 110 countries from a fish market in China in November or December; It is possible that it has been injected into flu vaccines since 2013 or 2014. Flu vaccines catalyze infection, and I am completely opposed to wearing masks, because if you carry this virus, and you put on the mask and You force yourself to manage that stress, with that fear, you can activate that virus thanks to the stress, of not having a job, for example. These viruses can reactivate even with the mask on. You're not going to make anyone sick, but you're going to make yourself sick, and it's worse for people with asthma." [...] "It is already known that the Spanish Flu was financed by the

---

12.   http://barcelona.indymedia.org/newswire/display/530720

Rockefeller Foundation. This virus is more contagious, but it is not more pathogenic" [...] "The coronavirus does not last more than an hour in the air, it does not spread through the air... anyone who demonstrates that they have antibodies must return to work now."

Regarding "false positives," Mikovits says, "right now two types of tests are done: 1) the polymerase charge reaction (PCR), which shows sequence reactions to cultures of other common viruses. These tests have become contaminated and no longer show exposure... the rapid, or serological, test does not detect the virus directly but rather identifies the IGG and IGM antibodies, present in our blood when we get sick. IGM refers to recent exposure to the virus, while IGG refers to past exposure, meaning that you are cured. The IGG is an antibody that you produce against a family of viruses... false positives, and one is used to confirm the other..." "In addition, the signature of inflammation must appear... a test is done with all viruses confirmatory..." "[What we are seeing] is all a propaganda agenda..." "the death toll is not supported scientifically." "all of this is nothing more than an act of corruption designed to steal the rights and freedoms of individuals to carry out the mass vaccination agenda."

From other content that I was able to save before being deleted from YouTube, where a doctor specializing in respiratory issues for more than 21 years speaks, I am going to paraphrase and summarize. He clarifies that what they say about the number of artificial respirators is not true. They are not even being used, contrary to what is said in the media. He maintains that all patients who come with different pathologies are integrated into Covid-19 lists – as if they had it – when clearly this is not the case, and that in all the time that the issue has been promoted they have only had one patient with respiratory problems. which was referred to the CDC, so the statistics they are promoting are not true. He adds that many of the patients are under investigation, but that they have never actually been tested, that the tests that are being performed on these people are sent for study and take 2 to 3 weeks until they arrive back (so it is false that the matter can be diagnosed in a matter of hours or days). He states that all the people who come to be studied and die, from anything – like cancer, or whatever – are entered into the registry as having died from COVID-19, "they put the numbers as if it were a football game to scare you." What they say and show about dead bodies in quantities is not real, "it has not happened", "all this is false." Regarding respirators, they have actually been prohibited from using them.

They leave them with the packaging and they are only for propaganda, because they do not want to be used in reality, since they have an air outlet that goes through the air and is distributed everywhere, and if it were real the virus would infect the entire population. hospital people "That is not the traditional procedure that we use," they first resort to other means before it becomes necessary to use any of those, which in the end are not even used, "we do not have permission to use them." It makes it clear that people who go to the hospital are not being tested for the virus, but for H1N1 (swine flu) and other conventional flu tests, RSB. That it is not true that they are testing the virus but rather an RNA sequence of a reaction to the virus. Then they do the PcR test, and at the slightest visible cellular damage they diagnose you as infected, when in reality this damage can be from anything, be it radiation or cancer itself, "it can come from a lot of things." There are companies like GM contracted to manufacture artificial respirators, and hospitals not only already have them, but they do not use them right now, and in addition the government already has companies that manufacture them. "Why do these companies start manufacturing different ones? What do these new respirators have?"... "and how much is each of these respirators going to cost the US, [which comes from taxpayer taxes]?" "What they are saying is not true." None of those patients under study have had symptoms of fever or lung problems.

Protective materials are used over and over again, packages are opened and used and everything is "contaminated" over and over again, "and as you see, I'm still here, we're all still here", they don't have any symptoms of anything. They are shocked by what is happening, but the deaths are not what they seem, H1N1 really was terrible. What they say about COVID-19 is not real, they are exaggerating everything. What is going to happen, like all viruses, like SARS, or ZIKA, or any other, is that you will see a high peak and then it will collapse, because that is what viruses are like. And yet I don't think this is a virus issue. The only thing they are going to achieve with vaccinations is to make people sicker. That man says to go and find out for yourselves. Ask experts, doctors... but be careful, because many doctors are as deceived as the people, because they have their job and they have their life, and they do not stop to check that the data they are told above is true, they don't stop to review the tests, because they don't stop to think that everything is a fraud. Question things, "these questions must be asked", question the facts they tell you. He adds, "I don't think Trump is behind this but rather he does what they tell him to do, that this comes from above, because we are doing the same thing as in France, Italy, etc. This comes from the Illuminati, from the Deep State, they are Shutting Down *the world,* and you must understand this (how it works): the world."

And finally I gather from his testimony: "Who is making the new respirators? Because? Who is reviewing them? If we already have it, and there are companies that already do it, why is this? "If they don't even let us use the ones we already have, they say they are overused and there is a great demand." This is just one example of many of them that echoed from the beginning of the plan-demic. What's more, on February 29, 2020 - when the quarantine had not yet been imposed in the Canary Islands, where I was based at that time -, several friends had a meal, and a friend who manages several areas of a hospital told us. He said that everything that was being said on television was being exaggerated, that there was no alarm or crisis, or emergency, that it was more what the news said than what was actually happening. We then saw, throughout 2020, recordings of people outraged by how a relative came in for a discomfort, sprain or check-up and they were no longer allowed to leave, and they said they had Covid and they couldn't see them. Doesn't it sound familiar to you? So many health professionals and scientists uploaded content online to tell the truth, and within days – then in a matter of hours – their content was censored, and finally their YouTube accounts were deleted.

Subsequently, Instagram and Facebook began to add Covid advertising labels to each publication made where the topic was discussed. But they didn't stop there. Facebook invented such "independent reviewers" who "proved" that something published was "false", or at best, "partially false". Now YouTube and Facebook censored you, prohibited you from publishing, penalized your account and even closed it. Twitter continued down that path, and to a large extent Instagram. Even websites, whether independent or government, were infiltrated. Things that were presented as public information on the US government website disappeared at the moment when Joe Biden was presented as the new president of that country.

POLITICAL PANDEMIC

Dr. Heiko Schöning, founder of Doctors for Truth, after his recent arrest in Great Britain, invited deep reflection. He points out that it is necessary to ask how this orchestrated "plandemic" could evolve. Meanwhile, a Chilean surgeon draws attention to the paradox of which the elderly are victims: to care for them, we have left them alone. In an article by Agustina Sucri, dated October 4, 2020, she writes: Heiko Schöning is a military doctor from Hamburg and one of the creators of the Extra-Parliamentary Committee for Research on Covid-19. Heiko Schöning is considered one of the most critical voices against the draconian measures adopted by the German government and so many other countries to manage covid-19. He is the founder of 'Doctors for Truth', which has the support of more than 500 health professionals and 200,000 collaborators, in the German country alone, and whose objective is to denounce the exaggerated interventions arranged to contain the coronavirus. Schöning maintains that this pandemic does not have a medical justification but a political one. So much so, that the professional has not limited himself to warning the population about this irregularity but is also co-founder of the Extraparliamentary Committee for the Investigation of Covid-19, launched on May 31 in Stuttgart in front of 5,000 protesters.

Through this committee, it is proposed to investigate the false notions that have spread around the coronavirus and that have been used as support to justify many of the unusual measures adopted. The media has not only turned its back on him or labeled him a "denialist." When last Saturday he participated in a peaceful demonstration in London and was arrested by the police, in addition to being detained for 22 hours, almost no media in the world considered it a scandal that even this resource was resorted to to silence him. "It was around 22 hours of an illegal arrest here in Great Britain," said the doctor in front of a group of people who applauded him after being released. "Of course, we will continue forward, telling the truth and we will never give in," said the representative of Doctors for Truth, who questioned where the United Kingdom is going and where the world is going "if one does not have the right to express oneself." . "Expressing yourself is not a crime. Even under these very dubious Covid-19 laws, this is not a crime to arrest someone. But you can see what happened yesterday in Hyde Park, at Speaker's Corner. People gathered peacefully, listened and the police came," Schöning continued. "I did not offer any resistance, but they quickly arrested me, handcuffed me, and took me away for talking to you and telling the truth, the truth about what is happening with Covid-19," he continued.

The German doctor recalled that he decided to found the Extraparliamentary Covid-19 Investigation Committee together with other professionals because the world's parliaments failed to establish an appropriate committee for this purpose. "We, the citizens, have the duty to do so. I invite you internationally to be part of this movement," he emphasized. He also said he was happy with the fact that doctors in different countries around the world have stood up to tell the truth and conduct research regarding the management of the pandemic. DIVIDE TO REIGN? "I need to emphasize that all those who officially said they would work for the people, like governments, police, army officers, must think that now is the time to be brave. Now is the time to speak. It is time to demonstrate that humanity is a family and that we will not allow ourselves to be divided: neither between races, as happened to us in Germany in the 1930s, nor between the so-called "sick" or the "vaccinated." This is a division. We are a family: humanity," Schöning highlighted. Along the same lines, he urged us to think about what is happening behind all this. "The police seized my phone, my computer and the book 'Coronovirus, false alarm'. They are afraid that we will communicate that is why they take away your phone. They are afraid of books because the scientific evidence is already established," he argued. The German doctor stressed that "there is no pandemic in medical terms" and that it is not necessary to be immersed in fear of a deadly virus. "All the data shows that it causes no more damage than the common flu," he added.

Schöning considered it necessary to ask how this orchestrated "plandemic" could evolve. In that sense, he referred to the financial crisis of 2008. "The financial system is dominating everything and this is its collapse. In 2008 it was clear that the banks and their owners were to blame for the crisis. Shall we repair the system? No. They put a lot more money into this insane financial system and bought time. Everyone said it. Now we are in 2020 and it seems that they have a plan: a big reset of the financial system. It has nothing to do with health. But who do we blame? Now they blame a virus, the coronavirus," he summarized. Finally, he anticipated that next Saturday they will hold a new demonstration in Berlin for peace and so that these injustices do not continue. He asked again: "Please wake up. Please, let's think of humanity as a family. Let's be peaceful. Let's go to our neighbors, to our family and just inform them." Schöning's case is just a sample of what happens with the "dissidents" of the official story. Never before have we seen so many entities - whose competence is unknown - that attribute to themselves the power to certify what is real from what is not, under the seal of "fake". Curiously, the largest number of stamps almost always falls on statements that deviate from what is stipulated by international health organizations.

In line with Schöning's statements, the Chilean surgeon Dan Macías Flores recently published an article in which he points to covid-19 as the "disease that has been instrumentalized to support the health and political measures imposed since March 2020." Macías Flores emphasizes that the elderly in Chile are not afraid of dying from covid-19, but rather "they fear loneliness and we ourselves have given them to it because of the love that we say we have for them." "There is a collective fear of death, which is latent in the human subconscious and which has been intentionally exacerbated by the hegemonic mass media," he writes and then questions: "Why would all the major television media coordinate and electronics to talk about death and fear, which nullifies people's reflective capacity: why are they concerned about the well-being of Chileans or because these media work for their own well-being?" Next, answer a series of questions worth reproducing:

- Is covid-19 a disease?
- TRUE.
- Is there a montage regarding this real illness?
- Yes, there is no doubt.
- Is the virus that causes covid-19 recently discovered?
- I am not aware.
- Do asymptomatic infected people transmit the virus?
- No, and my answer is supported by the WHO and also by independent scientific research; In addition, a study of how contagious an infected asymptomatic carrier of SARS-CoV-2 can be reported that a 22-year-old, asymptomatic hospitalized woman had contact with 455 people, which included other patients, family members and healthcare personnel. After their case was detected, all contacts were monitored and did not contract the infection, as demonstrated by the PCR tests performed on all of them on two occasions.

- What is the role of asymptomatic infected people?

- They make everyday human interaction safer, since an asymptomatic infected person is someone whose immune system successfully dealt with the virus and therefore did not develop the disease; Precisely, causing the disease in an individual (that is, generating coughing, sneezing, fever, etc.) is the mechanism by which the virus manages to spread, and an asymptomatic infected person is someone where the virus could not fulfill its purpose: an infected Asymptomatic is someone who stops the transmission of the virus, it is someone who, without even trying, is taking care of the health of others.

- Can covid-19 cause death?

- Of course, just like influenza and other respiratory diseases.

- What is the probability of dying from covid-19?

- In Chile, the average probability of dying is very low, 1% for all those under 60 years of age, so it is evident how disproportionate and irrational the measures announced by the WHO (such as vaccination) and those that have been implemented by the Government of Chile.

"I have come to embrace the idea that the worst-case scenario approach, instilled by the media and communication platforms, replaced the balanced assessment of risks, instilled by rationality, and that the worst-case scenario approach is motivated by the belief of that the danger we face is so overwhelmingly catastrophic that we must act immediately. In other words, this approach - which is a falsehood - carries the idea that we must launch a preventive attack and avoid the apparent loss of time that reflection entails," continues the surgeon, who clarifies: "I do not propose sacrificing the elderly to save the entrepreneurship of young people, nor sacrificing the young to save the elderly, nor do I promote the survival of the fittest. There is an ethical obligation to consider the expectations of the governed people when dictating public measures, and also when forcing the elderly to 'not die' from covid-19, because this could mean for them 'dying'. in-life' without having even been consulted regarding their preference. "The elderly do not fear death, but rather loneliness."

Doctors for Truth published an article in 2020 showing real tables and statistics from the government's own sources. It says, let's go to the Ministry of Health website by clicking here. Once inside the website, you must open the following link: You will see data that represents the number of deaths each year. Looking at this data, the question is: Where is the pandemic? If as of November 20, 328,499 people have died, in just over a month we will not reach the number of deaths from previous years. So the obvious question is: Where is the pandemic? BE CAREFUL WITH THIS DATA BECAUSE IT CAN LEAD TO ERROR! Let's prove it. If we compare the report of November 20, 2019 with the report of November 20, 2020 we will see the following: The first thing is that this year 2020 there are 62,086 more deaths than last year, as of November 20. The second thing we see is that in November 2019 there were 266,413 deaths and the 2020 report shows a cumulative total of 416,637 deaths in 2019. That does not fit. 150,224 people cannot have died in the month of December 2019. The third thing we see is that the deaths from previous years are increasing in the 2020 reports. Is it possible that the deaths from 2019 are increasing in the 2020 reports? If we compare the November 2019 report with the February 2020 report and the March 2020 report, we see the following: Evolution of the 2019 deaths in the 2020 reports.

The first thing we observe is that it is impossible that only 77 people have died in 2020 as of February 19, 2020, in a population of 47 million inhabitants such as Spain. The second thing we see is that the deaths in 2019 continue to increase in the 2020 reports. CONCLUSION TO ALL THIS DATA. The data from the Ministry of Health counts the deceased through the Civil Registry, at the time these data reach them; and these data take between 2 and 3 months to arrive from the time the person died. This means that the accumulated number of deaths in the reports has a delay of 2 or 3 months. For example: If someone dies in November 2020, their death certificate may reach the Ministry of Health in January 2021 or February 2021. And it is at that time that they count that death, within the accumulated 2020. Said Another way: If someone died last week, it won't be reflected in this report until a couple of months have passed, give or take. DATA FROM THE INE (National Institute of Statistics): The INE says that in week 41 of 2020, there is a cumulative of 384,618 deaths; while in week 41 of 2019, there are a total of 326,801 deaths. That makes a difference of 57,817 deaths. That is to say: We will very likely have about 60,000 more deaths this year 2020 compared to the previous year 2019, due to:

• Deaths in nursing homes due to neglect by their caregivers; who were afraid of contagion, inoculated by the media. These elderly people died alone, and most of them did not even make it to the hospital.

• Suicides due to economic desperation, due to the closure of their business, or due to the ERTE of the company where they worked and not being able to make ends meet, not even with the help of the state, which on many occasions did not arrive on time.

• Chronic and serious pathologies, which have nothing to do with COVID-19, and were postponed due to a supposed collapse of the health system. Late detection of serious illnesses because, since all medical care was by telephone, it was impossible to detect it in time. This ultimately causes deaths, which in any other health situation could have been avoided.

• Those who died from COVID-19. We do not deny that there have been some, but surely there are not as many as they would have us believe. Proof of this is that the detection of deaths from the flu disappeared the moment COVID-19 appeared.

The Carlos III Institute is part of the Ministry of Health. If we go to the official flu reports from the Carlos III Institute; In the situation reports section, we can compare this year's 2020 flu with the flu from previous years. While the flu in previous years has had a mortality rate of between 15,000 and 20,000 deaths. Here we can see that as of week 12 of 2020, flu detection practically DISAPPEARED. When COVID-19 appeared, the FLU disappeared. Who can believe it? If this were true, why is the Ministry of Health carrying out a flu vaccination campaign for this year 2020? It's more! Why has the flu vaccination campaign started earlier and is it reaching many more people than in previous years? Source: http ://medicos.porla Verdad.org/ministerio-de-sanidad/[13]

Agenda 21 was renamed Agenda 2030, but what it really means is outside of social perception. Agenda 21 was proposed at the United Nations in 1992 and signed by 180 nations, including the Vatican. It consists of controlling our lands, our water, our fields, our plants, our energy, our law enforcement (for law enforcement), our food production, our education, our animals, our resources, our minerals, and the population. Thus, the "Plan for Sustainable Development" was introduced into each nation, and in the US - with George HW Bush - a program was established to execute it with absolute power. Having ceded power to those led by the Agenda, the subversive capacity to

---

13.   http://medicos.porlaverdad.org/ministerio-de-sanidad/

achieve its goals at will no longer has limitations or setbacks (except for the small resistance that would subsequently be crushed). For the previous move of population control, deprivation of rights and privacy, and monitoring, they used the story of terrorism. Now they use the "bug", and take the medical infrastructure into their pockets, making those in whom the people put their health the ones who obey the criminal cartel and take away their physical well-being and life itself. I present an example of this now, showing how a case used until now, HIV-AIDS, has deceived the population. For 30 years people have been teased with something that was never isolated or photographed. This is an example of how those who dominate the institutions, the media, politics and corporations are the ones who invent the films that the people are about.

THE HIV MOUNT

In this section I add the transcript shared by one of my students from Mexico, about a documentary on the issue of tests and treatments based on HIV-AIDS deception. Medicine has been evolving, and so have the first chemical medicines. The first medicine was acetate, which was used for chemotherapy, for cancer. This is what the Burwell laboratory came up with. 30 years after it began to be used for AIDS, it was considered unauthorized, because it was super toxic. Everyone knows that any chemotherapy for cancer is toxic, that the immune system collapses, the red blood cells collapse, the person becomes anemia, the intestinal mucosa is destroyed, etc. With chemotherapy, tests are done before each cycle, but in the case of AIDS the medication was extremely high and there was no one left, they took everyone they could. The medication that is given now, antiretrovirals of that type and acetate, are still given, but at much smaller doses. Yet the problem is not the treatment. In the diagnosis, the first tests that were done were the Elisa test, but we must know that this was patented the same day that Dr. Gallo appeared with the Minister of Health before the television cameras to say that they already knew what it is. what was happening, that it was a virus that caused these diseases. On the same day the test was shamelessly patented. They are royalties. On the one hand, the money that is made from the Elisa tests, and on the other hand they give more than 80% false positives (according to the 'New England Journal of Medicine', which is the most prestigious journal of Western medicine, in a study of tens of thousands of US Navy applicants).

What's more, in England it is prohibited for being unreliable. Antibody agents test positive in more than 70 circumstances known to be documented in the scientific literature, ranging from having had many pregnancies to having had hepatitis, rheumatic diseases such as arthritis, for example, or having been vaccinated. Then came the virus tests. In reality, virus tests were done from the beginning, which are conventional, for viruses, but they were not done systematically because before viruses they might be done for hepatitis or for other things, since many times they came back negative even though people were was dying. So the fact that you were dying of AIDS or in terminal states and that you didn't have the virus was a small problem, so they stopped doing it, they even renamed the cases subject to disease control. From Atlanta, with Anthony Fauci, from the National Institutes of Health, they established an agreement whereby if you had AIDS but there was no virus in the virus tests, you no longer had AIDS, you had idiopathic CD4 lymphocytopenia. This, which sounds so nice, simply means that they had no idea why the CD4 lymphocytes had decreased, and they got the problem out of the way. Later came the viral load tests. Unfortunately, the TDIs began to find viruses everywhere. These viral load tests are based on the PCR test, the polymerase chain reaction. This technique was invented by Kary Mullis, and for this he was awarded the Nobel Prize in Chemistry in the 90s, but Kary Mullis said from the beginning that his technique was not useful for counting viruses.

Evidently, all this has meant that the detractors of the hoax have earned insults in the media, have had their publications boycotted, and the same thing that has earned all the AIDS dissidents, who have received attacks from all sides while the others They have become multimillionaires, and we must not lose sight of this. Now, those three tests mentioned are supposedly to detect the presence of a virus. All three are made from the assumption that a virus is a fragment of DNA genetic information, due to the type of virus, and that it is wrapped in proteins (this would be somewhat the official conception that biology has). Then, the tests are manufactured from these components, and there are two fundamental types of complex but fundamentally topics: there are two types of genetic tests, which are the famous PCR and the tests that have to do with proteins. Genetic tests consist of searching for fragments of the supposed genome of the virus in a sample obtained from the body. Others would try to locate a fragment of this genome and from there it is deduced that if the virus is present, it is inside the person, while the tests that are done with the proteins are somewhat more complicated, because they are based on a relationship which is supposedly produced by the person's immune system when a virus - or any other foreign element - enters the body, triggering a reaction called an antibody antigen, and this reaction can be detected through a series of tests.

It can be either in the antigens or in the antibodies, but in any of the three cases, be it the RNA, be it the antibodies, be it the antigens, it is an absolutely essential condition to have first isolated the virus that we later want to locate, because without having inhabited it We cannot know its components, and without knowing its components we cannot manufacture them or make vaccines. Therefore, if the virus has not been isolated, what is being detected is anything but a specific virus - which has not been proven to have been effectively isolated -, so you can give positives or negatives that will always be false positive. And the joke is that if you test "positive" you are "infected", but if you test "negative" it means that "you have not developed defenses". I mean, whatever you do, you're screwed: according to these people, yes or yes, you're sick. They always turn it around so that in the end it is something negative. Therefore, it is not that the tests are not detecting a complete virus and are not specific, not because they have a margin of error, because they are better or worse, because they have scammed us, because they have sold us some very bad tests, but until It is proven that the virus – any virus – has been isolated, the rest is pantomime. Kary Mullis in the preface to a book by Peter Docter tells how he realized, and that he believed that the AIDS virus caused AIDS, but they gave him a job and he started looking for where the original documents are, but those documents originals that proved that AIDS was caused by a virus did not exist.

Speaking even as a Nobel Prize winner face to face with Mr. Montagnier, with Gallo, with the highest authorities, he concludes, we have not been able to find any good reason why the majority of people on Earth believe that AIDS is a disease caused by a virus called HIV. There is simply no scientific evidence to prove this to be true. We know that to err is human, but the HIV/AIDS hypothesis is a diabolical error. In a live broadcast on the Discovery channel, concerning Health, titled 'Yes, The Farce Continues', it is explained that no one has ever isolated the so-called HIV, and therefore, there are no micrographs, that is, photographs taken with a microscope electronic of that supposed retrovirus. This has led to comments from numerous people who are surprised by the statement, claiming that a simple internet search is enough to find them. Then they evoke an electron micrograph of the budding of a virus that circulated after being isolated by Dr. Stefan Lanka in 1990. Viruses are stable entities that can be isolated and photographed in three dimensions. The same does not happen with cellular material with the so-called retroviruses for to obtain a micrograph of these particles, they must be fixed in resin and cut into ultra-thin sheets that are placed in the microscope. Different kinds of particles can be seen in the image, some of which are considered retroviruses and others not.

With the naked eye, no expert can distinguish them, which is a basic condition of any micrograph. The reference to the article describing how an HIV micrograph was obtained as it should be. What you see in the image is the scheme that Professor Hans Gelderblom, the world's leading expert in HIV micrography, proposed to explain its composition. In it you can see the genetic information, the enzyme retro transcriptase, the capsid and the protuberances that cover it and that it is said to use to bind to the cells that HIV infects. Like the rest of the retroviruses, it also has other characteristics: it measures between 100 and 120 nanometers, so it is essential that the micrographs include a measurement bar that allows it to be observed and 16 grams per milliliter are deposited in the density band 1 when centrifuged. in a sucrose density gradient. Finally, it is necessary that the micrograph's reference article has demonstrated its ability to infect and in the same or other complementary articles its genome sequence and proteins have been demonstrated, as Dr. Lanka's team did with the virus. An image that circulated in an article that appeared in Biology, where the sequencing of the proteins and DNA obtained from the isolated virus was discussed. The point is that almost 30 years since the supposed discovery of HIV, no one has ever shown particles that meet these characteristics, nor are there articles in the scientific literature that describe the isolation and purification of infectious particles with the characteristics of HIV. Likewise, no micrograph of particles corresponding to that description has ever been published, that is, particles with a diameter of 100 to 120 nanometers and with protuberances.

However, the images that can be found on the Internet and that are presented as photographs of HIV are drawings, diagrams, airbrushes, infographics, graphic recreations or 3D animations made using a computer, some of which can be seen in the images, that is, pure fiction. In some cases these are authentic micrographs, but they do not show particles with the characteristics attributed to HIV. In reality, these are endogenous retroviruses like the hierarch that appears in the microvesicular image behind cells such as those extracted from the prestigious manual Molecular Biology of the Cell, or other types of particles called retrovirus-like. Precisely because of his similarity to them, as can be seen by comparing this image of the supposed HIV with that of the leader. Another important detail to emphasize is that there is a lot of talk about retroviruses as causing diseases. These would be a type of virus, of which 4 are known to affect humans through T lymphocytes. This expanded or even deformed jargon is very common among scientists like Anthony Fauci or Robert Gallo, people associated with the Rockefellers. and his Agenda of deception. Since the Rockefellers have all the money in the world and own the banks that control the world, you can imagine how easy it is for them to buy from anyone. But as I was talking about retroviruses, it has been understood that in reality retroviruses - such as the alleged

Sars-Cov-2 - could simply be fragments of genetic information and proteins produced by cells under stress.

Put another way, these elite-bought scientists have come up with the idea of retroviruses and disease-creating bacteria. This is contrary to Hamer's Laws. Yeshua (Jesus) already said it two thousand years ago, <<it is not what enters that defiles a man, but what comes out of his interior>>, referring to his mind. The mind? Yes, the source of Beliefs, Emotions and Thoughts. This is what produces psychosomatic effects, which are the real reason for an illness or disease due to the nocebo effect, or healing due to the placebo effect. Yes, I mean suggestion. Due to this, it is shown that it is emotional states, beliefs and thoughts that produce a cure or a state of illness. If the mind is not affected, the body does not have any negative reaction. These "agents" of the body, to which diseases are attributed, are actually a consequence of a pathology, not the causes of them. You will see this when we talk more in depth about the effects of microtesla waves from 5G antennas, by stimulating agents in the body that are usually there QUIET, and are harmless. These are altered by the waves and react in a way that is detrimental to the system.

A GLOBALIST AGENDA

That's how it is. I will summarize it so that it serves as a basis for what I will later postulate, since it is crucial that at this point we really know what is happening with the people who are said to have been infected or killed by a type of coronavirus that, suddenly, became malevolent and anti-human:

1st. The vast majority of diagnosed cases are not of a virus called covid (which is not the name of a virus but of an agenda of the elite to establish their so-called New World Order), but of covid symptomatology. What is this 'covid symptomatology'? These are the effects caused by waves from 5G antennas.

2nd. Many cases of the symptoms attributed to the sars-cov-2 virus are actually the result of the scientifically called 'Electromagnetic Hypersensitivity' (or 'EHS', according to its acronym in English). This covers a wide number of microwave wave systems, microtesla, radio frequencies, wi-fi or the aforementioned 5G network system (and even 4G and 3G).

3rd. Another large part of the pathologies attributed to sars-cov-2 are different viruses, which are conveniently classified as covid. This is the case of the common flu, which since December 2019 has been categorized as covid.

4th. A large part of these diseases that are wrongly called covid are primarily things unrelated to sars-cov-2, primarily related to breathing. These are essentially respiratory diseases, such as Atypical Pneumonia, caused by bacteria such as Legionella pneumophila, Mycoplasma pneumoniae and Chlamydophila pneumoniae.

5th. The numbers of sick and dead people are inflated by governments, in turn inflated by hospital statistics, which are inflated for the benefit of medical centers, since governments give them subsidies and aid for doing this. The news, however, only promotes propaganda and makes people sick with fear.

6th. Similar to this parameter, many deaths for various reasons are referred to as deaths BY covid-19, when almost all of them died for completely unrelated reasons. These cases are people without relatives, beggars or poor, people who cannot complain or pay for lawyers, and only a certain number are people who have relatives who are paid – depending on the country – between €7,000 and €9,500. In the same way, hospital centers and clinics are paid for people who are declared dead from covid, for people who are put on a respirator, and for people who are vaccinated. It is a business.

7th. In extension of the previous point, they play with the death certificates, confusing people who do not understand, with allusions to death "by" covid, instead of "with" covid. It's as simple as if you crashed in your car, but you had the flu - and even a sneeze made you lose concentration and caused you to crash - then they say you died "from" the flu, when you died it was from a road collision. This play on words is one of the most used to make people believe that a bug is killing people. The same thing happens with words like "asymptomatic" or "active positive" that do not exist in scientific jargon, but invented to imply that someone can get sick from the most lethal virus in history, but not show any symptoms. Thus everyone is caught in the net.

8th. The real sars-cov-2 virus - whose modifications with two strains of HIV and one of TB (tuberculosis) - was created in US military laboratories, and later studied with them and Chinese scientists in Wuhan laboratories. The patent was registered in England in 2014, and 4 proteins were replaced through at least 3 deliberate alterations. However, this virus IS NOT TRANSMITTED THROUGH THE AIR, not even through saliva. It is only transmitted BY INJECTION, that is, only intravenously. This virus is IN THE FLU VACCINE, and had already begun to be introduced into the population in the 2019 vaccination campaigns, so that its effects would be seen later at the beginning of 2020. Now it is introduced in the so-called vaccine against C-19 (covid-19), and will also be put into the C-21 (covid-21) vaccine in summer 2021.

9th. Many viral pathogens that infected the European population at the beginning of 2020 were the result of Chinese sent by their government to Europe at Christmas to spread these agents everywhere.

10th. The compromised immune system allows any virus to kill a person. Older people are prone to any infectious agent that could knock them down, and therefore it is known that 94% of deaths are precisely the elderly and people with very poor health or with previous determinants of health problems. The fact that this group of the population is the most delicate comes from the subconscious belief system that they do not feel socially useful or productive, and already question their existence. On the level of the mind this is related to the Vshuddha chakra, or fifth energy center of the body (also called the blue ray). This affects the areas of the neck, shoulders, mouth, nose and ears. The connection between Vshuddha and the Anahata (or green ray) chakra is the path of emotions towards the desire to live. If you sow fear in the population, your immune system lowers. Through what procedure? The emotional one, since this activates or deactivates the potential of the green energy center, and goes to the throat. However, it is not a virus that is going to kill them, because nothing that enters contaminates a man, but what comes out of his mind contaminates him. It is your emotions, beliefs and ideas that destroy you. Below is an interview they did with Javier Villamor (a Spanish journalist).

- Questioner: Are we witnessing the creation of a New World Order?

- Journalist: What is called the New World Order (NWO) is being created. Although outside of conspiracy theories it is very simple to define it: the New World Order is nothing other than the implementation of a supranational power based, precisely, on those supranational organizations that have been created since the end of the Second World War, specifically as a result of of the Bretton Woods pacts, in 1944. We have the European Union (EU), the International Monetary Fund (IMF), the World Bank, the UN itself and all its subdivisions. And it is clear that what it seeks is to establish a new humanity, a single world, with a single government, with a single religion and a single economic system, but for that we have to eliminate the previous human being. Therefore, those pillars that are the fundamental ones, moral relativism, secularism, gender ideology, among many others, we can add abortion, now comes euthanasia, with the objective of deprogramming the human being that existed before and implementing a new code of values and to be able to begin to implement transhumanism, which is what we are going for.

"We are heading towards what they also call the "Fourth Industrial Revolution", which is the implementation of a robotic system, based on artificial intelligence that controls everything that was previously, in some way, sporadic in human beings. For this we need, as I said, to format, eliminate the old Christian civilization, Christian values, and implement a new series of values that allow the new youth to perfectly enter that "new reality" for this, is what they call, among other things, the 2030 Global Agenda or 21st Century Agenda [RT Noticias, video from Argentina: "The United Nations has promoted the 2030 Agenda and this must remain the Central Guide]. The surprising and striking thing is that everything is perfectly intertwined and everything perfectly connected, because, if we touch all the points, health, education, science, all of this will allow them to guide, let's say, everything in parallel, everything towards the same point. Although in reality we obviously know that there are national governments, in practice, a large part of these national governments are not working for the good of their nations at all, but are working, precisely, for the interests of these globalites. We have seen it with the Sánchez government, we are seeing it in other countries, for example, also in Latin America and the world we are going to, it is the result of social engineering, perfectly planned and perfectly implemented."

- Questioner: Will its implementation be solely ideological?

- Journalist: The first implementation is ideological. Ideology first serves to destabilize a nation. If we do not pay attention, for example, to Yuri Bezmenov, the former KGB agent who emigrated to the United States and who described, precisely, those processes by which a nation can be destabilized: destabilization, demoralization, crisis and normalization, we are perfectly living those crises, those stages. We have had a destabilization. Now we are in the phase of demoralization, which is, turning nations against themselves, endophobia, hatred of our Christian culture, hatred of the same biology, the same male-female biological reality to make the population completely confused and make it much easier to guide them to a new point. It's a herd mentality. Now, first is the ideology, second is the rest, social, economic, political, technological, environmental, health, nutritional implementation, all of this is perfectly designed on the World Economic Forum page, they have perfectly designed what the new world. They don't leave anything out.

- Questioner: Why are abortion, gender or environmental ideology pillars of this NOM?

- Journalist: Abortion is something that is in the 2030 Global Agenda, that is included, it is embedded in the DNA of globalists and they want to promote it at all costs. Abortion, so we understand it, is a state policy. Abortion has been applied since 1974 through Kissinger's report, which is preceded by a report from the Rockefeller Foundation from 1972, which is preceded by statements by Robert Mc Namara, who was Secretary of Defense under Nixon, and who in In 1968 he became President of the World Bank. What's happening? Obviously if we understand this as a State policy, obviously it cannot be sold to the rest of the population by saying: "You are going to stop having children because we are interested in the resources that you have." What is being done is political marketing, and this is how they are selling everything to us. Abortion is a State interest, it is a geostrategic interest, all the other proposals that we have today: gender ideology, ecology or this new environmental religion, all of that is the same, they are State policies that sell it to us for the large public with political marketing so that people accept it, because, for example, if we now understand environmental policies as, let's say, obviously necessary for all governments, within those environmental policies is the reduction of the population.

"They sell it to us as a necessary good, that is, if we continue to grow we are going to destroy the planet. Therefore, stop having children, because, if not, this rhythm is unbearable. They sell us the green ideology as something necessary, but, within that green ideology it contains all those State policies that they want to sell it to us to, obviously, control the population with the precise objective of destabilizing us in order to have complete control over us. There is nothing easier to dominate than a population facing each other. That is why it is so important to understand how they work in the application of policies? How do supranational elites work? "To be able to understand what type of policy is being applied to us at the national and local level."

- Questioner: What is the enemy to defeat? The human being? The religion?

- Journalist: The enemy to be defeated by this supranational or globalist elite is none other than the human being, that is, there is absolute contempt on the part of the elites for the ordinary human being. Not only in the supranational elites, we also have them in the national elites. And, obviously, to destroy that part of the population, not in the physical sense, but in the psychological sense, we must obviously attack their beliefs, their moral bases and in this case, first it is to destroy the nations, and obviously, the religion. . There is an objective that is to create a unique religion. Traditional religions are an obstacle for that NOM to achieve that political power. If we eliminate religion, we are obviously eliminating a very human escape route that, in some way, prevents you from reaching the mind control of people. We can control them physically, but religion allows these people to escape to another plane and, obviously, it also contains very firm ethical-moral codes that are completely opposed to the moral codes that they want to implant in us.

"In this case, the Catholic religion or the Catholic Church has been the enemy to be defeated for centuries. I am not only talking about Freemasonry, but about many people. That is to say, it is necessary to bring down that Christian civilization in order to establish a new civilization. The general objective when I talk about humanity is the absolute control of the population, but I am not only talking about, say, police control, but also control of what is consumed, what is thought, what is educated, what is seen. . More or less, I believe that everyone has this reality in their heads because it is a bit of what we are seeing, they censor us on social networks, they censor us in the media, they censor us even in the schools themselves, it is nothing other than put up barriers, so they need to put an end to all that to be able to have control."

- Questioner: What role does Soros play in this NOM? Are there other characters behind this globalist project?

- Journalist: Obviously when I talk about Soros as one of the main promoters of this New World Order, I make it very clear: "one of the main ones", or let's say "one of the visible faces". I believe that if we know Soros so much it is because Soros is allowed to show himself. What I want to say with it? With this I say that the truly powerful are in the shadows. Now, Soros works on the social side, I mean, in civil society. In other words, he is an expert in modifying consciousness. That's why he works at the Overton window. The Overton window is a tool that allows us to transform the impossible into a feasible fact, and there are several phases. Obviously first comes the propaganda, the ideology. For this, "think tanks", foundations, associations are created and financed, which generate supposed official scientific documents, studies, etc., which are then echoed by the media. These media reach the masses, the masses through repetition of these studies, these concepts, these ideologies, they end up accepting those ideologies or thoughts as their own, yes, accepting it, saying it as something that already exists and they see it for everywhere, it is something that must be accepted. Once, let's say that is the third phase, the fourth phase comes, which is that of the politicians. Politicians, obviously with the partisan interest of continuing in power, make a supposed echo of these supposedly "social" claims and, obviously, then the fifth, which is the transformation of laws, legislation.

"So, those five steps are what has been followed with many things. We have abortion, we have homosexual marriage, now we have – it has already begun – euthanasia, and the next step is pedophilia. And this is pure mathematics, it is political science, and it always works. So, if we stick to it, this is used to apply certain things. What has Soros done on a social level? Likewise, it has financed NGOs, associations, foundations, etc., it has financed media, it has financed politicians and it has even financed institutions such as, for example, the European Union, or the Europa Council Foreign Relations (ECFR), which is the European version of the North American CFR, which is the main lobby of North American foreign policy. In this case, in Europe, then, if you have the five steps, or four of the five steps in your hand, it is much easier to modify the reality of the citizens, precisely because it touches all those issues."

- Questioner: What role do supranational institutions such as the UN, IMF, WHO, etc. play?

- Journalist: If we go to supranational situations, what is the role of the UN, the EU, WHO, etc.? It is very similar, the World Bank obviously is global economic management, the same is similar to the International Monetary Fund when it comes to loans. Economic control and loans serve to economically blackmail nations. There are many African nations that have complained precisely about the economic blackmail of money, supposedly development aid, always depending on issues such as, for example, the implementation of abortion, the implementation of gender ideology, early sexual education for children, etc. The WHO has been fundamental to the implementation of the idea that there is a global pandemic, and if it had not been for the WHO, in this case for Tedros Adhanour, a global lockdown would not have been created or called.

"It is the first time in history that the citizens of this planet have seen how all nations followed the same steps, that is, nothing has been achieved before that there was truly coordination never seen before at a global level. Coordination that, although it seems like a lot to us, has generally been very suspicious, so to speak, is still not enough for this elite. According to them, "the challenges posed by future pandemics far exceed the management capacity of independent States." That is to say, since we have not known how to manage the coronavirus, it is necessary that we cede more of our sovereignty to these supranational entities, that they really know what we have to do: lead us to that "good path", to guide us as if they were a God, because we, as ordinary citizens, are too stupid to fend for ourselves."

- Questioner: Why do globalist elites control and censor the media and social networks?

- Journalist: Social networks have always been a fundamental tool in the field of communication, but, like all technological advances, they always have their heads and tails. Like all technological advances, they sell us that it is good to be able to talk to our families, to be in contact with people from all over the world, but the problem, the counterbalance, is absolute control. Not only the control of what we do, but even our thoughts, because many times, we say things on social networks, which, perhaps, were too private, and that is precisely where they are going now with the censorship issue. You have seen that in recent years there has also been a small revolution in social networks given that there are more and more conservative, anti-globalist profiles, more profiles of people opposed to the designs of this New World Order, and, if we were certainly in a free world , democratic – and I say this so that people realize that we do not live in a free and democratic world -, the free circulation of ideas and debates should be one of the main characteristics of the entire system, and we are together on the opposite.

"And the opposite is not fair because "de facto" you cannot talk, because before you could talk about many things. The problem is that the really powerful, those who control things, have realized that, if we allow certain ideas to circulate freely, and not their own, in terms of debate, those ideas win. It has been shown that they have more weight than others and, for example, with the issue of abortion, there are no longer scientific or medical arguments, now they are purely sentimental arguments: "a woman's right to choose her own body," because with They know that medical arguments cannot defeat them. Regarding arguments, for example, about information from the media, about how governments work, exactly the same, anyone who tries to make a constructive or negative criticism of anything is completely censored, but making a criticism to warn of what is happening. There is no debate of ideas in the media, but precisely because they are afraid of what may happen. Because, when it has happened that some people have gone to certain debates and presented certain ideas, people have realized that there is another line of thinking different from the one they had in mind. And, therefore, there is another way to reason things."

NUMBERS INFLADED BY THE CDC

What is the CDC? The Center for Disease Control, which, ironically, is not an independent agency. The CDC is also a vaccine company, owner of about 20 vaccine patents, and sells about $4.6 billion in vaccines each year, according to the complaints of lawyer Robert Kennedy junior, grandson of former President John F. Kennedy. Now let's look at a report from February 1, 2021 on how the CDC (Center for Disease Control) – who is increasingly said to have been bought by Bill Gates -, which would have been inflating numbers to instill fear: The CDC would have inflated COVID numbers by up to 1600% and are accused of violating federal law, from www.nationalfile.com [14]. The Centers for Disease Control and Prevention (CDC) is accused of violating federal law by inflating coronavirus death tolls, according to stunning data obtained by NATIONAL FILE. The CDC illegally inflated the COVID death toll by 1,600 percent while the 2020 presidential election was underway, according to a study published by the Public Health Initiative of the Institute for Pure and Applied Knowledge.

The study, "COVID-19 Data Collection, Comorbidity & Federal Law: A Historical Retrospective," was prepared by Henry Ealy, Michael McEvoy, Daniel Chong, John Nowicki, Monica Sava, Sandeep Gupta, David White, James Jordan, Daniel Simon and Paul Anderson. The CDC is now legally requiring Americans to wear face masks on public transportation, as globalists try to push the "double mask" concept on the population. Since the [US] elections, the World Health Organization admits that PCR tests are not completely reliable on a first try and that a second test may be necessary. This corresponds with the CDC's silent admission that it is mixing viral and antibody test results into its case numbers and that people can test positive for an antibody test if they have antibodies from a family of viruses that cause the virus. common cold.

Florida hospitals had so many accuracy issues that Orlando Health had to admit that its 9.4% positivity rate was recorded at 98%. "The groundbreaking, peer-reviewed research... alleges that the CDC willfully violated multiple federal laws, including the Information Quality Act, the Paperwork Reduction Act, and the Administrative Procedures Act, at a minimum." (Publishing Journal – Institute for Pure and Applied Knowledge/Public

---

14.   http://www.nationalfile.com

Health Policy Initiative) Most notably, the CDC illegally enacted new rules for data collection and reporting exclusively for COVID-19 that resulted in inflated 1,600% of current COVID-19 fatality totals, " the watchdog group All Concerned Citizens declared in a statement provided to NATIONAL FILE, referring to the Institute for Pure and Applied Knowledge study.

"The investigation shows that CDC did not request mandatory federal oversight and did not open a mandatory period for public scientific comment in both cases, as required by federal law before promulgating new rules for data collection and reporting. reports. The CDC is required to fully comply with all federal laws, even in emergency situations. "The investigation alleges that CDC deliberately compromised the accuracy and integrity of all COVID-19 case and death data since the beginning of this crisis, to fraudulently inflate case and death data," stated All Concerned Citizens. "On March 24, CDC released NVSS COVID-19 Alert No. 2, which instructed coroners and medical examiners to downplay underlying causes of death, also called pre-existing conditions or comorbidities, recording them in Part II instead of Part I of death certificates, since "...the underlying cause of death is expected to be COVID-19 more frequently." "This was a major change to the rules for reporting death certificates from the Coroners' Handbook on Death Registration and Fetal Death Reporting and the Physicians' Handbook on Medical Certification of Death. Deaths and Fetal Death Reporting and the 2003 CDC Physicians' Handbook on Medical Certification of Death, which had instructed death reporting professionals nationwide to report underlying conditions in the Part I for the previous 17 years."

"This single change resulted in a significant inflation of COVID-19 deaths by mandating that COVID-19 be listed on Part I of death certificates as the definitive cause of death, regardless of confirmatory testing, instead of be listed in Part II as a contributing factor to death in the presence of pre-existing conditions, as would have been done with the 2003 guidelines. The investigation draws attention to this key distinction, as it has led to significant inflation in COVID fatality totals. According to the researcher's estimates, recorded COVID-19 deaths are inflated nationwide by up to 1,600% above what they would be if the CDC had used the 2003 manuals, All Concerned Citizens stated. «Then, on April 14, the CDC adopted additional rules unique to COVID-19 in violation of federal law by outsourcing the development of data collection rules to the Council of State and Territorial Epidemiologists (CSTE), a non-profit entity, once again without requesting oversight and the possibility of public scientific review. «On April 5, the CSTE published a position paper entitled Standardized surveillance case definition and national notification for 2019 novel coronavirus disease (COVID-19). COVID-19)], which included 5 CDC employees as subject matter experts.

"This key document created new rules for counting probable cases as actual cases without definitive evidence of infection (section VII.A1 – pages 4 and 5), new rules for contact tracing that allow contact tracers to practice medicine without a license (section VII.A3 – page 5), and yet refused to define new rules to ensure that the same person could not be counted multiple times as a new case (section VII.B – page 7)," stated All Concerned Citizens. "By enacting these new rules exclusively for COVID-19 in violation of federal law, the investigation alleges that the CDC significantly inflated data that has been used by elected officials and public health officials, along with untested projection models." from the Institute for Health Metrics and Evaluation (IHME), to justify the prolonged closures of schools, places of worship, entertainment and small businesses that lead to unprecedented emotional and economic hardships across the country. "A formal petition has been sent to the Department of Justice, as well as all US attorneys, requesting an immediate grand jury investigation into these allegations," All Concerned Citizens added. Source in Spanish: https://tierrapura.org/2021/02/01/el-cdc-habria-inflado-las-cifras-de-covid-hasta-en-un-1600-y-esta-acusado-de- violate-federal-law/[15]

I conclude with this publication: In the West 'it is forbidden to heal and tell the truth', denounce Nobel Prize winners in medicine and elite scientists. With so many conspiracy theories being confirmed one after another, the establishment that controls the Western world has no choice but to undertake massive campaigns of censorship and discredit, and even seek to classify any dissident voice as "terrorist" for the simple fact of not being agree with the operating beliefs of the ruling oligarchy. Many brave doctors and scientists have reported the censorship and banning of effective alternative medications and treatments during the current health crisis. But fear is normal. Doctors are mostly aware that what is happening is unreasonable, and others still understand more and have documented themselves, and see the plot, but they have worked decades to get where they are and do not want to lose their jobs. Most love what they do and want to serve their fellow human beings. Hence there are those who do not apply vaccines but placebos, or give natural medications to their patients under the hood, or prescribe them to commune with nature and have an alkaline diet, even when

---

15.   https://tierrapura.org/2021/02/01/el-cdc-habria-inflado-las-cifras-de-covid-hasta-en-un-1600-y-esta-acusado-de-violar-la-ley-federal/

they do not earn commissions from this (because they make money by prescribing the drugs).

For their part, scientists, who have also dedicated decades of research, find themselves in a funnel that pushes them in the same direction. If they leave there, they do not receive help, and if they have a different opinion, they remain like weirdos among their colleagues, and in the end they lose credibility. They are afraid to tell the truth about what is happening so as not to lose research opportunities and funding for their studies. Below, we present the cases of three elite scientists nominated for the Nobel Prize, who exemplify how far the elites who pull the strings of the pharmaceutical industry in the West have been able to go in order to nullify alternative visions of medicine as a business and mechanism. of control. Dr. Luc Montagnier: Nobel Prize in Medicine (2008). COVID-19: Why the Atlantic Council calls the virologist and Nobel Prize winner Dr. Luc Montagnier a 'spreader of conspiracy theories'. The Atlantic Council (a tentacle of the British crown) has launched a smear campaign against Nobel Prize winner Dr. Luc Montagnier [1], for supporting the theory that COVID-19 was created in a laboratory and for having proposed an international program of electromagnetic wave therapy to treat diseases, instead of investing in vaccines.

Molecular biologist Dr. Richard John Roberts, winner of the Nobel Prize in Medicine in 1993, said the following in an interview [2] fourteen years after being awarded: "The pharmaceutical industry wants to serve the capital markets... If you only think about benefits, you stop worrying about serving human beings... I have seen how in some cases researchers dependent on private funds would have discovered very effective medicines that would have completely ended a disease... [but] pharmaceutical companies are often not so interested in curing you as in taking money from you, so that research, suddenly, is diverted towards the discovery of medicines that do not completely cure, but rather make the disease chronic and make you experience an improvement that disappears when you stop taking the medicine... Well, it is common for pharmaceutical companies to be interested in lines of research not to cure but only to make chronic ailments with chronicizing medications that are much more profitable than those that cure completely and once and for all. And you just have to follow the financial analysis of the pharmaceutical industry and you will see what I say."

Dr. Peter Gariaev: Nominated for the Nobel Prize in Medicine in 2021. Creator of quantum genetics says what Covid really is and dies nominated for the Nobel in 'the most crucial and precarious moment in the history of medicine'. Peter Gariaev, creator of quantum genetics who also said that Covid was created in the laboratory and proposed wave genetic therapy to treat it, was nominated in October 2020 for the 2021 Nobel Prize in Medicine, and died a month after receiving the nomination letter due to a brain aneurysm, as reported by some of his academic colleagues and other people who knew him and who "are concerned that his death at this time is unusual, since he was in excellent condition despite being 79 years old," in addition that "this great independent researcher and pioneer of the life sciences could not have died at a more crucial and precarious moment in the history of medicine." Months before his death, Dr. Gariaev published the following on the portal of his research center:

"[...] With traditional genetics and virology, we will always remain in the same place, wasting a lot of money on useless work. We urgently need fundamentally new genetics and virology. We have, first of all, Linguistic Wave Genetics (BTY), which we have developed since 1984, experiencing tremendous resistance from official science. And what can we offer from our wave genetics to combat the pandemic? The first and most important thing is the review and correction of the old model of the genetic code. The model is scientifically incorrect and, therefore, is an absolute mistake, even though it was awarded a Nobel Prize at the time. What is your mistake and how can correcting it help combat the pandemic? The mistake is ignoring the importance of everything linguistic (textual), as part of genetic coding, in the entire human genome, not just in the 2% that produces proteins and that is all that could be studied in the West. . They constantly deny the meaning of genes, as parts of texts with their components: words, the roots of words, prefixes, morphemes, phonemes, punctuation, declensions, conjugations, sometimes, probabilistic aspects of the meanings of genetic texts and everything. a world of things that would be very difficult to describe. The only way out of these rather gloomy circumstances that prevail is to immediately begin global research in the field of 'linguistic wave genetics.' We already have a great theoretical and experimental base in this area, the main part is that we can now operate with quantum copies of genes that, in the near future, will allow us to deactivate RNA genes and other pathogenic viruses, both RNA and DNA. In other words 'turn off' the genetic components in a quantum way, which means deactivating any pathogen." Source: https://www.mentealternativa.com/en-occidente-esta-prohibido-curarse-y-decir-la- Verdad-denuncian-premios-nobel-de-medicina-y-cientifico-de-elite [16]/.

But constantly, despite refutations, you hear many ask, "so what are people dying of?" And I answer them, "don't people die, are we immortal?" Dying is part of life. People are dying

---

all the time, and it has been like this since man was a man, as far as we know. Animals die, even trees die. But who tells you what someone dies of? The government, which has a great reputation for transparency and honesty, and they always tell you the truth... right? To find out the causes of death, an autopsy is performed, and since autopsies have not been performed since the beginning of 2019, it is not possible to know what people die from. So, where do they get that a certain number of people die and that they die from a certain bug that murdered them? Bribes. There have been many reports, complaints and trials in 2020 and 2021 due to the manipulation of figures and the modification of death certificates. In the end, in only a few cases could it be said that the dead people did not die for the reasons that they do every year. But it is true that there were some exceptions, when medical malpractice ended up killing the individual, when a cocktail of drugs they were given caused systemic collapse, or when they simply were not given anti-inflammatories, anticoagulants or antibiotics and they got worse, then the They were intubated, blocking their lungs, then their liver and finally their kidneys, causing their death.

So they come and say - the deniers of the truth -, and then what are people getting sick from? And I ask them, "do people never get sick?" If we reach the point where 270 symptoms encompass covid, then even the flu will be called covid, and thus they will stop talking about deaths – because now they die is due to pseudo- vaccines – and talk about "cases", "infections", "infections", "positive", "increasing numbers". according to whom? Based on tests for bacteria, unreliable tests, non-confirmatory tests, tests that determine that "something" you have had... something can be anything, it does not mean disease. Next, the defenders of the Covid ruling party argue, "but I had the symptoms, I lost my sense of smell, I was terrible."

And I ask them, "what did you have?" The description may fit one or more things. Why does it have to be covid, why do they call everything covid? They sprayed pathogens, germs, bacteria, abtrax, heavy metals and more from aerosols by airplanes in late 2019 and early 2020. The 5G antenna troubles began, starting in Wuhan and the city of San Marino, where it was said that everything exploded. Some virologists also postulate, and some of them with great confidence, that the 2019 winter flu vaccines had Sars-Cov-2, which was not and has never been transmitted through air or saliva, but rather intravenously. But above all, people get sick from fear, LITERALLY, and that is scientifically proven. A year of fear propaganda makes those who watch television and/or follow the current of social deception sick.

THE VIRUS THAT BREAKS THE NETWORK

Let's look at children's programming, which is for the most vulnerable. For example, to look at one of countless cases, I will tell you about my daughter and I's favorite animated film, 'Wreck It Ralph', from Disney, from 2012. Since the end of 2020, I had been finding a lot kinship between Anthony Fauci and the character there called 'Fix It Felix', who embodies the figure of the avatar who fixes the Wreck It Ralph game. It is negative primacy. People don't recognize it directly but their subconscious does, and they see someone coming to solve a problem and their mind tells them "yes, he fixes it", because there was a prior conditioning preparation through an image. That's called Stealth Programming. Another curious detail is that 'Felix Junior's job is to prevent the spread of a virus that Ralph unleashed because "he didn't want to be the bad guy anymore", he was tired of the monotony, of not knowing the world, of his life being robotic, predictable and limited to a small space, and, above all, being the one on the receiving end of constant humiliation. You want to be a winner and be recognized, so you look for a medal that honors you. In an accident in another game, a virus escapes and infiltrates Sugar Rush and threatens to destroy the entire game room. The person who helps Felix Junior is a secret operations "military" and his future wife. To accept this soldier's intervention favorably, they make her very attractive and in high definition, even with her dictatorial temperament. It is interesting that despite the chaos, there is no general board of directors to take action on the matter, but rather Felix and his "friend" (Sergeant Tamora Jean Calhoun, from the game Hero's Duty) take the job. of saviors for themselves.

The analogy here with the 'coronaplan' is evident: it is not the government that is actually in charge, but the medical and military cartel, led by the WHO (similar to the later footage 'The Emoji Movie' (2017), where the focus are "computer failures" (avatars that act differently from the standards, like you and me), the digital age, viruses, corporate imperialism and the police dictatorship in technocratic service). Now let's see, Vanellope, the girl in the game in danger, was a victim of mental programming, which in the game they define as "erasing her parent program", so that she does not know who she is, and they treat her as "a bug" that must be removed. Everyone in that game is a victim of brainwashing by their ruler, and lives in a world of "fantasy" and "candy", and is distracted by car racing - like television, sports, movies - until The problem is now unstoppable. They do not remember who they are nor do they know that they are being manipulated. In fact, they attack Vanellope and don't let her win the game to prevent the system from being "reset." The 'Reset' of the game is key to saving the machine room (of video games), which is an analogy of our world. What they introduce here is a key element that aims to say that the virus crisis can only be resolved with a complete "reset" of the entire system. And since Vanellope can't start the "gold medal," we have to assume that it's all about the economy. Everyone must pay, but she puts up the "gold" medal, a financial symbol by nature.

Curiously, through the film 'Zootopia', Disney presented another preview in 2016 about a "serum" (virus) that is injected into the "potential enemies" of society in SmartCities, making them "dangerous." Now, in Wreck It Ralph, both Vanellope and Ralph suffer from contempt and criticism and are intended to be eliminated by whoever controls the game. Turbo, who causes problems in one game (country, system) infiltrates "another" – like Bill Gates – corrupting the data of all the avatars – as a good computer and Trojan connoisseur knows -, and making himself the "king " (King Candy). Only the "bitter candy" – the resigned one – knows about the conspiracy and reveals the truth to Ralph through threats. They all use such beautiful names, to be accepted by the subconscious, even though the conscious area sees them as bad. Another aspect of the mental program here is that all people must accept their roles and limit themselves to "not leaving their corresponding games" (as is the case with 'Emoji, The Movie', where being "different" implies tacit elimination). The key phrase here is said by Sonic in an advertisement: "remember, don't leave your game, because if you die outside your game, you don't regenerate, goodbye." Here we see the newscasts represented in the famous figure of Sonic, and what Arcade lover would not pay attention to Sonic. Of course, the news is always presented as "now, all the information", "in seconds, you will have all the events that happen", etc., implying to the subconscious that you will know the outside world and the truth of what is happening around you. through the "truth" that they present to you, and as they present it to you.

Let's also see how Sonic introduces the idea that if you leave your game (your house), you will die. The idea of the game is that "you can die inside it", because you regenerate, but if you die outside, you don't regenerate. I could venture to interpret that this may even be a hint at globalist ideas of introducing transhumanism and certain drugs in the future, which will prevent people from getting old or sick (compare Rev. 9:6), but of course, those that have left at the end of the "planetary purification of the species". On the other hand, they indoctrinate you, "live your life at home, because you are safe there, no matter what happens, but not outside." Here is the letter that Disney had incorporated into this film 8 years earlier. We also see how bullying is essential against detractors and those who do not allow themselves to be brainwashed, even undermining their creativity and free thinking, as I already said they did with Ralph and Vanellope. But going back to the "reset", as I said, Ralph takes a gold medal (symbol of wealth, prosperity, economy) from the game Hero's Duty, and takes it to Sugar Rush where Vanellope enters it into the race.

The medal decomposes and becomes "data", whose value is translated into the registration to compete (in the future, a mere cryptocurrency, without which you will not be able to "run", or have a place in society). Here I interpret that they clearly suggest a change from physical to virtual currency, without which "you can't run", and running is, in Sugar Rush, the only purpose. Only if you run can you be chosen again, and if you win you are among those who can enjoy the benefits of the game's avatars. This is an analogy to the chip that would replace cash, and without which you will be nobody in the system, which will become a complete digital network.

Something a little more cryptic in this whole story is the fact that all the inhabitants of Sugar Rush, except for sour candy (King Candy's spokesperson), the king and the police, are children, "candy children" (clearly a reference to pedophilia, childhood vulnerability). Avatars serve the interests of the humans playing in the Arcade Machine Room, just as the masters of the world use our race, or the Reptilians and Orians use everyone else under them. These types of subliminal sexual messages are found in many places, especially in advertisements, and Disney has already had complaints in the past, and has had to pay millionaire fines in courts of law for the evidence against it that shows the merciless bombing of subliminal messages and sexual sigils in his films, especially in 'The Little Mermaid', 'The Lion King' and 'Pocahontas'. These types of concepts are not seen with the naked eye and are often hidden behind representations only understood among adepts, among those under Monarch mental control, or those who understand picaresque ideas. That is the case of a scene where Ralph leaves the PacMan game eating some cherries and when he sees orphan avatars (without a game) he gives them to them, already bitten. As reflected in the PizzaGate scandal, these ideas have a greater meaning behind them, but it doesn't take a genius to argue that two cherries are commonly used in SexShops as a cultural representation of testicles. We see the same example with a bitten apple, like the slogan of the Apple company, which is used to refer to "original sin", which are also sexual ideas and erotic or passionate temptation (adultery, fornication, prostitution, etc.). I only add that no one is demonizing sex itself, at all, but the perversion and degradation of values.

In 2018, Disney released the second part of Wreck It Ralph, called 'Ralph Breaks the Internet'. As if by chance, the film came out exactly one year before the decision of the US elections between Trump and Madame Clinton. The plot revolves around how Vanellope gets bored of the game and Ralph creates a new driving track. The player "breaks the steering wheel" while "fighting against the driver's rebellion" and now they must find a handlebar on Ebay to replace it, or it will be out of play. The message here evokes how there is a clash between the resistance and the elite, which forces a reset (if the helm is not replaced, the game will be withdrawn). Ralph and Vanellope oppose the elite and this poses a threat to the safety and subsistence of the Arcade game. The director of the room (Mr. Litwack) installs the internet (the digital world, the Internet of Things) and these two rebels escape to find how to fix the problem, find a "cure." Meanwhile, Fauci and the police state... sorry, I meant, Fix It Felix and Sergeant Calhoun, are in charge of "taking care" of all the "candy game children", now "homeless". From that point everything revolves around "raising the most money" to "defray the costs" of the steering wheel. Translated into our language, pull all the strings and make use of all "digital" means to "pay" for the "solution", which here essentially translates into the problem of unpayable global debt. The digital idea of the internet world suggests how society is embarking towards a completely virtual reality and entertainment.

Vanellope meets the fatherless feminists: the Disney princesses. They understand each other perfectly, independent of men, without parental relationship, without children, without family, without husband, in their own bubble and lacking general culture. They all coincide in an external beauty and an internal intellectual emptiness, not having grown up with a father figure, since this is an important strategy of Walt Disney to introduce into the minds of children, and part of the feminist agenda of the Rockefeller Foundation. Vanellope then meets another girl, a daring racer, played by Israeli actress Gal Gadot, and wants to stay in her high-resolution, multi-hazard car racing game, but Ralph gets jealous and puts a virus in that game. Yes, we are represented by the spoilsport Ralf, who does not want this new improved digital world. This is where it gets interesting.

Once again a virus threatens security, but this time it is no longer local but global. Once again the solution is a reset, now on a global and total scale. If we compare it with the covid agenda, first there was a quarantine of decapitalization to begin to destabilize the planet, and then comes a real virus, both biological and cybernetic, to restart the planetary structure, first financial, and then global and contextual. The virus actually spreads through **people's "insecurities," that is, their fears**.

And here is the ace of this deck: the real virus that attacks the world is fear, and thanks to this fear it spreads and achieves the goals of the creator of the "worm". Feminist independence wins (the anti-family and exclusive philosophy of the value of man), and the network is saved. What does it mean in Illuminati language? Reduction of world population, with viruses, sterilization and eugenics. Once again, society can continue in its virtual world and the masters can direct their avatars, but now in a "renewed" system. If there is one way the elite can use to tell you whatever they want and you won't realize it, it is through cartoons, and now with animation. And if you realize it, what are you going to say? Will you tell your friends that you see the intentions of the Illuminati because of "a cartoon"? It doesn't sound very credible. That's what it's about. Disney princesses, for example, are represented in practically all the films, and they are always instilling the same idea: worship of the monarchy. It is the "princess" who presents the kind and acceptable face of some type of royalty or caste. This is a success in England, where the royal house is almost a showbiz icon, more famous and admired than film or music stars. Thus they become untouchable, and their image remains well seen. How is it that in the 21st century we continue to feed parasites?

What purpose do monarchies have? But there they are, seen as an idol to love, care for and respect. It is so easy to introduce these ideas to children that there have been debates for years about the use of subliminal messages in young people, because it is known how susceptible and vulnerable they are to them. Advertisements are a clear example, and anyone who is a parent knows it well: their child comes after watching a spot and tells them they want that toy they just presented. Now imagine a Disney Channel putting girls daily in the trend of the Barbie series, and boys addicted to their hobbies, in a bubble and without interest in the outside world or culture (knowledge). Children are the objective of the elite in a crazy way, and that is why it is so common in Disney films to see orphans or children without one or both of their parents (based on the emotional imprint of the uprooting of one of them). In 2016, DreamWorks released the film 'Trolls', which is about some horrible, big people who want to "eat" the "little ones", those divine little heavens of love and colors. But I will not focus this book on the dark strategy of pedophilia, I only intend to give you an idea of what is not seen with the naked eye. Let's continue.

IX. THE INVISIBLE ENEMY

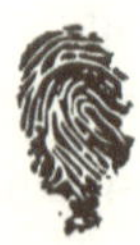

What is a virus, what is a bacteria, what is a fungus, what is a germ, what is a protozoan? The term "germs" refers to microorganisms such as microscopic bacteria, viruses, fungi and protozoa that are said to cause disease. Let's look at this carefully. We have bacteria, which are tiny single-celled organisms that obtain nutrients from their environment. In some cases, that environment is your child or some other living being. Some bacteria are good for our body: they help keep the digestive system working and prevent harmful bacteria from entering. We are talking about the most abundant organisms on the planet, which are said to also cause problems, such as cavities, urinary tract infections, ear infections or strep throat. Let's start by considering a detail: if bacteria are the most abundant organisms on the planet, everything around us and inside us is full of them. Would it be unreasonable to assume that statistically – if what the media sells us is true – our health and the rest of the planet's organisms would be in a Russian roulette game? I take myself as an example - hoping this doesn't sound like a preponderance - and how, to say the least, in about 3 years I have never gotten sick from absolutely anything. I have slept on the street, among cardboard, on the ground, under a bridge, I have gone days without eating, I have been exposed to the rain, wet, spending cold nights... where would statistics apply here, the probabilities of falling ill?

In total, it is estimated that there are approximately 5x1030 bacteria in the world. What do you do? For what purpose did

God, aliens, evolution or Mother Nature create bacteria? Have you ever stopped to think why ants, bees, cockroaches or flies exist? What purpose do animals, plants or trees have? Everything is part of a gear. Cockroaches clean organic waste on land like prawns (shrimp, doe, etc.) do in the sea. Oysters filter waste. Shelled marine animals essentially clean up the ocean floor. Fish without scales clean the surface of the water. Rats clean, eliminate garbage, reduce the exponential increase of insects. Cats prevent them from reproducing too much. There is a balance. Snakes do the same on the plain, and birds of prey hunt vipers. Trees, algae and plankton clean the air and aerobic organisms can live, and they feed on our waste when we breathe. The wind carries these currents through the air and under the sea through cyclic currents that travel around the entire planet. The water undergoes its hydrological cycle, taking by sublimation everything that the cloud condenses and moves to the mountains and plains and releases it, rehydrating the surface, and the channels return the liquid to the sea. If we think about canons of order and reason for being, bacteria could no longer be seen as we perceive them.

There are approximately ten times more bacterial cells than human cells in the human body, with large numbers of bacteria on the skin and in the digestive tract. Although the protective effect of the immune system would make the vast majority of these bacteria harmless or beneficial, some of them are considered pathogenic and cause infectious diseases, such as cholera, diphtheria, scarlet fever, leprosy, syphilis or typhus, although the most popular due to its danger is the one that causes tuberculosis. But let's analyze this carefully. These diseases are associated with circumstances where people have poor hygiene, consume dirty or directly contaminated water, and have a very poor diet. So the focus is going in the wrong direction.

You may be in very good health, but if you have a cut with rusty metal and you do not have something within reach to sterilize the wound, a disinfectant product, an anti-tetal injection and/or clean material or clean water to treat the cut, rest assured that it could take you to death in a few days. THE FACTORS must be ADDED, because in and of themselves, by themselves, they are not conclusive on a person's health. If Africans had good food, clean water and a hygienic environment, epidemic outbreaks would end. Pharmaceutical companies and vaccine manufacturing companies would go bankrupt.

We have been told since we were children that we should wash our hands thoroughly and it is often the best way to prevent germs from causing infections and illnesses. We still see this in the ancient law of Moses, even though, ironically, Yeshua (Jesus) refuted this postulate. Nature uses an "aggression-recovery" cycle to continually regenerate and get stronger. In industry, bacteria are important in processes such as wastewater treatment, in the production of butter, cheese, vinegar, yogurt, etc., and in the manufacture of medicines and other chemical products. In the case of yeasts, these germs are fungi that make chemical changes in the compounds. That's why we have wine, we have bread, we have pizza. Let us consider that many of the modifications in scientific principles in recent decades have come from a lucrative interest. I mentioned cavities... they talk about preventing the tooth from being punctured by cleaning the teeth well, but the most obvious aspects are overlooked. Avoiding a problem does not eliminate the problem, much less go to the root of it to solve it, but that idea is what companies sell. A healthy tooth is an unemployed dentist. Fluoride, which is promoted as a powerful dental protectant and cleaner, is actually a corrosive element. If you put a tooth in fluoride for 48 hours you will begin to see how it eats away. Tooth enamel is produced by salivation. The hardness of the teeth emulates the principle of crystals. The consistency of the teeth depends on the micronutrients consumed. So let's look at the equations: 1. You "protect" your teeth by brushing with fluoride cream and flossing, versus 2. The tooth is protected only by a diet high in essential micronutrients and good oral salivation.

We see more examples of how science seems to contradict itself, when we talk about "antibiotics," used to treat "bacterial infections." The word "antibiotic" means "against living organisms." The consumption of "prebiotics" and "probiotics" is promoted. ¿is not this a contradiction? When industries have vested interests, we see apparent contradictions of science. It is the intestinal microbiome that is mainly responsible for a well-protected system. An "antibiotic" is a nuclear bomb that falls on the intestine and pulverizes all these microorganisms responsible for the biodiversity of the intestinal flora. But we also see examples of this nature with other types of germs, such as fungi. This family of eukaryotic organisms includes molds, yeasts and mushroom producers. Some are very healthy foods, others are hallucinogenic, others are toxic. They come in various shapes and sizes. Many fungal infections, such as athlete's foot and yeast infections, are not dangerous to a healthy person. However, people with weak immune systems (from diseases such as HIV or cancer) can get more serious fungal infections. Back to the same. Current Western science focuses on causes, not effects. They promote expensive treatments, drugs and chemicals instead of getting to the root of the matter. Is it a scientific conspiracy? No. All this is known, but those who move the millions and millions of dollars promote what interests them. The rest of the scientific truths remain almost anonymous and are not usually even mentioned.

Then there are protozoa, which also consist of a great variety, with only some becoming parasites of other living beings, and many being part of the food chain. Protozoa are single-celled organisms, like bacteria. But they are larger than bacteria and contain a nucleus and other cellular structures, making them more similar to plant and animal cells. Protozoa love humidity. So intestinal infections and other diseases they cause, such as amoebiasis and giardiasis, are often transmitted through contaminated water. And as I said, some protozoa are parasites. This means that they need to live in another organism (such as an animal or plant) to survive. For example, the protozoa that cause malaria grow inside red blood cells and eventually destroy them. Some protozoa are encapsulated in cysts, which helps them live outside the human body and in harsh environments for long periods of time. If there were no contaminated water, there would be no parasites. End of the matter. What is cheaper, on the one hand a water filter and purifying tablets or bleach, or on the other, a chemical component from a laboratory, genetically modified, inoculated into the population? Who benefits and who harms one or the other? We all know the answer is too obvious. Africa is the main business cradle for the pharmaceutical industry. Consequently, it is enough to finance those who carry out "humanitarian" campaigns and movements, and that's it.

Finally we have another type of germ: viruses. Viruses are even smaller than bacteria. They are not even a full cell. They are simply genetic material (DNA or RNA) packaged within a protein shell. They are cellular waste. They need to use the structures of another cell to reproduce. This means that they cannot survive unless they live inside something else (such as a person, animal, or plant). Viruses can only live for a very short time outside of other living cells. For example, viruses in infected body fluids left on surfaces such as a doorknob or toilet seat can live there for a short time. They will die quickly unless a live host comes. However, it is said that when they have moved into someone's body, viruses spread easily and can make a person sick, but they cause minor illnesses such as colds, common illnesses such as the flu, and very serious illnesses such as smallpox or HIV. AIDS. That is the idea that is becoming popular. It is also argued that antibiotics are not effective against viruses, although antiviral drugs have been developed against a small and select group of viruses.

But let's analyze what a disease is. The definition of disease according to the World Health Organization (WHO) is "alteration or deviation from the physiological state in one or more parts of the body, for generally known causes, manifested by characteristic symptoms and signs, and whose evolution is more or less predictable. According to Wikipedia itself, <<Health and illness are an integral part of life, of the biological process and of environmental and social interactions.>> And there is something very illuminating, which was said at the time by the famous doctor Sebi in an impeachment court in the US, where he won against the State: By definition, <<there is only one disease>>, but the characterization and identification of various different processes and states of health has led to discrimination of a universe of different entities (nosological entities), many of them understood strictly as diseases but others not (cf. syndrome, clinical entity and disorder). In this way, diseases and substitute and analogous processes are understood as categories determined by the human mind. Being simply "sick", and has certain symptoms that affect it. An example is phlegm, the cause of natural obstructions made by the body, and consequently, the catalyst of any pathology. In 1884 Robert Koch, who established the etiology of tuberculosis, presented what would be the parameters for understanding diseases and viruses, Koch's postulates. In essence, its intention is to confirm the etiological role of a microorganism in other diseases. These postulates are the following:

- The pathogenic agent must be present in sick animals and absent in healthy ones.

- The agent must be grown in a pure axenic culture isolated from the animal's body.

- The agent isolated in an axenic culture must cause disease in a susceptible animal when inoculated.

- The agent must be isolated again from the lesions produced in the experimental animals and be exactly the same as that originally isolated.

THE PHLEGM PRODUCED by dairy products is not a reason for debate. Only in certain cases, when "things are already bad", the doctor advises removing dairy products from the diet. Why do we wait to see the adverse reactions to react? Because no government in its "sane mind" will remove milk, yogurt, butter and cheese from its markets. Doing this would mean a collapse in an essential part of the food and production supply chain. Thousands of ranchers would be left unemployed, without counting all those who are intermediaries, who are part of the mechanism of the structure of this production and marketing. So it is not about physical health, but financial health, one of the most essential parts of sustaining a country. The same happens with meats, which are already known to be carcinogenic, as their Heme iron damages the endothelial walls of the arteries and produces premature aging. Even Turkish scientific studies have said that the characteristics of an animal are passed to whoever consumes it, including the morphology of the section of the body that is consumed. That means that if you eat pork belly repeatedly, your belly will progressively look like that of a pig. It is notable that no one who eats animal meat would like to hear this. Muslims don't mind, because they don't eat pork in the first place. But what courage you acquire in the influence and memory of DNA by eating "chicken".

But my point is not to pick on carnivores. My point is to show that nutrition is not promoted from the most essential area: scientific. There is no talk about how the body works at a vibrational level, at an energetic level, at an emotional level, at an atomic level, at a molecular level. We only talk about myths that suit the food industry and the pharmaceutical industry. And as cruel as he usually is, a healthy person is a lost customer. The year AIDS appeared, the medical system in the US and Europe was about to collapse: there were no patients. What a coincidence. What would happen to the millions of doctors and health personnel around the planet if there were no sick people? What would become of the surgeons? Just think how many millions and millions and millions of dollars medical centers would lose without treatments such as chemotherapy. How much does the health system earn per Cancer patient... it is horrible to have to think like that, but numbers and common sense don't lie. So, with the current crisis, based on the interest of collapsing the current economic model, debt increases, the Chinese, medical and pharmaceutical business increases (and its agreements with governments), and experts who want to speak are censored. However, Koch's postulates are ignored. Hamer's principles are ignored – if modern medical students are taught at all.

Let's talk about coronavirus. These are pathogenic agents present in animals, since who knows when. Certain animals contract this virus in a specific category. Among them there are birds, mammals and humans. Yes, it seems that getting sick from coronavirus is not something new. What is new is that "something" that they have also called coronavirus, and that according to certain experts, is not easy to transmit: it is unlikely to cause infections, except in very complex conditions. Whether a coronavirus kills is just as complex. Just these days I shared a meme that showed the ridiculousness that the probability of an asteroid colliding with the Earth is 0.042%, while the probability of dying from "COVID" is 0.026%, that is, half, so now It was time for you to buy a helmet instead of a mask. A conventional coronavirus can cause respiratory and digestive diseases, which has a solution. How is he going to kill you? Either it is a chimera, or other conditions cause you to get very sick. If not, it does not make sense. A certain type of coronavirus occurs in humans, which causes the common cold, bronchitis and other types of pneumonia, Middle East respiratory syndrome (MERS) or severe respiratory syndrome (SARS). But if the issue is breathing, let's start by giving anticoagulants and anti-inflammatories for the lungs. No! They prohibit that. Because? Because you cut the drama, the movie ends. If the person arrives with the flu or pneumonia and you give them a pill and they come home healthy, how does the government, the medical system, the pharmaceutical industry, Chinese industries, social security or health personnel benefit?

Who benefits from having a marijuana infusion relieve your muscle spasms? To you. But who does it harm? Who benefits from using chlorine dioxide? To you, but who does it harm? Of the more than 30 coronaviruses officially identified, 3 or 4 are those that cause "infections" in humans. But what is an infection? A strange people in the organism. Well, if it is foreign, the body has its well-organized system to repel it if it does not suit it. What is acquired immunodeficiency syndrome? The so-called AIDS, which is said to consist of the immune system not doing what it should do. However, it does not kill you, but rather it allows whatever enters your body to do so. We have a body that is only affected if our mind allows it to be affected. If she determines it, anything will be a funnel or channel for an experience, since illness is a form of experience, an exercise in learning and forgiveness. So they tell us that the SARS-CoV type coronavirus is, along with MHV (mouse hepatitis virus), known as betacoronavirus (previously defined as betacoronavirus group 2 (CoV-2)). This, and the alphacoronavirus, would have the bat friend as a host. So, scientists maintain that there are 7 strains of related coronaviruses: human coronavirus 229E, NL63, OC43 and HKU1 (MERS-CoV), SARS-CoV, MERS (Eastern respiratory syndrome) and the famous SARS-CoV-2, which covid-19 is attributed to it. Curiously, if people with power wanted to make a population sick, without leaving traces, they would use this type of virus, which has been studied, precisely in relation to its reaction in humans, and at first glance does not raise suspicions.

When the matter of the coronavirus that infected the Chinese came out, it was known that the first cases that were said to have occurred had no relationship with the Wuhan seafood market. But the strategy of the invisible enemy has been widely disseminated for the globalists to achieve their ends. This strategy is notorious in many cases when someone wants a goal and wants to find an excuse that allows them to achieve it. In these times the invisible enemy is "the bug", just as "terrorism" was the last 30 years – especially the last 20, with the trigger of "extremist attacks" and such "weapons of mass destruction" –.

Although, there is a great mythology around what society calls "viruses" and the idea of "diseases". Since the works of Sigmund Freud and his friend Carl Gustav Jung, much progress has been made in the analysis of the mind and its relationship with biological behavior. The "psychosomatic" aspect (psycho = mind; soma = body) plays a fundamental role in the body's reactions, and yet it is not the only one. The mind not only operates on the organism but on the "quantum space" and its "field of possibilities-probabilities", which is increasingly accepted, integrated, taught and expanded by quantum physics. This means that everything that happens to a person, whether in the body or in their environment, and even in their life, has its genesis in their mind.

The mythology of viruses is a mixture of scientific elements of biology and chemistry in a soup lacking certain essential seasonings and vegetables to give it the correct flavor, or meaning. Matter cannot be separated from the psyche, since they are strictly dependent. Nothing happens in matter that does not have its functional motor in the non-physical area, that is, psychic. The mind has four levels, three of which are the most popular or accepted in psychology: the conscious area, the subconscious and the unconscious. There is another one: the superconscious. In analogy with these 3 conventional sections there are the 3 brain areas of response and memory, and there are also the 3 levels of reception and reaction. We would have to go to Hamer's Laws and the multiple studies carried out in the field of neuropsychology, neuroemotion and psychosomatic activity, and the purpose of this book is not that. However, I will only address this matter in a cursory and superficial way, defining in the introduction of this chapter the mechanisms by which a person is really healthy or sick. It should be understood that this science is not expressly limited to the case of the body, but, as

I have said, is perennial to all existential development. It could be said that a person's destiny is conditioned in the mind, which includes both their goals in life and the experiences they live. In other words, if you get sick, it's because you had to get sick; If you were rich, it is because you had to be rich; If you suffered abuse, it is because you had to suffer abuse. However, I will explain what is behind this because I know that there will be several questions that you are seriously asking yourself at this moment regarding these statements.

In Kabalah methods we teach that there are two realities: the spiritual and the material. The material is embedded within the spiritual. By spiritual I mean that it is not based on the laws of matter nor does it have a material form or is measured by physical instruments. To give an example, we know that there are laws of the universe due to the behavior of phenomena, but we cannot put them in a box or review them like a laboratory mouse. This universe is a mental holographic projection within an Infinite Collective Mind (see my book, 'In the Beginning God Created a Hologram'), and in it there is identical behavior between the human brain and the cosmos, when we see the neural network and synaptic impulses. Communication within the brain is immediate, and acts instantly on the body's cells. The same thing happens in this universe. Everything is interconnected. Everything belonging to the etheric and psychic realm is not dominated by time or space. You will think, "well, matter is." The truth is that no, it is a mere perception. It is that "perception" of the mind that makes it "seem" that things are what they are, or that phenomena are arbitrary, pragmatic in time and immovable.

The mind is distributed in fields, in the same analogous way that molecular structures are distributed in groups. If we observe what exists, we see objects composed of tissue structures and microscopic beings. What are they? In the long run, molecules. These are what we call "living organisms". But whether "living" (biological) or "inert", they are all molecular structures assembling fields in space: forms (holograms). And what are molecular structures? Complexes formed based on unions of atoms. And when I say "unions" we have to consider that in reality nothing in the cosmos is truly united. Everything is kept "connected" by energy fields called "magnetism". Now, what are atoms? Electric charges". They are energy charges, whether positive or negative. And what is a positive or negative charge? A magnetic force of attraction or repulsion. And what is a magnetic force? A polarity fluctuating energy principle. And what is that? Strictly speaking, "something" that "consciously" does something similar to "pushing" magnetic energy to both sides of the same thing, creating a principle of polarity. And what is that "something"? Awareness. That consciousness operates in the universe just as a brain operates in the body. The "nervous system" of the body, operated through "impulses" is the same as consciousness operating in infinite space through an "invisible energy" called VIBRATION. This vibration produces a wave field oscillation that creates energy at its peak lengths, and these "sparks" travel as particles of consciousness or information such as brain information in the nervous system. This "information" is the basis of light, and is known as a photon.

Having made this introduction as clarifying as possible, I now move on to explain what the mind is like. Just like the example I have given about atoms, so is the mind. All visible and invisible matter is a network of atomic structures that are simply fields magnetized by an Infinite Mind. Our mind is the same. What we call "I" is a mind (similar to the atom), part of another structure of minds (similar to molecules), called 'Collective Mind'. This Collective Mind can vary in its breadth depending on the network of consciousnesses that make it up. Consciousness retreats into the universe in sections of different vibrational scales. We see the most elementary scale in "inert" matter, a more developed (conscious) level in plants, and so on, passing through trees to various animals. When we reach the human being we find another higher level of consciousness, however, a higher level of vibration. At first glance, the mineral, plant-animal and human kingdoms seem equally "solid". That's right... at first glance. Likewise, there are other states of higher vibration that escape the retentive and retention capacity of our senses of this density-dimension. Ergo, we are individualized consciousnesses wrapped in a vibration field relative to our state of consciousness. All the highest parts of Infinite Consciousness are organized as "souls", "angels" or "thought-forms". These "spiritual" bodies have an envelope that in certain dimensions requires another envelope or clothing: body. The coating of the spiritual being requires a whole gear to function, and this is where your consciousness links the "matter" of that state with that of your spirit: that is the secular mind.

Consciousness is a Mind. Just as there are individualized consciousnesses, there are minds that are part of the framework of consciousness. So you have your mind and I have mine, but both are connected, just as neurons are through synapses (connection and communication without physical contact). A network of consciousnesses-souls-minds create a Social Consciousness, a Racial Consciousness and a Planetary Consciousness. At the scale you want to take it, the framework expands. That is why it is true when it has been said that "we are all one." Your mind is yours, but it is part of a 1) Social, 2) Racial, 3) Collective, 4) Planetary, 5) Galactic, 6) Universal and 7) Infinite Mind. It depends on the level and proportion we are talking about. Just as we are connected as souls, as minds, as consciousness, we are connected in the fabric of the probabilities-possibilities of the space-time, and time-space continuum. The Infinite Mind created the various universes, their dimensions, planes, worlds, laws, beings and races, as well as the "script" of their existence. I have already talked a lot about this in conferences, webinars, articles and books, but what I want to incorporate here is the understanding that there is a pre-established destiny or script, and our existence develops according to it.

Everything was created by Consciousness, the Infinite Mind, and was co-created by the other portions of it as they became aware of themselves. This is the law of creation. The so-called 'Law of Attraction' follows 3 principles: 1. Every object attracts that which resembles itself; 2. What I think about and what I believe in, or what I hope for, is; 3. I am what I am and I am willing for others to be what they are. We can call these 3: Law of Attraction, Science of Deliberate Creation and Art of Allowing (basic principle of Taoism and Buddhism, known as 'principle of non-intervention': doing is not doing). We see that the Mind creates automatically, and that everything responds to the magnetism of thoughts. This is nothing other than intelligent energy operating throughout the Infinite, which is, in turn, "intelligent." You may be wondering if this is indeed the case, how come you don't have everything you want. Well, there are 2 reasons: time and mind distortions. Where space and time exist, phenomena are conditioned to a "process" in "time." This only accelerates or disappears when a necessary experience has been integrated. This is called 'miracle'. Regarding the "distortions" of the mind, we speak of "programs" acquired from ancestors, from previous incarnations, from the fetal process, from childhood or from traumas already in adulthood (strong emotional impacts).

The Mind operates in the script according to its Higher Self, or Supraconscious aspect, but at the level of form and time-space the experiences are lived according to the acquired programs. Everything is stored in memory unconsciously, subconsciously or consciously. In this way, the "system of beliefs and convictions" is built, which is an extension of the "thought system", our ideas about things and existence. However, 3 energetic forces drive the magnetism that attracts or repels: Beliefs, Emotions and Thoughts. They in turn develop the projections that occur in our lives respecting the "hermetic principles" (Laws of Hermes), which are the mechanisms of the script or destiny of the universe. Now, the Mind communicates with the body through 7 light channels that you may have heard of by the name of "chacras", which are the channels of the individual's consciousness. In the development of the growth of the being (as an evolving consciousness) the Mind maintains a connection with the experience "outside of time", that is, it obeys the particular script (Dharma), collective (plan of Redemption) and general (Destiny of the Universe), all of which enter the so-called 'Script of the Holy Spirit', whose basis is the detachment of the ego to return to the Source. You can see the Mind as a biomagnetic field in a toroidal shape (whose color has been called 'Aura') that sends relays to the brain and this to the organs.

But the Mind not only sends relays to the brain, it does so to its field of possibilities-probabilities of quantum reality or space of experiences. This is how everything you do, think, feel and believe magnetizes your environment and your body. So think at this moment if it is plausible that a "bug" could bite you, or enter your body and make you sick. If your mind magnetizes the disease, and it is arranged in the script of your personal growth, it will arrive with a mosquito, with waves from an antenna, with the infection of an unsterilized cut, with a bacteria in the water or with cancer. Essentially, your subconscious will put together the movie for this to happen, and it will use the means at its disposal that require the least energy to expend. If society believes in a deadly virus, it will be easier for your mind to use that argument as a way to lead you to the experience of a serious health process. In other circumstances it will create another scenario, but it will always look for the simplest, which is usually what is socially most likely to be thought of: a war, an epidemic, famine, robberies, rapes... it depends on what most attracts/ creates a social conscience. Clearly Yeshua said that <<it is not what enters... that contaminates>> the being, but <<what comes out>> of his mind, what is inside, in his beliefs, emotions and thoughts.

Therefore, what is said about viruses is mythology. Not only because misfortunes, illnesses, ailments or the moment of death are conditioned by our Mind and the script of destiny, but because the conception of viruses, in itself, is incorrect. And it is incorrect partly because the body itself is immune to viruses, and partly because such viruses are incapable of fighting an organism without the help of favorable conditions. If your blood pH is high (alkaline) no virus will be able to have any effect on you. Now imagine what your mental state is like: your emotions and thoughts. If they are high and energetic, your body is "enlightened," so to speak, and nothing can affect it. However, the component of "beliefs" is the treacherous one here, because we have countless stories stuck in our "heads," and until they are reviewed and modified, they are the ones that will direct the circumstances that arise in our lives. and that includes pathologies. Now understand why it is so important for the elite to CONVINCE the population about the existence of a "virus" and its supposed mortality-lethality. If people do not believe the

story, the story does not work, but when society believes it –
and they believe it en masse – it lowers their vibratory state and
also induces their body to predispose itself to being affected. Of
course, many do not fall for the hoax, but not because they do
not believe in "the bug," but because they do not have repressed
feelings of guilt. It is because we feel guilty "since Adam and Eve",
that we want to be "punished", and our subconscious attracts
"whatever" that expiates that supposed guilt.

The unconscious feeling of guilt has been with us since the
dawn of humanity. Whether you are religious or not, it is
memorized in your DNA, it is hidden in the unconscious of
your mind, it is breathed in the air of society. It is because of
this feeling of unconscious guilt that pain, suffering, illnesses,
accidents and so-called death exist: we attract it. As long as we
do not forgive ourselves, we cannot get out of that vicious circle.
As long as we do not understand that the beings of this universe
feel guilty for something that is not real, they will continue to
experience the consequences of a separate mind, dualism will
continue to prevail. You are not guilty of anything. You are not
of what happened thousands or millions of years ago, nor are
you of now, nor is it the fault of your parents or your neighbors,
teachers or government. It's all part of the Holy Spirit's script
in line with your own Higher Self, which chooses the most
important experiences that will make you bring out the best
in you, forgive yourself (because you are holy and innocent
(without guilt)), become the best version of yourself. yourself
and perfect yourself in love. That is the objective of the script, the
culmination of which is to return to the Source: the ONE.

MASSIVE DESTRUCTION WEAPONS

What are real viruses? Those created in the laboratory. What
are the lethal ones? The mental and psychological ones. Nothing
outside the being can harm the body. If something happens to

our body, our psyche or our environment, its trigger and fuel is ALWAYS in our mind: the source of all things. For this reason the elite uses mind control technology to reach all areas where the sr can be harmed. Damage the mind and it will damage the being, damage the body and it will regenerate (as long as the mind is balanced and upright), or it will simply be immune to attacks. The stronger the psychological attack, the deeper the structure of the being will be disrupted, even creating alter egos (misnamed 'multiple personality syndrome'). This is achieved through a combination of various elements, especially shock (physical pain).

We see examples of the most powerful models of mental control over living beings in the area of sexual harassment, sodomizing another person. Millions of children who suffer sexual abuse, mostly in elite pedophile networks, are victims of mind control and "empty vessels." We are adults, so we have to say things openly, as they are. The "adult entertainment" industry presents images to weaken mental and psychic strength, as well as to wear down the Ki of the being and reduce the micronutrients of the marrow. This is also seen with brothels and prostitution, white slavery, homosexuality and other unnatural sexual activities, from promiscuity itself. This is extensive to address but if you read 'Naked Sex' (2018) you already know what I'm talking about. Dictators like Adolf Hitler and Francisco Franco banned pornography, and that is strange for tyrants. Ironically they considered these as elements of social and psychological degradation. Israel, for its part, used the secret service to introduce pornography into Muslim countries, for exactly the same reason: to weaken their minds. Israel has acquired the psychology and cunning to weaken the psyche and energy of its enemies. However, pornography responds to archetypes and conceptualizations of the subconscious mind, but since the majority is a victim of them, it achieves its effect on them, who have a weak mind and are prone to projecting their energy outside, in images, in the illusion of projections of matter.

In the "adult entertainment industry" there is little "entertainment." It is actually a mass mind control network. Those who are filmed are prostitutes and studs who come from traumatic experiences, abandonment, sexual abuse, mistreatment, father absence, drug addiction or, in the best of cases, serious financial debts that lead them to this. Many of those who are in that world are actually being sexually abused, going so far as to sodomize their victim in horrendous ways, but those images are retouched, or the actors are threatened with not paying them if they do not finish the shoot. Some lose consciousness in the middle of filming due to the physical pain inflicted on their body, even though the majority enter the scene drugged or, in the best of cases, intoxicated, to resist the treatment to which they are subjected. This is the part that is seen of how psychologically affected people feed back on this state and present this type of sex as "entertainment". The mind that does not see it with these eyes believes that this is normal for pleasure and passionate games. This is the visible part of a mind control structure. The saddest is what is done to babies and children, especially orphans and kidnapped people. Those who are stronger are not physically touched but are used for programs like Manequin, where mostly Latino children are part of projects to develop extrasensory abilities for military purposes. Those who do not achieve this are used as dolls of relief and satisfaction for the most powerful people on the planet.

Those children are dead in life. Many people who have been through similar situations and/or physical, psychological and/or verbal abuse and the same antecedents mentioned above are dead in life, ending up accepting to live among some cardboard, under a bridge and digging for resources in containers and garbage bags. Mind control is the most malevolent machinery ever designed. For decades it has been cleverly used in the "children's industry" of cartoons and 3D animation. Disney has had to pay high fines decades ago after being found guilty in US courts for putting subliminal sexual messages in its films. Clearly the company, cleaning up its reputation, has paid for all legal controversy in this regard to disappear from the internet. However, this has been well known for a long time and these are scenes that cannot be hidden. We grew up watching them. But whether it is Disney, Warner, Nickelodeon, Cartoon Network or any of its affiliates or subsidized companies, they have promoted sexual secrecy, feminist tendencies, values of social degradation, "gender" ideology, destruction of marriage, degradation of the home, family rebellion, apathy. family, childhood ignorance, social ignorance, vanity, idolatry, economic materialism and the cult of the very "industry" that indoctrinates them. You might wonder, how does doing this benefit these companies? All of them are part of the corrupt, satanic and pedophile elite. Its banner is sexual degradation, a symbol of the lowest and most twisted diabolical values.

But you don't have to go that far to see how a society is brainwashed. You can use advertisements on television to make them believe that they need to buy things, which in reality they don't. You promote campaigns or social and philosophical movements that touch their main sensitive fibers and they will run after them and defend them to the death. You play with beautiful feelings like love, romance, passion, and flirting, in movies, soap operas, books, magazines, advertising spots, music videos, television series, radio programs and songs. You disguise sexual courtship with the label of 'LOVE', and from there true love is confused with sexual passion. The love of a parent for a child no longer makes sense, because the love of an adult for a minor translates into sexual desire, into intercourse. Exactly, that is one of the strategies of 'gender ideology' and the 'LGTBAEIOU movement...', which will soon include the 'P' (pedophilia), because there is no age for "love". So altruism, selflessness, empathy, serving others, and natural affection are defined as "chemical reactions." On the other hand, the alteration of neuropeptides, disorders and insecurities, repressed emotions and abuse traumas are described as love. There is no longer love in marriage, home, family, friends, neighbors or divinity, because "sexual passion" - and even "post-traumatic psychological disorder" - is replaced by the sacred word, love.

<u>THE HISTORY OF VIRUSES</u>

Continuing with the scientific documentation of these matters, I turn to Sayer Ji, whose publication is shared on GreenMedInfo LLC, August 24, 2020. Here he maintains: Innovative research indicates that most of what is believed about the supposed properties deadly viruses like the flu, in fact, is not based on evidence, but on a myth. Germ theory is an immensely powerful force on this planet, affecting everyday interactions from a handshake, all the way to national vaccination agendas and global eradication campaigns. But what if there has not yet been fundamental research into what exactly these 'pathogens' are, how they infect us? What if much of what is assumed and believed about the danger of microbes, particularly viruses, has been completely undermined in light of radical new discoveries in microbiology? Some of our readers already know that in my previous writings I discuss why the concept of "germs as our enemies" has been decimated by the relatively recent discovery of the microbiome. For more detailed information on this topic, read my previous article, "How the Microbiome Destroyed Ego, Vaccine Politics, and the Patriarchy." You can also read 'Profound virome implications for human health and autoimmunity', to better understand how viruses are truly beneficial for mammalian health.

In this article I will take a less philosophical approach and focus on influenza as a more concrete example of the Copernican paradigm shift in biomedicine and life sciences that we are all immersed in today, even if the medical establishment still has We have to recognize it (a topic I cover extensively in my book 'REGENERATE: Unlocking Your Body's Radical Resilience through the New Biology'). Deadly flu virus: vaccinate or die? The hyperbolic way health policymakers and media pundits talk about it today, the flu virus (or COVID-19) is an inexorably lethal force (note: viruses are obligate parasites, in worst case scenario, with no internal driving force to actively "infect" others), against which all citizens, of all ages 6 months and older, need the annual influenza vaccine to protect themselves, lest (are said) to face deadly consequences. Worse still, those who have religious or philosophical objections, or who consciously oppose vaccination, are known for harming others by denying them herd immunity (a concept that has been completely debunked by a study careful of the evidence, or lack thereof)). For example, in an interview, Bill Gates tells Sanjay Gupta that he believes that those who do not vaccinate "kill children."

But what if I told you that there isn't even a "flu virus," in the sense of a monolithic disease vector that exists outside of us, conceived as is the predator-prey relationship? First, consider that the highly authoritative Cochrane Collaboration recognizes that there are many different influenza viruses that are not, in fact, influenza A, against which influenza vaccines are directed, but which may nonetheless contribute to identical symptoms. to those attributed to influenza A: "More than 200 viruses cause influenza and influenza-like illnesses that produce the same symptoms (fever, headache, aches and pains, cough, and runny nose). Without laboratory tests, doctors cannot differentiate the two illnesses. Both last for days and rarely lead to death or serious illness. At best, vaccines could be effective only against influenza A and B, which account for about 10% of all circulating viruses". (Source: Cochrane Abstracts)." [Emphasis added] This creates a picture of complexity that powerfully undermines health policies that presuppose that vaccination equates to bona fide immunity and, by implication, requires the herd to collectively participate in the ritual. of mass vaccination campaigns as a matter of life or death social necessity.

Even using the word "immunization" to describe vaccination is very misleading. The moment the word is used, it already presupposes efficacy and makes it seem like non-vaccinators are anti-immunity, rather than what they really are: pro-immunity (via clean air, food, water, and sunlight)., but reluctant to subject themselves or their healthy children to "inevitably unsafe" medical procedures with only theoretical benefits. Why doesn't the flu virus exist (as we were told)? But the topic becomes even more interesting when we consider the findings of a 2015 study titled "Conserved and host-specific features of influenza virion architecture." This was the first study to plumb the molecular depths of what the influenza virus is actually made of. Surprisingly, given the long history of vaccine use and promotion, full characterization of the proteins they contain and where they are derived from has never been done before. It is difficult to understand how we invest billions of dollars annually in influenza vaccines and how we have created a global campaign to counter a viral enemy, the basic components of which were not even known until a few years ago. However, it is true.

The study's abstract begins with this highly provocative line: "Viruses use virions to disseminate between hosts, and therefore virion composition is the primary determinant of viral transmissibility and immunogenicity." [Emphasis added] Virions are also known as "viral particles" and are the means by which viral nucleic acids can move and "infect" living organisms. Without the viral particle (taxi) to carry the virus DNA (passenger), it would be harmless; In fact, viruses are often described as existing somewhere between living and inanimate objects for this reason: they do not produce their own energy nor are they transmissible without a living host. And so, in this first line, the authors make clear that the composition of the virion is also the main determinant of how or if a virus is infectious (transmitted) and what effects it will have on the immune system of the infected host. Influenza viral particles... This distinction is important because we often think of viruses simply as pathogenic strands of DNA or RNA. The irony, of course, is that the very things to which we attribute so much lethality, viral nucleic acids, are not even alive and cannot infect an organism without all the other components (proteins, lipids, extraviral nucleic acids)) that, Technically, they are not of viral origin, they participate in the process.

And so, if non-viral components are essential for the virus to cause harm, how can we continue to maintain that we are dealing with a monolithic disease entity "out there" that "infects" us, a passive victim? It is fundamentally absurd, given these findings. It also clearly undermines the incessant, let's delve into the study's findings. The next line of the summary addresses the fact with which we opened this article: namely, that there is great complexity involved at the level of profound variability in virion composition: "However, the virions of many viruses are complex and pleomorphic, which makes it difficult to analyze in detail. But this problem of great variability in the composition of the influenza virion is exactly why the study was done. They explain: "Here we address this by identifying and quantifying viral proteins with mass spectrometry, producing a complete and quantifiable model of the hundreds of viral and host-encoded proteins that make up the pleomorphic virions of the influenza virus. We demonstrate that an architecture of "Conserved influenza virions, which include substantial amounts of host proteins as well as the viral NSI protein, are made with abundant host-dependent characteristics. As a result, influenza virions produced by mammalian and avian hosts have distinct protein compositions."

In other words, they discovered that the flu virus is made up of both biological material from the host that the virus 'infects' and the viral genetic material of the virus itself. So how do we differentiate the influenza virus as completely "other"? Since it would not exist without "own" proteins, or those of other host animals such as birds or insects, this would be impossible to do with intellectual honesty intact. There is also the significant problem with the production of influenza vaccines. Currently, the human influenza vaccine antigen is produced by insects and chicken eggs. This means that virus particles extracted from these hosts would contain foreign proteins and would therefore produce different and/or unpredictable immune responses in humans than would be expected from human influenza viral particles. One possibility is that the dozens of foreign proteins found within avian influenza could theoretically produce antigens in humans that cross-react with self-structures resulting in autoimmunity. Safety testing, at present, does not test for these cross-reactions. Clearly, this discovery opens a Pandora's box of potential problems that have never been sufficiently analyzed, since it was never understood until now what "influenza" was.

Are flu viruses really "hijacked" exosomes? Finally, the study identified something even more surprising: "Finally, we observed that influenza virions share an underlying protein composition with exosomes, suggesting that influenza virions form by subverting the "production" of microvesicles. What these researchers are talking about is the discovery that virion particles share striking similarities with the naturally occurring virus-like particles that all living cells produce called exosomes. Exosomes, like many viruses (i.e. enveloped), are enclosed in a membrane and are within the 50-100 nanometer size range of viruses (20-400 nm). They also contain biologically active molecules, such as proteins and lipids, as well as information-containing molecules such as RNA, exactly or very similar to the types of content found in viral particles. When we start to look at viruses through the lens of their overlap with exosomes, which as RNA carriers are essential for regulating the expression of the vast majority of the human genome, we are beginning to understand how its function could be considered neutral as "information." Carriers, if not beneficial. Both exosomes and viruses may be responsible for communication and regulation between species or between kingdoms within the biosphere, given the way in which they can facilitate and mediate the horizontal transfer of information between organisms. Even eating a piece of fruit that contains these exosomes can alter the expression of vitally important genes within our body.

In light of this post-germ theory perspective, viruses could be described as chromosome-seeking pieces of information; is not inherently "bad," but in fact is essential for mediating the genotype/phenotype relationship within organisms, which must adapt to ever-changing environmental conditions in real time in order to survive; something that the glacial pace of genetic changes within the primary nucleotide sequences of our DNA cannot do (for example, it can take ~100,000 years for a sequence of a gene encoding a protein to change rather than seconds for the expression of a gene encoding a protein is altered by modulation through viral or exosomal RNAs). This doesn't mean they are "all good" either. Sometimes, given many conditions outside their control, their messages can present challenges or misinformation to the cells they are exposed to, which could result in a "disease symptom." These symptoms of illness are often, if not invariably, attempts by the body to self-regulate and ultimately improve and heal itself.

In other words, the virion composition of viruses appears to be the byproduct of the cell's normal exosome (also known as microvesicle) production and trafficking machinery, although it is influenced by influenza DNA. And like exosomes, viruses may be a means of extracellular communication between cells, rather than simply a pathological disease. This could explain why a growing body of research on the role of the virome in human health indicates that so-called infectious agents, including viruses such as measles, confer important health benefits. [See: The health benefits of measles and the healing power of germs]. Other researchers have made similar discoveries about the relationship between exosomes and viruses, sometimes describing viral hijacking of exosome pathways as a "Trojan horse" hypothesis. HIV may provide such an example. Concluding Remarks: The remarkably recent discovery of the host-dependent nature of influenza virus virion composition is really just the tip of an intellectual iceberg that has not yet fully emerged into the light of day, but is already there." sinking" ships; paradigm ships, if you will.

One such paradigm is that germs are enemy combatants, and that viruses do not play a critical role in our health, and should be eradicated from the Earth with medications and vaccines, if possible. This belief, however, is unsustainable. With the discovery of the indispensable role of the microbiome, and the subpopulation of viruses within it, the virome, we have entered a completely new view, based on the ecology of the body and its surroundings that are fundamentally inseparable. Ironically, the only thing the flu can kill is the germ theory itself. For an in-depth exploration of this, see the lecture below on the virome. I promise you that if you do, you will no longer be able to hold germ theory as a monolithic truth. You may even begin to understand how we might consider some viruses "our friends" and why we may need viruses much more than they need us. Source: https://www.greenmedinfo.com/blog/why-only-thing-influenza-may-kill-germ-theory [1].

100 years ago we had a world stage that went around the planet, and from which media reports rely to sell fear. Let's now look at a brief postulate from Dr. Thomas Cowan on this matter: In 1918, after the massive Spanish flu pandemic, Rudolf Steiner was asked about the possible causes. He said: "Viruses are just the excretion, the waste of cells that have been poisoned. They are pieces of DNA or RNA with other proteins that are expelled from the poisoned cells. "They are not the cause of anything." The cells are poisoned and try to clean themselves by expelling their waste that we call viruses. Different current theories consider them "exomes". Every pandemic of the last 150 years coincides with a quantum leap in the electrification of the Earth. In the fall of 1917 and 1918, radio waves were introduced around the world. When living beings are exposed to a new

---

1.   https://www.greenmedinfo.com/blog/why-only-thing-influenza-may-kill-germ-theory

electromagnetic field, they are poisoned. A few die and the rest go into a kind of hibernation, living longer but sick. Then the Second World War began and with it a new pandemic due to the introduction of radars throughout the Earth, which was completely covered by the electromagnetic fields emitted by the radars. It was the first time humanity was exposed to this.

In 1968, the Hong Kong flu occurred. It was the first time that the protective cover of the Van Allen belt - whose function is to integrate radiation coming from the Sun, Moon, Jupiter, etc. - was affected. – and distribute them to all living beings on Earth. In those days, a number of satellites were launched into space that emitted radioactive frequencies in the Van Allen belt. And six months later a new viral epidemic took place. Why viral? Because people were poisoned and, therefore, expelled toxins equivalent to viruses. It was thought to be a flu epidemic. In 1918, the Boston public health department decided to investigate contagions in epidemics. So, believe it or not, they took hundreds of people with the flu, took samples of their nasal excrescences, and injected them into healthy people. None got sick. They repeated the practice again and again, but were not able to demonstrate contagion. They did the same with horses that apparently had the Spanish flu. They put bags over their heads, so that they would sneeze inside. Then they put the bag on the heads of other horses and they did not get sick. You can read about this in a book called "The invisible rainbow" by Arthur Firstenberg. He has studied the different stages of electrification of the Earth and how, within 6 months, a new flu pandemic occurred throughout the world. And there is no other explanation.

How could it spread from Kansas to South Africa in two weeks, so that everyone has the same symptoms? In addition to that the mode of transportation (in 1918) was horse and boat.

They found no explanation: "We don't know how it occurs" was the conclusion of that test. But let's think about all these radio waves and other frequencies... that some of you have in your pants or in your hands and that can send a signal to Japan that arrives instantly. Thus, even if you do not believe that there is an electromagnetic field that interconnects the entire world in a few seconds, there is no need to discuss it; It is a fact that we experience daily. And I will finish by adding that a dramatic quantum leap has been made over the last 6 years in the electrification of the Earth. I'm sure many of you know what it is. It is called 5G and it will have 20,000 satellites emitting radiation, like those emitted by your cell phones, and they are used continuously. This is not compatible with health! Sorry to say: It is not compatible with health! It is an aspect that destructures water.

And if anyone thinks: "Well, we are not electrical beings, we are just physical matter!" So why are they going to have tests like electrocardiograms or electroencephalograms or reflex tests for drivers? Because we are electrical beings and chemicals are just the waste of those electrical impulses. And I end with a riddle: What is the first city in the world completely covered by 5G? Wuhan. Exact. So when you start to think about this: we are in an existential crisis here and now, of a magnitude never experienced. And I don't want to play at being an Old Testament prophet but this is an unprecedented event: the placing into orbit of thousands of satellites in the Earth's own protective layer. And by the way, as I wanted to say before, this relates to vaccines. This concerns me because a year ago I had a patient in great shape who practiced surfing. He was an electrician-electronic technician who installed Wi-Fi systems for very rich people (this profession has a high mortality rate). Despite everything, he was fine; But one day he broke his arm and had to put a metal plate on it. Three months later, he couldn't get out of bed. He had arrhythmia and total exhaustion. Our functional stability depends on the amount of metal we have in the body, as well as the quality of the water in our cells.

Therefore, if they start injecting aluminum into people, they become receptors that absorb electromagnetic fields in an amplified way. And this is a perfect storm that can explain the type of ailments that our species experiences today. I want to end with a quote from Rudolf Steiner from 1917: "It was a different time. In the era when there was no electric current, when the air was not subject to electrical influences (we are talking about 1917) it was easier to be human. For this reason, in order to be fully human today, it is necessary to develop much stronger spiritual capacities, stay in harmony and thus overcome them, remember we are omnipotent beings of light, connect to your divine origin. Namaste." Psdt: there are videos on YouTube where they show tips on how to avoid wireless radiation, I hope all this helps you. But waves are one thing and chimeras are another. If you combine both, you have a deadly cocktail. In that order of things, there are reports of Barack Obama, Melinda Gates and Anthony Fauci visiting the Wuhan virus experimentation laboratory in 2015. The creation of chimeras has been in the hands of the US for decades. They have combined the technological changes of wave paradigms with the introduction of more or less lethal chimeras.

On December 14, 2020, the following article was published – by Anna von Reitz – which stated that Australia has become the first country in the world to scrap a $750 million Covid-19 vaccine project, after that volunteers in the tests tested positive for HIV, which according to the mass media are cases of "false positives." However, the reality is that the vaccine does contain fragments of HIV and more, as American judge Anna von Reitz explains. In fact, it has been shown that the "novel" coronavirus 19 that has the world upside down has 4 HIV1 subunits in its genome. If one investigates the virology and genetic manipulation involved in the development and the patentability and copyright of the "functional gain" that was the subject of the development of the Covid-19 virus, it is evident that the increase in infection rates was achieved using the same sequences that promote HIV infection. That was exactly Anthony Fauci's area of study and experience. And through his position at the NIH he funded research in Wuhan, China. Oh my God. The monsters among us took the common cold virus and "modified" it by adding fragments of HIV, to make it more infectious. And then, of course, any vaccine also has to have HIV fragments in it, to sensitize the victim's immune system.

The crazy thing about vaccines is that you inject yourself with "dead" copies of a bacteria or virus to provoke an immune response, which will then be ready to attack the real thing. However, since a virus is already dead, any vaccine for a virus is actually a pre-infection by a false copy of the same virus. You are actually getting infected in the hopes of building a stronger immune reaction... and in this case, the vaccine virus contains HIV sequences. Even the Silly Bunnies acting as United Nations Administrators of AUSTRALIA had enough sense to stand down and consider responsibility for the forced vaccination of millions of people with an HIV-containing vaccine (in Brazil, to say the least). , injections were recently forced on "risk groups", and what is that? What Hitler would define as the undesirable elements of the population: prisoners, the elderly and the destitute). The known and public danger of such idiocy is obvious and needs no further explanation. It's an indie disaster in the making, but wait, the genetic engineers responsible for developing these heinous new patented inventions are squealing like pigs. And there is more. Not only will people naturally "test positive" for HIV after being vaccinated, but there are other "treats" incorporated into this cocktail of poisons and gene fragments, and they are designed to interfere with the coding of proteins necessary to develop an infection. healthy placenta. Women who are injected with this will no longer be able to have children. They will undergo an abortion after an abortion after an abortion, since the placenta does not fully form.

You may be wondering, as I am, how come these clearly criminal patents have been allowed, and why, exactly, are people like Anthony Fauci and Bill Gates still walking around free? That's a great question that deserves an answer. And the answer is that they are being protected by the United Nations and UN CORP—the hypocrites who call themselves defenders of "peace," although in reality they are waging war against their favorite targets: babies and ignorant women. Just as the Bible says about the end of times, the United Nations will say "peace, peace" but there will be no peace, because these insane criminals are hypocrites as well as greedy and praying. We Americans, and the US State Assemblies, have business to settle with the US Patent and Trademark Office (USPTO) — Big Business. Unpleasant business. It is our right to extract the patents and destroy the corporations that have done this to profit, and it is our right to punish the SERCO patent officials and employees and agents responsible for this outrage against humanity. Sources: Business Insider — Australia abandons vaccine attempt, after the shot wrongly gave some people positive HIV test results. Anna Von Reitz / Paul Stramer LincolnCounty Watch — Yes, the Vaccine Contains Fragments of HIV and More: https://www.mentealternativa.com/si-la-vacuna-contiene-fragmentos-de-vih-y-mas-australia-   abandon-your-project/ [2].

Let's now go to another report, in this case by Anna Von Reitz, titled 'Welcome to the Boer War', about Antony Fauci and Glycoprotein 120, where we return with the deceptions, that man – the highest paid official in the United States – and the CDC (mostly owned by Bill Gates): First of all, consider these facts: the CDC, i.e. the Center for Disease Control, is a private organization in the vaccine manufacturing business. And, Dr. Anthony Fauci, the same CDC expert who appeared on camera with President Trump, and his cohort, Dr. Birx, have been working on the HIV culprit glycoprotein 120 that has accelerated this pandemic since 1986. No one knows more about HIV glycoprotein 120 than Dr. Fauci. And no one will benefit more financially from this pandemic than Dr. Fauci and the CDC, except perhaps Bill Gates. In the words of my friend, Noonie Bomblast, "Coo-ee Bono." When this whole mess started, I wrote articles about the sensitivity of people who suffer from porphyria to electromagnetic radiation, and how this is caused by the radiofrequency sensitivity of the entire class of pigmented proteins known as porphyrins that are a fundamentally important part of hemoglobin. SARS viruses are also known to be sensitive to EM radiofrequency.

In light of the 5G flood in Wuhan, China, it all seemed like too much of a coincidence that we would see patients die from what appeared to be "altitude sickness" -—hypoxia -—also known as oxygen deprivation -—and was. SARS is an acronym with a double meaning like ESF. It may mean "Severe Acute Respiratory Syndrome" or alternatively it may represent "Sensitivity to Specific Absorption Range." Now add the word "Virus" and it will describe the same kind of virus in two different ways: one, the effect of the virus, and the other, the

---

2.   https://www.mentealternativa.com/si-la-vacuna-contiene-fragmentos-de-vih-y-mas-australia-abandona-su-proyecto/

character of the virus. All SARS viruses are radiosensitive and so are the porphyrin rings that act as cages enclosing the iron atoms that form the "Heme" group in hemoglobin. In Covid-19, the corona virus of the SARS family attaches to the porphyrin ring and releases the iron atom of the Heme Group into the bloodstream. This does two things: (1) it cripples hemoglobin's ability to transport oxygen throughout the body, causing oxygen deprivation, clinical hypoxia; (2) causes iron poisoning of the bloodstream, which in turn drives the bone marrow into hyperdrive to produce new hemoglobin to capture loose iron and carry out its oxygen-carrying functions.

This is how Covid 19 patients die, deprived of oxygen like a fish out of water, drowning in their own blood. Now it's your turn, Dr. Fauci. And Bill Gates too. This all started during the Boer War, when one of the Rothschilds, Lord Pirbright, took advantage of this new science of virology, and what else? A weapon of war, which he turned against the hapless Boers, the Dutch farmers who colonized South Africa. This is also where the concentration camps began. Nazism was not first practiced by the Germans. He was born in Westminster. And that is where it must end as well. Perhaps with a real atomic bomb and the world's exposure of every little detail since 1840, when England was sold to the House of Wettin? That's why and how the Pirbright Institute is involved in this current pandemic, and so is the Wellcome Trust. In 1986, Dr. Fauci and Dr. Birx, his colleague at the privately run and funded CDC, began working on HIV glycoprotein 120. Glycoprotein 120 coats the HIV virus, like a chocolate-coated pill, instead of recognizing and rejecting it completely. This glycoprotein 120 coating gives the virus easy access to begin proliferating, and the right radiofrequency kicks that proliferation into overdrive.

It takes 885 pairs of precisely sequenced amino acids to encode the production of glycoprotein 120. Read that -—there is no way in hell that the presence of HIV glycoprotein 120 would simply "appear spontaneously" in a coronavirus. It was deliberately designed in the corona virus. And who better to design it than world-renowned experts: Dr. Fauci and Dr. Birx? If they didn't do it directly, they helped and assisted those who did: Bill Gates, the Pirbright Institute, the Wellcome Trust, DARPA, all the usual DIA corporate and Nazi eugenicist social engineering suspects. And for what? To reduce the population and thus avoid paying the debts these people have, collect the victim's life insurance and make a lot of money for themselves and their cronies by selling vaccines mixed with poisons and RFID chips. It's time to round them up and try them under the Code of Military Justice and hang them all.

This afternoon, I received a threat from them, saying that they will use STUXNET and cause a series of nuclear explosions. I responded that any such action on his part will result in the immediate worldwide release of the entire USB Receipt Book, all 13 parts, and the Kill Order to eradicate all members of the thirteen bloodline families. Including all the bastards we can track. Once and for all, zum Ende. It sucks to be on the receiving end. Source: http://www.paulstramer.net/2020/04/welcome-to-boer-war-antony-fauci-and.html [3]. Now I will share another report, titled, 'The flu kills more than the COVID-19 coronavirus to date', published a year ago (February 1, 2020), Mario Viciosa.

The COVID-2019 coronavirus outbreak has coincided with the epidemiological peaks of influenza in the northern hemisphere, because in reality the flu has been supplanted, like

---

3.   http://www.paulstramer.net/2020/04/welcome-to-boer-war-antony-fauci-and.html

many other pathologies, and slowly more and more things are labeled as covid. The most common types of flu (flu A, in Spain) leave more deaths globally than the coronavirus, waiting to see its behavior in the coming weeks. According to Marta López, researcher at the National Center for Biotechnology (CSIC), "the problem with the flu virus is that it infects many people. It can reach 20% of the world's population, which is why it causes many more deaths," says the doctor who did her thesis in Spain studying the SARS coronavirus and worked in the US, unraveling the flu. According to the infectious diseases specialist and researcher at the Barcelona Institute for Global Health (ISGlobal), Oriol Mitjà, he believes that the new coronavirus has caused alarm because it is new and not because it is serious, since this virus "is very mild and there is no "risk for the entire population," according to statements collected by Efe on February 13. [The Johns Hopkins CSSE Institute published an article on "'Fictional' increase in new cases with the new counting system"].

The SARS-Cov2 coronavirus and the influenza (flu) virus are different. Not only because of its genetic characteristics. The first is new and the second is an old acquaintance, the cause of pandemics, and whose strains can coexist every year, making it almost impossible to eradicate. But we compare them because the syndromes they produce may be similar. And because, although SARS-2 is genetically very similar to SARS-1, its impact and mortality are clearly different. The symptoms of COVID-19 are generally similar to those of this common flu illness or a cold, accompanied by fever and fatigue, dry cough and difficulty breathing. More than 95% of people who get sick recover. Although the flu usually affects part of the body's muscles and, unlike flu symptoms, it does not seem to usually cause severe sore throat or diarrhea. But it can lead to pneumonia. Another striking element: it seems that children under 10 years of age rarely present symptoms, despite having been infected by this new SARS-Cov2 coronavirus, unlike what happens with the common flu. There are no deaths in that population section.

Since the beginning of the year, Spain has emerged from its eighth week of intense flu, saying goodbye to the epidemic. Five flu outbreaks have been reported in three autonomous communities. In all of them, the type A virus was identified, in three of the outbreaks, the same as that of the 2019 pandemic. In recent weeks, type B has prevailed. Three of them occurred in health institutions, and the other two in geriatrics. The median age of affected patients is 62 years in health institutions and 88 years in nursing homes. The cumulative hospitalization rate of patients with confirmed flu has fallen to 12.2 cases per 100,000 inhabitants. The highest proportion is recorded in the 64 year old group (40%), followed by the 15 to 64 year old group (35%). "One of the influenza A viruses that we have now is derived from the 2009 flu that led to a pandemic," says Marta López. That is to say, neither that one nor this one were necessarily fatal. And some studies focused on influenza A in 2009 gave really low lethality figures (deaths among infected people).

What are people really dying from with the flu? According to the latest report from the Influenza Surveillance System in Spain, the majority of people who die in our country, admitted and infected by the flu virus, die with the following risk factors. In adults, the most prevalent are:

- Chronic cardiovascular disease (32%)
- Chronic lung disease (26%)
- Diabetes (26%)

In those under 15 years of age:

- Chronic lung disease (7%)

- Chronic cardiovascular disease (3%)
- Chronic kidney disease with immunodeficiency (2%).

Deaths among the population with previous illnesses in the case of the new coronavirus are similar. Lethality, technically, differs from mortality, a term that is usually applied to people who die from one or more diseases in the total population. In this sense, it will be necessary to attend to the development of a disease, COVID-19, for which there is no specific treatment or vaccine, at the moment. Since the beginning of the season, the fatality rate among serious cases hospitalized with flu is 13%, with 79% of cases concentrated in those over 64 years of age, according to the National Flu Surveillance System. In the case of the coronavirus that causes COVID-19, the lethality in severe cases is similar in hospitals in China. The WHO has indicated that about 10% of those who develop severe pneumonia from the coronavirus die. The latest data indicate that 81% of confirmed cases are mild. To compare (which is difficult) with other viruses, in the flu this February it is at 13%. Ebola has a fatality rate of around 40 to 50%. That is to say, the seasonal flu is not particularly deadly for the population as a whole, nor does the new coronavirus seem to be at the moment. But in absolute terms, things change.

The figure is somewhat higher than that of seasonal flu, although this varies depending on where and when it is measured. However, hospitalized flus that lead to complications – especially in the elderly population or those with immune problems – do have a high lethality, which increases in populations with limited resources or in overwhelmed hospitals. A pandemic, "with a fatality rate of 2%, already gives us a significant number of deaths," says López, hence the importance of containing the outbreak, in reference to the new coronavirus. The number of deaths/total infected by this ranges between around 2% since the beginning of the outbreak, depending on when and where it is measured. In its latest report, the WHO Global Prevention Monitoring Board made it clear that we are not prepared for a global epidemic of something as everyday and recurring as influenza. And there the countries with fewer resources bear the brunt. And a child dies every 39 seconds from treatable pneumonia in the world. Source: https://www.newtral.es/la-gripe-mas-letal-que-el-coronavirus-ncov-hasta-la-fecha/20200201/ [4]. In another report we can see a WHO inspector caught on camera revealing manipulation of the coronavirus in Wuhan before the pandemic. Its posted by Taiwan News Staff Writer Keoni Everington on January 18, 2021. In the video are Vincent Racaniello and Peter Daszak.

A video taken just days before the start of the coronavirus pandemic shows a current World Health Organization (WHO) inspector discussing testing of modified coronaviruses on human cells and humanized mice at the Wuhan Institute of Virology (WIV), just weeks before the first cases of COVID-19 were announced in the city of Wuhan itself. In a video originally taken on December 9, 2019, three weeks before the Wuhan Municipal Health Commission announced an outbreak of a new form of pneumonia, virologist Vincent Racaniello interviewed British zoologist and president of the EcoHealth Alliance Peter Daszak about his work at the nonprofit to protect the world from the emergence of new diseases and predict pandemics. Since 2014, Daszak's organization has received millions of dollars in funding from the US National Institutes of Health (NIH), which it has funneled to the WIV to conduct research on bat coronaviruses. In the first phase of the research, which took place from 2014 to 2019, Daszak coordinated with Shi Zhengli, (◇◇◇), also

---

4.   https://www.newtral.es/la-gripe-mas-letal-que-el-coronavirus-ncov-hasta-la-fecha/20200201/

known as "Bat Woman", at the WIV to research and catalog bat coronaviruses in China. EcoHealth Alliance received $3.7 million in NIH funding for this research, with 10 percent funneled to the WIV, NPR reported.

The second, more dangerous phase, which began in 2019, involved gain-of-function (GoF) research on coronaviruses and chimeras in humanized mice from the laboratory of Ralph S. Baric at the University of North Carolina. Funding for the program was withdrawn by the NIH under the Trump administration on April 27 amid the pandemic. At the 28:10 mark of the podcast interview, Daszak states that researchers found that SARS likely originated in bats and then set out to find more SARS-related coronaviruses, eventually finding more than 100. He noted that some Coronaviruses can "enter human cells in the laboratory," and others can cause SARS disease in "humanized mouse models." He warned ominously that such coronaviruses are "untreatable with therapeutic monoclonal [antibodies] and cannot be vaccinated against with a vaccine." Ironically, he says his team's goal was to try to find the next "spillover event" that could cause the next pandemic, just weeks before COVID-19 cases began to be reported in Wuhan.

When Racaniello asks what can be done to deal with the coronavirus given that there is no vaccine or treatment for them, Daszak at the 29:54 mark appears to reveal that the goal of the GoF experiments was to develop a pan-coronavirus vaccine for many different types of coronaviruses. Based on their response, it is evident that just before the start of the pandemic, WIV was modifying coronaviruses in the laboratory. "You can manipulate them in the lab quite easily." What he then mentioned has become the telltale feature of SARS-CoV-2, its spike protein: "The spike protein drives a lot of what happens with the coronavirus, zoonotic risk." Daszak mentions WIV's collaboration with Baric: "and we worked with Ralph Baric at UNC [University of North Carolina] to do this." As advocates that SARS-CoV-2 is a lab-made chimera have suggested, he talks about inserting the spike protein "into the backbone of another virus" and then doing "some work in the lab."

Providing evidence of creating chimeras for the sake of a vaccine, he states: "Now, the logical progression of vaccines is that, if you're going to develop a vaccine for SARS, people are going to use pandemic SARS, but let's try insert these other related diseases and get a better vaccine." Based on Daszak's statements, it appears that just before the start of the pandemic, the WIV was using GoF experiments with chimeras in an attempt to create a vaccine. These experiments appeared to have included infecting mice genetically modified to express the human ACE2 protein with these chimeras. In a presentation titled "Coronavirus Threat Assessment," which was given four years before the pandemic in 2015, Daszak notes that experiments with humanized mice carry the highest degree of risk. Demonstrating his close ties to the WIV, he also included the lab as a collaborator at the end of the presentation. Controversially, Daszak has been included among a team of WHO experts finally allowed by Beijing to investigate the origin of the COVID-19 outbreak, more than a year after it began.

Scientists such as Richard Ebright, a molecular biologist at Rutgers University in New Jersey, are condemning Daszak's participation due to conflicts of interest "that unequivocally disqualify him from being part of an investigation into the origins of the Covid-19 pandemic," he reported. the Daily. Mail. In light of the WHO trip to Wuhan, a researcher using the pseudonym Billy Bostickson and his colleagues at DRASTIC (Decentralized Radical Autonomous Search Team Investigating COVID-19) have created a petition demanding that the international research team respond 50 key questions about the outbreak in Wuhan. Among the questions is a request to access the facility's database and lab records, which are purported to go back 20 years and include a look at its safety procedures, safety audit reports and safety reports. security incidents. Source: https://www.taiwannews.com.tw/en/news/4104828 [5]. Lastly, for this chapter, but not least, is the transcription that one of our ProjectMagen collaborators made for us of a very complete audio, made by a Spanish researcher:

In principle, you have read the headline correctly, those people who have followed me on another profile, which was the one that had innovated in the face of censorship with an anonymous name in the sense that it is not mine but they have put a certain "Rafael Paradas Moreno" You can follow me there, I have been warning for days that I was evidently telling them that when they were going to administer this new medicine that they have called "VACCINE" and that it is not really a vaccine because of what I am going to say next, because really the deaths that are being caused of the new patients, the new deaths in the United Kingdom, really correspond to the medication of what they have called "VACCINE" and we have also been saying that in several days little by little, I told them, that here in Spain they were going to say That the new one knows was already here in Spain, well they have already said it today, they have already said it that they have confirmed that through I don't know what PCR because they were not specific because they did not have isolated and sequencing the supposed virus that causes this new disease when they are already telling them to change before they have added 4 confirmed cases of the new vaccine in Madrid, which means, well, it means that they are going to administer it, they

---

5.   https://www.taiwannews.com.tw/en/news/4104828

are going to make it coincide with the administration of the vaccine.

Understand, you are going to match the disastrous and light deaths initially but very deadly in the long term with what they have called the vaccine, you can stay with my opinion in this case of more than 6000 hours of research with university professors that we have interviewed live, that we are in daily contact with medical graduates such as Dr. "Alejandro Sousa" with graduates and doctors in genetics such as Dr. "Luis Marcelo Martínez", president of the genetics medical association of Argentina, with the doctor in immunology "Rosana Bruno" or with the professor we interviewed who diagnoses "María José Martínez" and check to break that mental laziness with everything I am telling you. What they have called a vaccine is not a vaccine as such, it is not a reduced traditional or classic vaccine or people's attenuated pathology, it is a genetic vaccine, it is introduced with biotechnologies or with gene therapy, it is genetic engineering and I am going to talk to you of the consequences of that vaccine in the long, medium-long term that have not been studied but that there is a scientific study and that I have had the opportunity to look at and when I say look I mean study in depth and corroborate with other professors. That vaccine that they call a vaccine, which consists of introducing messenger RNA into the body, when they tell you that this messenger RNA actually stays at the level of the ribosome and that it does not participate in the protein assistance to alter your genome, it is a lie and I am going to say at least 2 mechanisms by which this happens:

First, it is called insertional mutagenesis, which means this in a simple way so that you can understand it, simply when the messenger RNA enters the body through what they have called a vaccine, when if they really cure it, it goes inside a capsule. , a polymer, an amino acid, biodegradable proteins in the bloodstream, that means that it will fractionate at a certain moment and do or not do the function that it initially thought it would do, which it is not going to do, so I am also going to say it, those fragments by molecular affinity as a sequence of nuclei that are going to seek affinity precisely with another synthesis of protein and amino acids of their own genome and in that sense they will alter it through a process called "INSERTIONAL MUTAGENESIS", insertion of the synthetic point of view and foreign to the organism, this means that when you start cell proliferation as a multicellular organism that is, what is called the phenomenon of APOPTOSIS appears, this means that you really try to kill the body, its immune system literally an abnormal or strange cell proliferation but unfortunately you will not achieve it and even more so if they are when they give you 2 doses or 3 a year for all the years, this means in other words cancer, neoplasms, cancerous tissue, metastases, etc.

This is one of the main consequences in the medium term, it could be 8 or 9 months, 1 year or 1 and a half years, but it is much more, I have talked to you about this mechanism, the cell is not always covered from the point of view or shielded in the nucleus so that the nucleotide chromatid is present in the nucleus in a diffuse or agglomerated form. Rather, in some cellular processes, especially in cell reproduction and multiplication, they appear in a diffuse form, so that it is accessible by the Messenger RNA, that nucleus can also alter your genome, as I'm telling you, far beyond what I'm telling you, those experiments have been done on animals completely with a feline population with hundreds of them, and they literally ended up dead more than 95 % of them, at 7 or 8 months when they faced their natural virus, which is the wild feline virus, that is, if their natural interspecies coronavirus, ours would be "THE SEASONAL FLU" this is what is called the augmented disease syndrome, this is said directly by the

"CDC" of the United States, the "United States Center for Disease Control and Prevention" this is the same as or what is called the antibody-dependent immune enhancement system , it simply means that when you face a common cold once you have been vaccinated with this or a seasonal flu, your own immune system will end up killing you due to these two simply consequences that I have told you, the probability is that you will survive the inoculation of this vaccine is barely around 15% or 20% between now and a year or a year and a half in the long term.

If you are really waiting for people to put them on and wait, they will have to wait at least 1 and a half years to see the results, be careful with what I am saying far from the very serious serious adverse reactions that have already been described even by the own laboratory "PFIZER" as adverse to encephalitis, all inflammations ending in "ITIS" "West syndrome" "Bell's palsy" I think it was called, are all normally paraplegia that are also irreversible apart from anaphylactic shocks that they can really give him because you can do something ironic and that he does not know it and that he has to have, as the "PFIZER" laboratory says, a resuscitation or resuscitation system in case of inconsistency or in case a syringe with adrenaline and a device of electroshocks that you obviously do not have, do not expose your life and physical integrity to that risk to this transgenic experiment with the entire world population simultaneously, be really aware of what we are facing, we have told you all this: there are many more very serious adverse effects including death than what we are telling you spontaneously on board.

The fact that, for example, infertility and the vaccine itself are introduced as a consequence of the maximum expression of the angiotensin-converting enzyme 2 in the testes of men, but also in the ovaries of women, this is precisely what is It aims to reduce the world population in the most disgusting way possible and with deception implemented through this type of genocidal and clearly eugenic organisms. Reducing the world population directly due to high mortality above all, especially in the medium term, even if there is an initial mortality like any medicine that tells you that there is a new strain is obviously a "LIE" that is why we could foresee it a long time in advance. Despite the censorship, what else can I say! I already told you about this vaccine as such, it is not a vaccine, it is not the "Edwuar Jenner" vaccine of 1796, nor the ones that you already knew, even the flu vaccine with all the negative statistics that may have has nothing to do with that, because it does not have any type of genetic sequencing, isolation, purification, washing, centrifuging, of a new pathogenic agent that causes the disease.

Look at the official viral theory, virology that is barely 80 years old is obsolete, what we call viruses as such do not have pathogenic capacity, especially those that are transmitted with "Flügge droplets" through the air, they do not have pathogenic capacity. a transmissive capacity of genetic information to help, to help, that the environmental disturbance of the environment where that person was subjected and who has transmitted that information, is an interspecies information that is warning him precisely of the danger and the new danger inclusion this year already You know what it is that we are going to talk to you about a little later, when there are environmental disturbances such as a slight or sudden change, especially in temperatures that affect the environment. The body gets sick, the damaged cells release a microfiber exosome that they talked about Cham and that is precisely what which we know as genetic consequence or a type of coronavirus, for example, the person who receives this information does not nurse if he does not put the same environment, staying cold at 15° below zero, for example, another environmental disturbance can be a sudden alteration of the PH which also makes it sick and also releases those somas.

Another environmental disturbance can be a significant chemical pollution and especially for this year a new electromagnetic disturbance, in 2018 with 4G plus that technological implementation that considerably increased environmental electricity already caused 15,000 direct deaths from what they called a flu. In Spain and specifically in the world, 1,050,000 deaths were caused by 4G plus in 2018, a figure very similar to this one that already has a mortality rate of 1 and a half years. When the 5G trials have been implemented, we are seeing that the virus of the official version is traveling as the technology advances and where those autonomous communities and those countries where they implemented it are putting it, think that Wuhan was the first pilot sample city of this where They introduced the first experimental failure of 5G and it was precisely where this happened and the time series coincide exactly, think that in Africa apparently in North Africa there is no Coronavirus and yet there is in South Africa because it is industrialized and maintains a telephone network the problem In principle, what we can have is that they discredit us from the point of view that we are saying that the antennas cause the Coronavirus, they do not cause it, they do not spread it, I mean, they do not spread any type of virus, they spread the pictures, the pictures cause the pictures. symptoms and prologues of the disease.

There are more than 1,200 scientific studies by peers that are being discredited independent of doctoral theses that actually demonstrate that all temporary conditions can be caused by and in fact are caused by electromagnetic proliferation at various frequencies, dyspnea, nuclear thrombus as a consequence of Initial dyspnea since oxygen is removed electronically by radio frequencies does not supply the set of biochemical reactions of the body, in that case the body, faced with the apparent definition of oxygen, what it does is supply that definition by increasing the level of Hemoglobin in the blood that, like you You know, it is a protein that transports oxygen in it, it increases so much that it forms coagulant thrombi and the famous thrombi that we already have with Covid-19 appear. We have demonstrated in a study of more than 150 residences that all of them had been radiated in proximity to those antennas. Some of you have seen all of these works before they were censored and you know perfectly well what we are talking about: the tinnitus, the tinnitus, the hives, edema, inflammation are a consequence of the impact of these electromagnetic fields at different frequencies, I am not going to go into much more detail about the mechanisms by which electromagnetic fields cause all the flu symptoms that have been called.

For example, bilateral or symmetrical pneumonia as a result of a direct exposure to electromagnetic radiation and not precisely a biological agent, it is never the biological agent that makes the person sick, it is the sick person that launches an agent of non-biological genetic information, inert, dead matter, it is not a bacteria, it is not tuberculosis, it is not leprosy, it is not cholera, which is also transmitted through surfaces and the air through aerosols or particles, it is not that, we must change Literally the entire theory of contagion, not only do I say it, I rely on Doctor "Arthur Firstenberg" on Doctor "Thomas Cowan" in biology in one with audio, as well as on Doctor "Miralles Boye" with whom we are in contact daily this It is the beach bar that they have set up with anti-viral vaccines, they already had it set up, that is why anti-viral vaccines like the flu never work and far from not working, they not only do that but they have implemented the introduction of heavy materials or metals such as mercury. or aluminum with a series of very undesirable effects to cause chronic diseases and continue to profit over time such as autism linked precisely to aluminum stored in the bloodstream completely in the brain or mercury also stored in children in the thimerosal format.

You have to be aware that unfortunately there is a pharmacy that moves billions of euros, they knew perfectly well that by implementing this type of technology they were going to cause these flu symptoms and they wanted to make the population see why these somas were going to be released and that All of this was a biological agent that caused the severe Covid-19 disease, this is not the case, it is the electromagnetic disturbance that causes the severe Covid-19 disease, it is the electromagnetic disturbance that causes the severe Covid-19 disease. especially catalyzed or that dose of radiation is forgotten much more quickly with the certain detergent introduced in the vaccination period completely the chiromas R vaccine as demonstrated by the Barbastro report, because the chiromas R, because it contains polysulfate 80, is a detergent that permeabilizes the cell membrane, it is a detergent that permeabilizes the cell membrane that is made up of phospholipids, what a detergent does is dissolve the fat of that membrane to allow the entry of the reduced viral load of the vaccine, the strain they carry, to enter the nucleus of the cell and the body converts it or releases antibodies more easily, which means that by doing this it also dissociates it, alters the transmembrane potential, a small potential difference or voltage that we have in the cell, which acts as a shield precisely against these electromagnetic radiations.

It is as if, for example, when we say that polysulfate 80 or the Chiroma vaccine is a catalyst for the association of microwave electromagnetic radiation, 5G, for example, or 4G plus or 4G, it is also the same as if we say that alcohol if you get drunk the body with alcohol you are a catalyst for the absorption of ultraviolet electromagnetic radiation from the sun which is exactly the same. In principle, they classify certain ionizing from ultraviolet radiation toward x-rays and gamma radiation, which is the end, and non-ionizing from ultraviolet radiation toward the back, along with infrared, something visible, infrared, microwaves, which is where it would be. that technology but that does not mean that it can ionize you in the long term as we are seeing with the extensive case of cancers where there is one of these antennas and above all the most important thing, we do not care whether it transmits heat or not that is not it, it is simply what that we see from the official point of view the fact that they can burn or not. It is not that, it is electronic excitation the fact of making certain atoms of matter sing, vibrate or excite at a certain frequency, really of living matter, of carbon systems. For example, we use microwave technology, we bombard them with microwaves. food when we introduce it into a receptacle by vibrating at a specific frequency, which is 2.42 GHz, the hydrogen atoms of the water molecules that occur when we vibrate so quickly enter a degree of excitation that heats the food.

They heat food, but also at other frequencies, for example, at 60 GHz, the oxygen atoms can be excited. If you breathed that oxygen, it would apparently have the saturation of 100, which the health workers who have naively seen an extraordinary disease believed, in fact we cannot. doubt, but that oxygen does not really supply the set of biochemical reactions because it is altered, it is electronically excited, when it joins the metabolic pathway with the respiration complex it will have the consequences that we are seeing, the process is much more complex but he does not want to enter into a technical debate because what he does not want is for you to open the door for you to investigate, especially because we have little time, I say that we have little time because we are facing the largest genocide in the history of known humanity, at least after the Spanish flu, which was something similar.

We are facing the greatest genocide that your children may have seen, especially soon, and it will be precisely when they have the finishing touch or the finishing touch with what they have called Vaccine, these are authentic criminals, if not all of them have interests, including economic ones, if not Those who are ignorant, illiterate, politically speaking, are totally ignorant of the scientific point of view, and as I have said many times, the roundest thing they have seen has been a shoe box because they do not have enough room for more, and at the very least they have economic interests, such as For example, the wife of Mr. "Juan Marmorino", the president of the Andalusian board, who is my turn, and who is the institutional relations manager of Bidafarma, which is the same company that is going to market the million-dollar lots of vaccine in Andalusia, from which they obviously benefit, do not be naive, do not be stupid, because I really see myself with the moral and ethical obligation to try to help human beings. Think about the thousands of hours of research that we carry out apart from the information and the regulated university academic training that we may have.

Think about what we lose and that we gain nothing by telling you this and how much interest these types of pharmaceutical companies and corporations really have, but not only economic interests but interests of a clear eugenic nature and a clear demographic nature of the population. We no longer know how to alert part of the censorship that we are suffering, we do not know how they will be tomorrow. Let's hope that tomorrow is not too late and that this information reaches the greatest possible number of people. They will be judged in one of the trials like the one in Nuremberg. tried and it will not work to say I was following orders any more than it did in 1945 or 1949 when those trials took place, they will not work, obviously there is no airborne transmission, there is in any case airborne transmission of useful genetic information and precisely the use of the mask The only thing it allows is to avoid that type of information, which also does not even achieve all the inconsistencies that you have seen are answered with the reiteration of electromagnetic fields and none.

None has an answer to the point of view of the official version when you have actually seen a biological agent that causes tooth loss in what they have called persistent Covid-19, how a persistent biological agent can do if it really or the body of that immunity ends the life of the host but those say that there are consequences, of course there are consequences of the electromagnetic radiation, these people, thousands of them who are following our advice without any type of medical protocol, although there are doctors working with us, they have simply withdrawn from the disturbing focus once they have located it and have improved in a matter of hours we can go on for hours talking because especially the urgency, there is a special prize and that is that there are many lives at stake many people that you innocently know and that your parents naively go to wear and just as they have put a mask on their children, they are going to take them to have them administered or inoculated with what they have called a Vaccine, they are going to literally end up dead, they will end up dead due to the process of incersional mutagenesis, or due to the immunological improvement syndrome antibody-dependent, or what is the same, the enhanced response syndrome of the "Plasmapheresis" disease.

What's more, in what they have called a vaccine, we are aware that there is silencing of genes, they are going to silence genes, biotypology has advanced a lot but not in the face of society, precisely this is seen in the military field, although you do not think about it, the silencing of genes As the VMAC2 Gene is practically annulling your will, that is, the population is practically enslaved because you are already telling them that not even with that vaccine they are going to do 3 doses a year, at least 2 or 3 doses depending on the laboratory, everyone is going to do it. Over the years you are going to continue wearing a mask and on top of that you are not going to avoid swimming, think and be intelligent, even giving credibility to the figures that they handle from the official point of view of one and a half million (1,500,000) deaths, knowing full well that have been overestimated and that all the cases of common seasonal flu and all the normal cases of pneumonia, the pneumococcus infection that have been eliminated have evidently been caused by Covid-19 with a PCR diagnosis that is not a valid diagnosis.

We could also talk about the PCR but we have already lost too much time if you slip right now, split your head open and have a head injury and die 2 hours later and you had a positive PCR you end up dead from COVID that is the diagnosis that is being made using and there is no type of autopsy, then the million and a half deaths are not such either, there has been an extraordinary illness yes, with atypical bilateral pneumonia, yes, but caused by a biological agent, no, caused by electromagnetic disturbance, it is a million and average number of deaths really, probably not, they are much less, they are overestimated, even the CDS itself, the reaction control center of the United States, said that 96% had died from other pathologies, do you really think about a disease that in 90% of the cases you don't even find out that you have it, you are asymptomatic in 5% of cases, at most you will have a cold, the symptoms are similar and in 3% or 4% of cases you will go to the ICU if they are people older people have previous pathologies, have cancer, diabetes, etc. How can you subject yourself to this risk to that benefit-risk equation relationship in what there is and in what we are talking about? What I am telling you has been told to you by all the people I have mentioned before, including the former vice president of the laboratory. PFIZER", who together with the former president of the European health council, Mr. "Wolfgang Wodarg", epidemiologist and doctor, who has already denounced the apnea flu.

They have denounced and asked for the urgent stoppage of this vaccine, we have to be intelligent, people of this vaccine, be intelligent, your own laboratory is not going to directly throw dirt on your roof, they are going to tell everyone that this is already Wonderful, the economic issue is already covered because the vaccines have already been paid for. Now only transhumanist ideas of a clear eugenic nature come. If you are an official from outside the state security force, police, civil guard, local police, national police, you continue, You health workers, nurses, as many as you are talking to dozens of us because you don't want to put that on, delay the administration of this transgenic experiment as much as possible when we read the 48 pages of the "PFIZER" laboratory itself, the report they have released has no scientific validity whatsoever, it is tested in absolutely healthy people without any type of previous pathology, that is to begin with when they describe the phenomenon of insertional mutagenesis that I have told you about, because only 2 months have passed, there is no time for experimentation in humans and there is no time for experimentation in animals. I have already told you, and by the way, they did in mice about 97% of them ended up infertile in the positive control group, so please, even giving credibility to those figures of one and a half million that are clearly overestimated, think about it. malaria that kills 2,600,000 million people a year, tuberculosis that kills 2,500,000 million people a year, and they are bacteria that are living organisms that are not the virus and the context of what we have about a virus at the moment.

Think about the pneumonias that kill 3,000,000 million people a year from infection by Pneumococcus, which is another bacteria a year in the world, figures much higher than this, even think about the seasonal flu that killed a million people in the world. 2018 and 700,000 thousand people every year and never under any circumstances have they forced you to get vaccinated, people are normally living an artificial reality, a holographic Matrix that they implement in the mass terrorism disinformation media that are currently bought in 4 or 5 corporate media groups by these globalist elites, communists, capitalists whatever you want to call them, the objective is clear to reduce the world population to the maximum is the development of the 2030 agenda, a 2030 sustainable development agenda and it will be sustained precisely by removing the people in the middle, be intelligent, be intelligent with simply the figures, you don't even believe the electromagnetic disturbance, just look at it and really believe that this is a biological agent, look at the figure really and study it like other diseases And then ask yourself why, where is the urgency, there is no type of epidemiological emergency, there is no type of epidemiological emergency, there is no type of new strain, much less has the first one been isolated as they are going to have the new strain isolated in the new United Kingdom.

How are they going to know that the 4 people from Madrid have been isolated in a PCR, but what PCR you are intelligent, use reason, use rationality and if not you have no knowledge of biology or what we are really talking about if you do not have it, use your intuition, which is the deepest knowledge that your intuition really told you because the barrier to what you think about that intuition is deception and lies or life and not death, it's that easy and please try to talk to as many as possible. possible of people, warn those around you, lose your shame and pride because after this do not open up neither pride nor shame because you will not really be there to tell it if you have really undergone what they have said they call a vaccine, which is never a vaccine, they play with the concepts, they play with the concepts and call it a vaccine so that people, the population, really believe that it is an effective medicine and that it will cure them, it is not a vaccine, it is not a vaccine nor a new concept of vaccine, it is a syringe I am going to leave it here, because now I am going to enter a meeting precisely with other doctors and I do not want to enter this environment either but the impotence is very great, very great for the majority as long as they do not censor this channel of María, through which It is still broadcasting now and they have let it broadcast again starting today for a while coming out here and if you don't see me then don't be surprised that something has happened to me because they are doing it directly with other people.

But you will see me on the Facebook profile called "Rafael Paradas Moreno", okay, a photograph of no one appears, that is, a kind of holographic, there is whatever it takes to mislead, there is no other way, on YouTube I have also opened a channel that we are the fifth column 2 that I want to remind you that it is 20 censored and we are putting that information. Doctor "Alejandro Sousa" who has a degree in medicine and surgery from the University of Santiago de Compostela is giving the same information, the professor proceeds clinical diagnoses "María José Martínez" in which we interview and are in contact daily with given this same information, also a graduate in medicine, Dr. "Luis Marcelo Martínez", the president of the genetic medicine association of Argentina, probably the most important geneticist in the world as well. has given this information and much more, Dr. "José Luis Sevillano" with a degree in community medicine has also given this information, Dr. "Natalia Prego" with a degree in community surgery medicine has also given this information.

Yes, of course everything, everything that really does not appear on television and is not the 4 purchases that appear on your television in each of the countries where you watch TV, remember that right now there are 100,000 thousand doctors, 700,000 thousand people and 30,000 thousand epidemiologists who are against this thing that they have called a vaccine, at least as far as we know, at least remember that and put it on a scale, you are really fine, if you are fine, you do not need any type of medication and when they really tell you that They are going to oblige but of course they are not obliging us but temporarily we are obligated but otherwise we will not have our immunity card or passport to be able to travel and so on we will see. [End of audio] I did not want to move on to the next section without first sharing this publication from October 28, 2020, which sheds light between the postulates of Pasteur and those of Béchmap, which are not wasted. For those unfamiliar with the ideas of Louis Pasteur, have you heard of "pasteurized" milk? Well, the issue with Pasteur goes back to the origins of the theory of Evolution and Darwinism, for which I invite you to read my first book, 'Creation vs. Evolution' (2010). Now, below I quote the text in question from the debate between these two postulates:

For 150 years, Pasteur's erroneous germ theory has led us to an endless sea of drugs and diseases. When a lie can create billions of dollars and is taught to each next generation as a fact, it is a pretty serious matter; In fact, it is a revolutionary act to confront it. Even the worst lie can be clothed in a cloak of respectability if it has not been publicly exposed for a considerable time. There was a time when Pasteur did not enjoy the divine respect accorded him today, and instead he was considered a failure in almost all of his experiments, causing death and immense financial losses to those who followed his beliefs. Today, the germ theory of disease, including vaccination and pharmaceutical intervention, has survived to become the basis of the disease industry. It is interesting to note that we would have inherited a very different world, if those who were in favor of Béchamp had been able to offer something profitable to the then emerging business with the disease. Instead they said: "It's the health of the cell that's important, not the germs."

Today, germs are important and the health of the cell is so unimportant that no university is dedicated to it, while billions are being invested to learn everything about germs and in this we are successful; Yet we don't even know how to describe health except as the absence of disease. A truly confusing world, deliberately kept that way. "Germs cause disease"... We could have avoided modern epidemics of unnecessary diseases, such as cancer, diabetes, heart disease, if only civilization had followed Bechamp instead of Pasteur. The work of French biologist Antoine Béchamp (1816-1908) demonstrated that disease causes germs; Louis Pasteur, Béchamp's contemporary (and former student), announced that his studies proved that germs cause disease. A man has been forgotten by history; the other is considered the father of modern medicine. Pasteur's work, unlike that carried out by his professor, delighted the emerging pharmaceutical industry. "If germs are external attackers that invade the body, then we can develop and market an endless arsenal of weapons with which to kill them. But, if damage or imbalance with the body causes germs, then we simply must restore the balance to remove the conditions on which the germs feed." Instead of introducing poison, we would need to introduce only the missing natural elements.

Pasteur's germ theory of disease gave birth to the pharmacological era. If medicine had adopted Béchamp's germ theory of disease, and the subsequent work of Drs Brewer, Warburg, Pauling and others, it would be common knowledge that disease symptoms are prevented or reversed by nutrition at the cellular level. . Today, thousands of researchers and doctors know that we were deceived, but the end result has been so catastrophic that even the very concept of truth has been momentarily damaged as we move through the 20th and 21st centuries. Men of apparent moral rectitude are afraid to admit that no amount of toxicity can heal, and instead they follow a creed they know is wrong. It seems that a long time ago, we made the most incredible of mistakes and knowledgeable and sophisticated men would die before admitting that they have been foolish and failed to recognize the obvious. Now in the 21st century, an enlightened public and a few brave investigators dare to lead the expose of a mafia empire, so corrupt that it doesn't even care that we all have discovered the truth. Believe us - says the allopathic drug industry - and we will clean up our own act... really.

But the pharmaco-allopathic empire is already in an advanced state of irreparable damage, caused by several generations of ignorance, clothed in arrogance. There is no sign of a genuine desire for reform, and those few who try to practice true healing are viciously attacked by their own peers. Nowadays, it is truly hell to try to practice real healing, because if you do not use the most toxic poisons to apply them where they cannot possibly cure, and instead use a natural alternative method, other doctors and the drug industry drugs label him a "charlatan."

Pasteur vs Béchamp: Is it possible that a seemingly advanced society could be living in a state of total delusion, always trying to achieve something that is doomed to failure, simply because we don't know enough about ourselves to make the right decisions? It certainly looks that way in the healthcare area. Could it be that even living in the 21st century, the entire modern disease industry rests on one of the world's biggest lies? Germs cause illness.

Antoine Béchamp (1816-1908): The French biologist demonstrated precisely the opposite: disease causes germs. He proved that "all natural organic matter (matter that once lived), absolutely protected against atmospheric germs, invariably and spontaneously alter and ferment, because they necessarily and intrinsically contain within themselves the agents of their spontaneous alteration, digestion." , dissolution. Bechamp was able to prove that all animal and plant cells contain these tiny particles, which continue to live after the death of the organism and from them, microorganisms develop. In his research, Bechamp laid the foundations for understanding pleomorphism (the ability of organisms to change). Whenever there is something in nature that is dying, beginning to decay, something appears and eats it, as its particles become microbes that come out of the tissue cells to clean up any toxins or decaying matter that is left behind. found in the body. That's what microbes (germs) are for. They are the result, not the cause, of the disease.

While a blood sample placed on a glass plate for microscopic observation (stage) ages in a day or two, tiny organisms can literally be seen moving as they emerge from the blood cells, organisms changing into more degenerate forms and more pathological as the process progresses. When the process of decomposition or putrefaction is over, when there is nothing more for the newly formed viruses, bacteria and fungi to eat, they are destroyed, disappear, and return to the form they had. They can be observed doing this through the microscope at x100 or more. "While the microsomes of the destroyed bacteria also live, what follows is that these microsomes are the living end of the entire cellular organization which, in turn, become all living things, beings, organs, everything. They are the end and the beginning of all physical life. "All cells, organs, all living forms are built from these small bodies." When you break an element into smaller and smaller pieces, you end up with one atom of that element. When you break organic matter, physical life, into smaller and smaller pieces, you end up with this particle, no matter what form of living organic matter you started with.

Professor Bechamp's results were buried, ignored and distanced from subsequent generations of students, who today do not even know that Béchamp was the top scientist who worked with patience and order in the laboratory, while Pasteur received praise for a work which was plagiarized, and often altered, in the most unscientific way. This was discovered when in 1901 his notes were finally made public for people to read. Today we have discovered all this, but an industry built on Pasteur is not going to give ground. Instead, we must work in two different spheres. What Béchamp discovered was that the cells of our body are not attacked by external disease-carrying germs, as Pasteur's theory suggests, but rather our cells deteriorate, degenerate and are damaged by the stress of daily life or by introduced toxins (physical or chemical) and degenerate to a point where they become weak, poisoned or sick. Under this condition, its acidity increases, which destroys its own degenerative tissue, through the use of what he called microsomes, always present in the cell. Basically, Béchamp discovered that the cell self-destructs if it becomes contaminated or degenerates. Pasteur said that external germs enter the body and destroy cells. Béchamp's theory says that if we keep the cell healthy and strong, it will perform well, but if not, this will allow the small microsomes, which react to the poor acidic conditions of the cell, to ferment or eat it.

Pasteur's theory says that regardless of whether the cell is healthy or not, external germs enter and cause death or contamination of the cell. This was immediately accepted as an explanation for all diseases, and thus grew the gigantic industries we know today as drugs, medicines and vaccines. Along with them, the theory of getting rid of symptoms by cutting them, burning them with radiation or heat, and poisoning them with toxic substances evolved. Today these methods seem to have reached the maximum of what they can be applied and the diseases that germs are supposed to bring us still continue to appear, as if they were not being treated at all. This has generated a lot of research in our times because it is becoming more and more obvious that we use erroneous theories in current medicine. The most important discovery that science (today) has made is that toxins do not cure. It seems that the more we poison our cells with chemical cures and pollutants, the sicker we get. Many researchers have returned to Béchamp's discoveries and after reading his reports, we discovered that we knew the solution, but it had been very cleverly hidden so that the disease industry could flourish, based on the destruction of microbes suspected of causing disease. .

However, cells cannot resist disease if they are allowed to become weakened or poisoned. The current method of treating the disease is to ignore the biological or nutritional needs of the cells and at the same time, attack them with toxic substances, in the hope that the germs die and the cell lives. A nutrient-deficient cell is poisoned at the same time. This is standard procedure. Professor Pierre Jacques Antoine Béchamp was a physician, professor of chemistry and pharmacy, and one of the leading researchers of the 19th century, the same period as Pasteur. Béchamp conducted experiments that found that the bacteria grow inside the body as tiny, granulated evolutionary forms that live inside the cells of all living forms. He called these microsomes and believed that they could be found in all healthy living tissue. These microsomes are physiologically and chemically active, and are the builders of our cells, in addition to being agents of decomposition after the death of a cell in our tissues or organs. Béchamp discovered that microsomes developed into bacteria when the body's tissues were poisoned, damaged or unable to function. From his research comes his statement that the bacteria is a product of the disease, not its cause.

People get sick because their cells are compromised, which unbalances them and makes them susceptible to the growth of bacteria from within, instead of being invaded from the outside, according to what Pasteur expressed. His philosophy was based on preventing an invasion of bacteria from outside the body, while Bechamp was based on preventing the growth of bacteria from within the body. Over time, we have found out who was right, but an industry built solely on toxic substances, which requires a fortune to remain viable, is not going to change or get its claws out of the world's largest wallet. Béchamp's method would have allowed us to develop cell health. Pasteur has allowed us to develop all kinds of toxins to attack invading germs. Healthy cells do not need to be protected by toxins. Toxins cause healthy cells to become sick, and as Bechamp discovered, they self-destruct when they can no longer function. "If I lived again, I would dedicate my life to proving that germs seek their natural habitat, diseased tissue, instead of being the cause of tissue disease; "Just like mosquitoes look for stagnant water, but they

are not the cause of stagnant puddles." Rudolph Virchaw, father
of pathology: Even the great scientists of our time were able,
at some point in their careers, to admit that modern medicine
has been taken for a ride. Pasteur admitted when he died that:
"Germs are nothing and the tissue in which they grow is
everything."

Lies are heavy baggage when we face death, and money is no
longer a motivation. Nor is it a consolation when summarizing
the meaning of our lives. What are the basic differences between
Pasteur and Béchamp? Germ Theory – Pasteur (as taught to
modern students):

- The disease arises from microorganisms outside the body.
- In general, we must protect ourselves from microorganisms.
- The function of microorganisms is constant.
- The shapes and colors of the microorganisms are constant.
- Each disease is associated with a particular microorganism.
- Microorganisms are the primary causative agents.
- The disease can attack anyone.
- To prevent disease we must kill microorganisms.

Cell theory – Béchamp (as taught to Pasteur and others
during this era)

- Diseases arise from microorganisms within the body's cells.
- These intracellular microorganisms normally function to build and assist in the body's metabolic processes.
- The function of these organisms changes to assist in the catabolic processes (disintegration) of the host organism when it dies or is damaged, which can be both chemical and mechanical.
- Microorganisms change their colors and shapes to reflect the environment.
- Each disease is associated with a particular condition.

• Microorganisms become 'pathogenic' as the health of the host organism deteriorates. Therefore, the condition of the host organism is the primary agent.

• Disease is built from unhealthy conditions within the cell.

• To prevent disease we must create health.

Source: https://canal7salta.com/2020/10/28/internacional-pasteur-vs-bechamp-diez-mil-mentiras-trabajon-ocultar-una- Verdad [6]/.

The biggest fraud in history has been perpetrated using money. When you have all the capital necessary to achieve what you want, you bribe whoever, and if they don't let you, you hire a hitman to get them out of the way. The real virus was never even isolated. What is it that is "killing" people? First of all, people die every day, that's part of existence. People are catching a virus, they say, when has that been a novelty? If the news counted how many people got the flu, they would be in a greater state of alarm. The only people who to date at the beginning of 2021 had Sars-Cov-2 were those to whom it was given intravenously through an injection, that is, through a vaccine. And what skeptics usually say, that if that is so, how are the "so many" deaths in hospitals justified? In hospitals, to begin with, they are used to people dying. At the beginning of the pandemic there was so much corruption to earn money from the government that in many countries dishonest things were done to get those bonuses.

Next, someone dying "from" Covid, at least before the 2020-2021 winter vaccination waves, was almost unlikely. Whether someone "with" covid dies is debatable, especially after these waves of vaccination. Already there we could say that there is that high probability. By saying that it is "debatable" I mean

---

6.   https://canal7salta.com/2020/10/28/internacional-pasteur-vs-bechamp-diez-mil-mentiras-pueden-ocultar-una-verdad/

that someone can have "covid", but die from something else, and even "covid" may be the "trigger", but the problem itself was never "covid". If you are old and sick or weak, it makes no sense to blame death on "covid", because if not then we would have to apply that to tuberculosis, flu, hepatitis, AIDS, pneumonia, etc., etc. This would be creating misinformation and misrepresentation of behavioral and empirical facts. The problem is not the virus, it is the person's situation. But the virus that is being talked about is not killing people. The 5G waves make people sick with symptoms such as flu and pneumonia, and when they do a PCR test (which gives a false positive in 80.22% of cases), they say it is "covid." So the entire structure of the approach is adulterated. To make matters worse, they do not perform autopsies, consequently there is no way to know for sure what the causes of death were (in fact, the corpses are treated as type 2 (radioactive) not as what they should be, type 1 (functions due to a biological agent), and no dead person sneezes, so there are no such Fluge droplets that transmit anything. Not even after showing that the PCR test has been positive in papayas, cola-cola, goats... it is a bad joke.

But that's not the point, the protocol itself about this whole story is anti-scientific and anti-constitutional. Dr. Stefan Lanka expressed in an interview on May 23, 2020 that what the Sars-Cov-2 tests find are substances produced by "the human body's own metabolism," not a virus. There were 3 publications that gave rise to the montage worldwide, two of them supposedly demonstrate the discovery of the new coronavirus, and the third establishes the protocol for detecting the virus. There are 11 scientific criteria to determine a scientific publication, like the one that said we were in a "pandemic." Of these 11 criteria, all three meet the requirements for a scientific work, first; second, in only two of these three was the peer review carried out with external experts, since the third was published WITHOUT REVIEW; third, other possible causes of the problem were not considered, that is, non-viral origin; fourth, no pathogenic agent was isolated, which in itself is a cornerstone that has been blatantly ignored; fifth, the biochemical characterization of such pathogen was not carried out; sixth, it could not be demonstrated that a pathogen was causing the respiratory tract problem; seventh, there is no evidence of the transmissibility of such a pathogen (much less can it be said that it is in the air and therefore you should wear a mask in open spaces); eighth, there is no proof of the existence of a new pathogen called covid-19, but rather it may be the sum of other types of clinical conditions; ninth, it has not been demonstrated that the genetic material of said virus is present in nature, humans or plants; tenth, there is no reliable detector; Eleventh, the studies with adequate control groups were not corroborated.

In the eighth point, it must be clarified that experts have stated that the "genetic information" of the supposed virus is actually material from the human body itself that has been "completed" in a "computational" way. In other words, what should be a complete structure of a gene, its RNA and DNA information does not exist, and since it does not exist, it was artificially manufactured for that matter. They do not design it in the strict sense of the term, but rather they present it in a configuration like someone inventing the identification number of someone who does not exist, but since it appears in a database, it seems as if they did exist. The body or person does not exist, but in a record it appears as if it existed. In this way, the genetic map of such a new coronavirus is a construct where our material, typical of the human being, is mixed with an arrangement carried out by a computer system, in order to assemble what appears to be an isolated virus. The real Sars-Cov-2 chimera is known to those who created it, but what the media and politicians talk about is not that chimera, because if the truth came to light there would be an international problem between the US, China and Europe for use of biological weapons. Likewise, what "kills people" in 2020 is not a virus but the mixture of various things, in some cases even isolated from each other, without any relationship, but who proves it? And it proves it, who makes it known? And if you make it known, how much propaganda will you do and where? On the contrary, what they say was isolated as a virus, for political and media purposes, is a genetic pattern that does not exist in nature but in a computer program, from which it came so that they believe it exists.

Furthermore, in a more recent article (March 2, 2020), titled, 'the links between the coronavirus, the Pilgrims Society and the Pirbright Institute of the British Crown' - which leads me to remember a scene from 'I, Pet Goat II' where Obama has a royal "crown" coin under his foot, and is sweating from nerves – says that the coronavirus was invented by the Pirbright Institute in elegant and well-located laboratories located on the outskirts of London. According to research published by Americans for Innovation, this Coronavirus was invented by the Pirbright Institute in elegant and well-located laboratories, located in Woking, Surrey, England, just outside the M25 outer belt of London. The Pirbright Institute (UK) was awarded 11 US patents, including US Pat. No. 10,130,701 of Coronavirus. The Pirbright Institute is controlled by the Queen's Golden Share along with SERCO and QinetiQ. Pirbright's controllers can be traced back to SERCO, QinetiQ and Sir Geoffrey E. Pattie, President Marconi and the British Intellectual Property Institute. Currently, British SERCO runs the US Patent Office (evidence shown below), US FEMA Zone 02 and Region 04, the Obamacare, OPM, GSA and SPAWAR websites from the US

Navy, Virginia, New York, 63 US city air traffic controllers, and more. SERCO used its control of the US Patent Office to grant its British biocompany a patent on the Coronavirus in record time, which is a scandalous fraud that nothing is known about for the simple reason that the Pilgrims Society controls to the Western press.

The Pirbright Institute, a company owned by the Queen, holds US Patent No. 10,130,701 on CORONAVIRUS. Pirbright can be traced back to SERCO Group Plc and QinetiQ Group Plc, which have contracts with the US Patent Office. Outrageously, SERCO essentially runs the US Patent Office's patent application process (under the Department of Commerce)! In our opinion, this "unequal conduct" in patent legal terms is fraud and invalidates the claim as the world fights this emerging pandemic inspired by the British-American Pilgrims Society. See THE PIRBRIGHT INSTITUTE, Co. No. 00559784. (January 7, 1956). Certificate of incorporation and related records. Companies House (UK). Queen Elizabeth II is the long-time Patron of the British-American Pilgrims Society (1902-present) . Sir Henry Solomon Wellcome, pharmacist-propagandist-spy, was a founder member of the Pilgrims, along with Winston Churchill, propagandist John Buchan and the Daily Telegraph and Daily Mail Messrs. Burnham and Northcliffe. See The Pilgrims Society of Great Britain, United States, Profile Books, London (2002,2003) (January 2002, p.1: "As Patron of Pilgrims it has given me great pleasure to support the unique contribution that the Society has made to Anglo-American relations over the years. See Pilgrims Society controls the press. Pirbright Institute Donors:

- Founder member of Wellcome Trust Pilgrims Society (1902).

- GlaxoSmithKline (Wellcome clone).

- Bill and Melinda Gates Foundation.

- Department for Environment, Food and Rural Affairs (Defra).

- Defense Advanced Research Projects Agency (DARPA).

- World Health Organization (WHO).

- European Commission (EU).

- United Nations (UN).

- UK Research and Innovation (UKRI).

- Biological Sciences and Technology Research Council (BBSRC); formerly Science and Engineering Research Council (SERC), White Paper, also known as SERCO Limited (the trading spin-out controlled by Monarch's Golden Share).

Pirbright Institute Trustees:

- President, Professor John Stephenson.

- Ian Bateman, UK-NEA.

- Ian Black, London School of Economics (LSE).

- Jon Coles, Brunswick Group, Apple, Pizza Hut, Western Union, Bloomsbury and Macmillan.

- Professor Vince Emery, Surrey U.

- Roger Louth, Avrico.

- Dr Venessa Mayatt OBE.

- Dr. Sandy Primrose.

- Sir Bertie Ross, KCVO, FRICS, Savills, Court Member of the Worshipful Company of Farmers

- The City of London, Pilgrims Society (Prince Charles confidant, Charles is also the Pilgrims Society and its next Patron).

- Professor David Rowlands, Wellcome Fndn.

- Jane Tirard, Pfizer.

The American and British patent offices are completely coordinated factories of theft and weapons manufacturing for the Pilgrims Society: the source of technology for continued warfare: SERCO has controlled the processes of the US Patent Office from 20006 to the present. That's right, a BRITISH company controls the AMERICAN Patent Office, where America's best and brightest are fooled into thinking it's a fair process. In fact, as we will demonstrate below, the British and American PILGRIMS SOCIETY media, intelligence and banking are putting together everything they touch. See AFI. (November 22, 2017). The application of social media should concern us all. Americans for Innovation. The Coronavirus was invented by the Pirbright Institute in elegant, well-located laboratories in Woking, Surrey, England, just outside London's M25 outer belt. The Pirbright Institute is a British charity (Co.

No. 00559784) which has a charter from the Queen. It is controlled by the UK Government's Biological and Biotechnology Research Council (BBSRC). In turn, UK Research and Innovation oversees BBSRC.

BBSRC was created in 1994 by taking over the life sciences activities of the Science and Engineering Research Council (SERC). In 1986, SERC was funded by Sir Geoffrey E. Pattie, Minister of State for Industry and Information. He simultaneously incorporated a commercial SERCO and merged RCA into it. He later took control of Marconi, then merged it with GEC.

Sir Geoffrey E. Pattie, Society of Pilgrims, Keeper of the Monarch's Golden Shares, founder of SERCO. On 22 June 1994, Pattie became the president of the British Institute of Intellectual Property Law with founding members including well-known American corruptocrats including GEC, Glaxo Holdings (formerly Pirbright financier Wellcome), Thorn EMI, Unilever, Wellcome Foundation (Pirbright funder), Wellcome Research (Pirbright funder), Zeneca Group (Dame Bridget Margaret Ogilvie is a director of the Wellcome Trust), Amersham, Dyson, McDermott, Microsoft (Bill Gates, Pirbright funder), Wilmer Cutler Pickering Hale LLP (Robert Mueller's witch-hunting firm), Finnegan Henderson, Morrison & Forester, BAT, IBM (thief of Leader Technologies' social media inventions). See AFI (November 22, 2017). The application of social media should concern us all. Americans for Innovation. Our research has traced Burroughs Wellcome & Co.'s involvement with fake vaccines since their experiments on 60,000 black and white people in British concentration camps during the Second Boer War which was promoted by Cecil Rhodes disciples such as Viscount Alfred Milner, Winston

Churchill and John Buchan, among others, all founders of the Pilgrims Society in London (1902), then New York (1903).

Viscount Alfred Milner, co-founder, Pilgrims Society (16 July 1902). On July 20, 2005, Sir Geoffrey E. Pattie formed the Strategic Communications Laboratory public relations firm, the parent of Cambridge Analytica and a key antagonist in the Trump-Russia plot hoax. On May 17, 2006, the United States Patent Office under the administration of George W. Bush (a member of the Pilgrims Society) awarded processing of all patents to SERCO, a company controlled by the British Crown. Those contracts have been renewed and are currently in operation. See SERCO's 2015 press release. George W. Bush, Pilgrim Society; progenitor of The Patriot Act, where basic rights in the Bill of Rights were suspended following Pilgrim Society fears conjured and stoked by MSM Pilgrim propaganda after his false flag attack on 9/11. Numerous whistleblowers have confirmed that Bush, Cheney, Rumsfeld, etc., knew the attack was coming... because they ordered the CIA to organize it for their Pilgrim Society brethren in Britain and the US on December 28, 2006, Pattie formed Terrington Management LLP and immediately acquired clients including BEA, Lockheed, AWE and SERCO. Lockheed and SERCO control the Atomic Weapons Establishment (AWE), controlled by the Queen's Golden Share. On 28 February 2014, Rupert Soames, OBE, became CEO of SERCO. His brother is Sir Nicholas Soames, who is also a confidant of Prince Charles.

On January 6, 2015, SERCO CEO Rupert Soames was discovered on the "Little Blacklist" of human trafficking pedophile Jeffrey Epstein. Rupert C. Soames, Pilgrims Society; CEO of SERCO, human trafficking client of Jeffrey E. Epstein's "Lolita Express" passenger plane to "Pedophile Island" in the Caribbean. As of May 4, 2018, SERCO had received $5.52

billion in 15,699 contracts from the US government. 5,000 of those contracts were PRIME CONTRACTS. This does not include contracts with several US states such as New York and Virginia. Jeffrey E. Epstein, Pilgrims Society blackmailer for MI6, CIA and Mossad; human trafficking advocate for the Pilgrims Society. Tellingly, SERCO, Inc. was not incorporated in the United States until December 29, 2008, during President-elect Barack Obama's transition, just after Pilgrims Society member Larry Summers took over. National Economic Council, during the banking "crisis" of 2008. Clearly, SERCO did not have a corporate position to begin managing the US Patent Office in 2006, therefore the records have undoubtedly been obscured using some cheap "national security" excuse. SERCO, a British company controlled by the Crown, runs the US Patent Office. Stay tuned. More about sister corporation QinetiQ controlled by the Crown, and sister to SERCO. Hint: Former CIA Director George Tenet was director of QinetiQ shortly after leaving the CIA and while retaining his top secret clearances.

SERC-O formed the Pirbright Institute which submitted its Coronavirus invention for US Patent, having received funding for this work from the Bill & Melinda Gates Foundation (Microsoft), the Wellcome Trust (fake sold to GlaxoSmithKline), the European Commission (EU), World Health Organization (WHO), Defra, DARPA. In just 17 months, SERCO-run patent examiner Bao Q. Li issued the Coronavirus US Pat. No. 10,130,701 to Pirbright with almost no objection (that means it was probably a rubber stamp). This process typically takes three or more years. Neither Pirbright nor the US Patent Office disclosed their conflicts of interest in issuing this Coronavirus patent. On the British side, everything about this Coronavirus goes back to the Crown, the eugenics-loving Pilgrims Society, the Crown Agents and their corrupt Privy Council courtiers (the Pilgrims Society sucks). The connection between the coronavirus and the Anglo-American monopoly on war, trade and culture. Source: https://americans4innovation.blogspot.com/2020/01/ coronavirus-traced-to-british-crown.html [7]. You can see much more evidence, with the official reports and records in another link, which reflects added details of this relationship of DARPA, Bill Gates, Defra, the British Welcome Truth and the European Commission with the creation of the Wuhan-400 chimera, and its true intentions, as well as the intervention of the Pirbright Institute, here: https://patriots4truth.org/2020/01/28/corona-virus-is-a-globalist-bioweapon/ [8].

At minute 1.33 of 'I, Pet Goat II' we see that Alice drops an apple that rolls and reaches Barack Obama's right foot and opens in two, and two branches emerge from it that join together and form a flower pink lotus The most striking issue is that under Obama's shoe there is a coin, and it coincides with the British "crown coin." Certainly when I did the videoconferences related to this topic in the winter of 2015-2016, I did not suspect that this had anything to do with a "pandemic." Now I see it clearly. They chose the name "crown", and not "crown" to tell us that this comes from the "crown", without saying it in the common language: English. When someone is a genius at something, his art does not last long in anonymity, he wants his name to be known. This is what makes big thieves caught: they want to be recognized. The ego does not let them hide their activities, their merits. The real corona virus is not from a bat, it is from the British crown. There are other monarchies, but the House of

---

7.   https://americans4innovation.blogspot.com/2020/01/coronavirus-traced-to-british-crown.html

8.   https://patriots4truth.org/2020/01/28/corona-virus-is-a-globalist-bioweapon/

Windsor is the most powerful of all. Obama sweats when he sees that coin (economy) because it could have been his turn to "burden" it. He got rid of that weight. Although the House of Windsor released a commemorative coin in 2017, there is one that is more in line with the one that appears in 'I, Pet Goat II', for example, the 1928 King George V silver coin, or from 1927.

George V, grandson of Queen Victoria, comes from the House of Wales, where the current British royal house is from. Ironically, his brother dies and he remains the direct successor to the throne, then Victoria dies and then his father and he remains sovereign of the British Empire. The "coincidences" add up, because being also sovereign over India, the IGM (World War I) breaks out and his cousins die: Tsar Nicholas II of Russia and Kaiser William II of Germany. In 1917, George became the first monarch of the House of Windsor, the name with which he renamed the House of Saxe-Coburg-Gotha. The name 'George', it is worth saying, has a long significance, and comes to the United States to call a father and son who were not long ago presidents of the United States. There are researchers who maintain that there is a link genetic between the Bush family and the Windsor family, as well as with the famous British double agent and Satanist Aleister Crowley. This King George V, according to Wikipedia, <<His reign saw the rise of socialism, communism, fascism, Irish republicanism and the Indian independence movement, which radically changed the political landscape. The Parliament Act of 1911 established the supremacy of the House of Commons — whose members are democratically elected — over the House of Lords — whose members do not have to go through elections. In 1924, he appointed a Labor prime minister for the first time and in 1931, the Statute of Westminster recognized the dominions of the

Empire as independent kingdoms within the Commonwealth of Nations.>>

It is curious that George V declared war on Germany, where his first was Kaiser and from where the Illuminati-Jesuits had been expelled. It is curious that George V did not want to give asylum to his own first cousin Nicholas, and when the Tsarist Revolutionary War stopped he was assassinated (Nicholas II) by the Bolsheviks. I like to be misunderstood, because the apostle Paul said well, <<we are not ignorant of the machinations of the devil>>. The Windsor-Mountbatten family, formerly German-British Saxe-Coburg-Gotha, was clearly seeking world monopoly, British imperial power controlling everything. Returning to the "corona" plan, it is not at all unheard of that the British monarchy pushed this plan. In my previous books I have talked a lot about the connections of the Windsor family with the Arthurian "prophecy" of the Merovingian-Jewish-Mason messiah. The Windsors and Mountbattens are in effect part of the dynasties that rule the world and control the banking system. They are great allies and friends of the Rothschilds, Zionists with whom it is said that they even acquired family ties. All this leads us to deduce the possible relationship between the corona-plan and the Illuminati agenda. Let us remember that Illuminati is originally the name given to the secret high level of Freemasonry, in honor of the 13 families that dominate the world: Astor, Collins, Freeman, Reynolds, Bundy, Kennedy, Du Pont, Russell, Onassis, Rockefeller, Li, Dan Guyn and Rothschild. They are the top of the Illuminati, and above them is the House of Windsor, that is, currently the most powerful lady is Queen Elizabeth (Elizabeth). Below them are other families in order of influence power, economic power and purchasing power, where they are in the top 20, for example, the Bush.

It is crucial that everyone does their own research work, to begin with studying what the cofactors are. A virus does not kill. A series of things together lead you to death. It depends primarily on your age and previous health status. If you are over 70 years old, you are one of those who are on the list of possible casualties, and that is well known. If you have previous pathologies, obviously, anything else is going to make the situation worse. The rest will be done by fear, the water you drink, the food you eat, the drugs you take, the physical activity you do - or don't do -, the level of air you breathe - and its state -, the baths you take. you give – especially in the sea or in a pool -, the amount of sunlight you get. Those are the cofactors. There is no evidence of airborne transmissibility, so use your intelligence and connect with nature freely. Don't hide in an absurd bubble of disinfectants. Which gets sicker, a dog from the street or one from the house? Soak up germs, so your immune system strengthens. Get rid of the television. Don't let them brainwash you.

X. EXPERIMENTAL GENE THERAPY

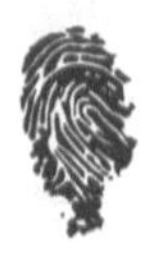

We are faced with an active component, weapons of mass sterilization. Do you know what EP3172319A1 is? A Google patent from 2014 (https://patents.google.com/patent/ EP3172319A1/en [1]), registered at the European Patent Office, relating to the "coronavirus" used as a "vaccine". Exactly, 7 years ago the coronavirus was already patented as an agent for use in vaccines for "various" cases. So we have to present it as a vaccine before being known as a "deadly disease." Where and on whom is it used? Is this reported? India distributes a kit of zinc, doxycycline and ivermectin pills to homes at a modest cost of $2.65 dollars, to heal from "coronavirus." The vaccines have been specially composed of MRC-5 (cells from aborted fetuses) and heavy metals such as aluminum and mercury (thimerosal, merthiolate), among other chemical compounds and drugs, which is logical that it leads, in the first instance, to a reaction Iatrogenic. The human body does not combine with metals. We have elements of a "metallic" order in ephemeral portions, necessary for various processes. If not, there would be no talk of treatments as beneficial as those performed with colloidal gold or silver. However, gold and silver are different from mercury and aluminum, starting with how they act within an organism.

Reporter Lou Collins' group sent a demand to the Irish Department of Health for several months asking for proof of the existence of Covid-19. Having no response, they went to the

---

1. https://patents.google.com/patent/EP3172319A1/en

offices of Tony Holohan, on Back Street, in Dublin. Holohan suspiciously left his position as Head of the Medical Office on July 02, 2020, allegedly due to family matters. At the end of that year Lou Collins asked Tony Holohan, and Steven Dundley, Minister of Health, directly at the offices of the HSE (Health and Safety Executive), or National Public Health Emergency Team, why they refused to respond to the freedom of information request (right to petition), which they had imposed months ago, regarding the existence of this Sars-CoV-2. By violating the constitution, refusing to give that information by the required date, Lou Collins made a live broadcast on his program that caused quite a stir and pressure in the HSE offices, after which they sent them a letter, responding to what at the level scientist and his criteria was a clear denial of the existence of Sars-Cov-2 (https://rumble.com/ved83t-departamento-de-salud-recognized-que-no-existe-el-covid-covid-doesnt-exist.html [2]). In a lawsuit in Court, they had also asked if there was evidence that the Quarantine and the use of masks had a true function of resistance to the spread of the "virus", and they could not give it to them, because it does not exist. I talk about social distancing and such infections. All these issues have already been said ad nauseum: they are anti-scientific. They fulfill a function that is more of a dictatorial nature, of controlling the population.

This is a letter about the COVID 19 Vaccine, from HE the Most Reverend. Mons. Dr. D. Pablo de Rojas Sánchez-Franco, Founder of the Pious Union of Saint Paul the Apostle, with whom I would like to begin this chapter of the book. Dr. Don Pablo de Rojas, Bishop, wrote this letter on December 24, 2020, <<which we could call pastoral, to be read in all private chapels

---

2.   https://rumble.com/ved83t-departamento-de-salud-reconoce-que-no-existe-el-covid-covid-doesnt-exist.html

where married couples, collaborators and sympathizers attend. Given the uncertainty that threatens us due to the so-called coronavirus, SARS COV-2, which produces the disease known as COVID 19, based on Catholic morality and the science of renowned doctors, Prego Cancello and Martin Salvaraccin among others, I see myself in the obligation to prohibit all those who freely submit themselves to an unworthy servant as a bishop by applying the epiqueya and using responses presided over to similar problems by the holy office in past times under penalty of mortal sin and impediment to administer and/or receive the sacraments . Get vaccinated against the aforementioned anomaly, for the following reasons: The so-called COVID 19 is not classified or recognized as a new virus because it does not meet the VOC requirements, and could be a laboratory creation with such "perfidious" purposes as enslaving the created society. For God's sake, I don't need to name the already very advanced New World Order and the 2030 agenda.>>

<<It should be noted that the common and vulgar type A flu in Spain has caused more deaths last year than the so-called COVID 19. Therefore, we can deduce that the goals that are moving scientists worldwide are not those of describe the reason for the pandemic and create a vaccine, but rather implement the long-cherished desires of Marxist and communist Judeo-Freemasonry, to diminish and subject society to their empire under a single New World Order. Humanity has faced plagues and pandemics for millions of years, the Black Death, the misnamed Spanish Flu, and smallpox. They left millions of deaths in their wake, for example, the 1918 flu pandemic known as the Spanish flu, it is known with certainty that it was a pandemic caused by an outbreak of the influenza virus Type A subtype Hn1n1. The first thing that the scientists and doctors of the time did was to make sure what had caused the pandemic and

what type of virus it was. Unlike other flu pandemics that affect children and the elderly, its victims were also young people and adults in good health, as well as like animals.>>

<<This is the most devastating pandemic in human history so far. Since in a single year it killed 40 million people. Doctors, even knowing the type of virus that had caused the pandemic, were not able to create an antidote, since it takes between 5 and 10 years. And yet society was not paralyzed, much less were the healthy locked up or the economy stopped as they are doing now and the middle class was sentenced to death, social injustices increased and the growing separation between the different classes of society increased. society. Creating a humanity subjugated to the new world order that is progressively being established, fulfilling its agenda where the new rich are getting richer and the new poor are getting poorer. An example of this progressive and accelerated implementation is the elimination, through scandalously fraudulent reader methods, of the only one who could stop the evolution of this agenda, even for 4 more years, the also Jewish Donald Trump.>>

<<How is it possible that in less than a year without knowing if it is a virus since, as I have indicated, it is not cataloged or recognized as such since it does not meet the VOC requirements, they have already been able to create several vaccines. It is impossible for them to have found an antidote to something they don't know about without having passed a reasonable amount of time, which according to Gaby's CEO Sir McCley would take between 5 and 10 years. The global vaccine and immunization alliance has made it clear that to get a vaccine the disease must first be diagnosed, which is why it is impossible for so many vaccines to have been found against something that is unknown in 4 or 5 months. Furthermore, to prove its effectiveness, when creating it they have to experiment and test it

on animals to see its side effects for a long time before supplying it to the population, which has not been done. And knowing as we know Pfizer Biotech, Cansino Biology, Oxford Johnsons University, University of Pittsburg, Immunity Bio, among others, to name some laboratories that are scandalously profiting from the creation and sale of them. They use cell cultures of human origin among their components, making the use of these vaccines obtained by morally execrable and repugnant methods objectively and intrinsically sinful.>>

<<My obligation as a Catholic bishop is to ensure not only the health of your souls but also that of your bodies. And that is why, according to Catholic morality, agreeing to be vaccinated under these current conditions is immoral and totally condemning. And in addition to the illicit means used to obtain it, its use violates the 5th commandment of the law of God. Well, the consequences on human beings in the long and short term that they may have are totally unknown. Since the See of Peter was vacant, only the Roman Pontiff could speak and bind the Universal Church, there being no jurisdiction for the Roman Catholic and Apostolic Church, as a consequence, only Catholics not having subjects. I insist that they hardly adhere to a server, and can prohibit, under penalty of mortal sin, from receiving the vaccine even if they force us to do so. This successor of the apostles doing his duty exposes Catholic doctrine and condemns errors. These are difficult times for Catholics, but our way of speaking has to be clear and express the truth. Well, the salvation of our soul is lost in it. That is why, in turn, I call, as far as possible, for an uprising against the new plans of the World Order in which the rights of God, the Church and the individual themselves are increasingly instilled. And if necessary we will offer our lives rather than commit a mortal sin...>>

Robert Francis Kennedy Jr., American lawyer and environmental activist, author – and since 2020 mostly vocal anti-vaccinationist – and son of Robert F. Kennedy (and nephew of former President John F. Kennedy), states the following in a 2020 publication: To all my patients: I would like to urgently draw your attention to important issues related to the upcoming Covid-19 vaccination. For the first time in the history of vaccination, the so-called next-generation mRNA vaccines intervene directly in the patient's genetic material and therefore change the individual genetic material, which represents genetic manipulation, something that has been prohibited and until now considered criminal. This intervention can be compared to that of genetically manipulated foods, which is also very controversial. Even if the media and politicians are currently trivializing the problem and even mindlessly clamoring for a new type of vaccine to return to normality, this vaccination is problematic in terms of health, morality and ethics and also in terms of genetic damage which, unlike The damage caused by previous vaccines will now be irreversible and irreparable.

Dear patients, after an unprecedented mRNA vaccine, you will no longer be able to treat the symptoms of the vaccine in a complementary way. They will have to live with the consequences, because they can no longer be cured simply by removing toxins from the human body, just as you cannot cure a person with a genetic defect such as Down syndrome, Klinefelter syndrome, Turner syndrome, the disease genetic heart disease, hemophilia, cystic fibrosis, Rett syndrome, etc.), because the genetic defect is forever! Clearly, this means: if a vaccination symptom develops after an mRNA vaccination, neither I nor any other therapist can help you, because the damage caused by the vaccination will be genetically irreversible. In my opinion, these new vaccines represent a crime against humanity that has never been committed in such a large way in history. As Dr. Wolfgang Wodarg, an experienced doctor, said: In reality, this "promising vaccine" for the vast majority of people is actually banned because it is genetic manipulation!" The vaccine, developed and supported by Anthony Fauci and financed by Bill Gates, used experimental mRNA technology. Three of the 15 human guinea pigs (20%) experienced a "serious adverse event."

Note: Messenger RNA or mRNA is the ribonucleic acid that transfers the genetic code from the DNA of the cell nucleus to a ribosome in the cytoplasm, that is, it determines the order in which the amino acids of a protein will be joined and acts as a template. or pattern for the synthesis of said protein. Resource: Robert F. Kennedy, Jr. (https://en.m.wikipedia.org/wiki/ Robert_F._Kennedy_Jr [3]). CLARIFICATION SO THAT THE POPULATION IS NO MORE DECEIVED: DOES THE CORONAVIRUS EXIST OR NOT? CLARIFICATION FOR THE CONFUSED:

1. DOES THE VIRUS EXIST? Yes, just like many more viruses.

2. DOES IT HAVE A CURE? Yes, if you use the appropriate medicines and do not leave your health in the hands of corrupt, commercial health systems.

3. ARE THERE GOOD DOCTORS? Yes, and many, some are acting in a low profile giving appropriate treatments, others have been braver and there are many videos on the networks that talk about these treatments and many have already been threatened, disqualified or silenced.

4. ARE THERE SCIENTISTS RESEARCHING? Yes, and there is a worldwide union convened and calling for more doctors and scientists called Doctors and Scientists for Truth, to

---

3.   https://en.m.wikipedia.org/wiki/Robert_F._Kennedy_Jr

expose the falsehood of the handling they have given to the issue of the bug.

5. IS IT A PANDEMIC? No. The WHO changed the term referring to pandemic before the bug emerged in order to call it a pandemic.

6. IS IT CONTAGIOUS? Yes, just like any flu.

7. IF I GET THE VIRUS, DOES IT MEAN I WILL DIE? No. If you get symptoms, you just have to take the appropriate medicine from the first day (boost your immune system, take anti-inflammatory drugs and anti-flu) and heal yourself at home.

8. CAN IT BE PREVENTED? Yes, being clean as you should always be and maintaining a high immune system, you also have: Ozone Therapy, Chlorine Dioxide with the preventive protocol.

9. ARE THE NUMBERS OF CONTACTED AND DEATHS FROM THE VIRUS TRUE? No. In the USA it was discovered that any figure given would actually be 10% of that figure because they have passed off cases of deaths from other diseases due to the virus and the tests are not reliable, they give false positives.

10. ARE ASYMPTOMATIC CASES REAL POSITIVE CASES? The human being has many microorganisms and viruses in the body and that does not mean that you are a sick or infectious person or that you have the virus, however the viruses that are supposedly "so aggressive" show some symptoms in patients because the body releases alarms of an intruder (fever, headache, vomiting, etc.) and according to Koch's theory the answer is NO.

11. WAS THE VIRUS CREATED? Yes, in a laboratory.

13. FOR WHAT PURPOSE? Be the excuse to restrict freedoms, change the current economic system for a more oppressive one / enslave you, frighten, blind flock obedience.

14. Are many countries part of this evil plan? Yes.

15. WILL WE GET OUT OF THIS? Yes. And all those who have contributed to the deaths and the NWO plan will fall and pay what they have to bear.

16. SHOULD I BE AFRAID? No. Fear lowers your immune system and makes you a mentally controllable person.

17. ARE THE MEDIA PART OF THE PLAN? Yes. The owners of the media are the same, the cabal controls the pharmaceutical industry, health, the media and they put everything together as they need, this is called mind control.

18. WHAT SHOULD I DO? You protect yourself and if you get sick you already know how to cure yourself, at home or with your trusted doctor, not committed to the abandonment protocol.

19. SHOULD I GET VACCINED? No. You don't need it if you stay healthy, vaccines bring chemicals, heavy metals and a series of "bugs" that will only further affect your health in the medium and long term both physically and mentally. It is your body and it is your right to decide about it and your physical and mental health. Would you trust a vaccine after a virus has been created to eliminate humanity?

20. IS THIS A WAR? Yeah! And we will be victorious, let's stay united and wake up other people by giving a lot of information.

Copied...pasted Do it too!!! "Forced to cover myself, but not to shut up." [End of article]. For example, Mr. Mike Yeadon, who served as vice president of Pfizer Pharmaceuticals, publicly said that this "pandemic" does not need a vaccine. And it does not need a vaccine because it has a very low mortality rate, which is 0.2% and, furthermore, the cure is achieved with medications that already exist. 99.8% of people infected with COVID-19 survive. When Pfizer claims that the vaccine is safe, it must be remembered that this Pharmaceutical Company has in the past paid billions of dollars in fines for LYING to medical doctors, and has also had to pay millions of dollars to compensate people whose health was harmed by THE MEDICINES produced by this Company. There is a lot that I can contribute here about the so-called vaccines, but I will leave it in the hands of the experts to delve into this issue, limiting myself only to making some additional comments when appropriate. Do your part, being an intelligent being, and connect the dots. Start by "guessing", what do the vaccine manufacturers get out of it? Millionaire profits. What do governments gain? Dictatorial power and training of the masses who will no longer be rebellious after the supply of these components in their blood.

John of Jerusalem prophesied about these pharmaceutical companies around the year 1100 AD. C., <<When the year one thousand begins, which follows the year one thousand, hunger oppresses the bellies of so many men and the cold will chill so many hands, that they will want to see another world. And **merchants of illusions will come who will offer the poison**. But this **<u>will destroy the bodies and rot the souls</u>**; and <u>those who have mixed poison with their blood will be like wild beasts caught in a trap, and they will kill, and rape, and plunder, and steal; and life will be an everyday Apocalypse</u>.>> The issue of vaccination was planned a long time ago, since for the elite it is the most efficient way to achieve the two most important objectives of their philosophy: 1. Reduce the population, 2. Idiotize the survivors. Everything else revolves around these two essential elements. You will have seen – and will continue to see – that viruses have never been a problem, and despite this this propaganda has been used to inoculate the masses with real poisons from laboratories that have orchestrated serious epidemics on a global level. In addition to this, by now you will have understood that viruses and chimeras alone cannot do us any harm if there are not 2 essential elements: 1. A conviction at the subconscious level of the mind, and 2. Functional collateral factors (poor diet, heavy metals in the blood, an already compromised immune system, and stimulating waves, among others). In fact, if you convince people that they should be afraid, they will lower their state of vibration and magnetize a doom. Then you poison them with heavy metals and hit them with low and high frequency waves from all directions, then even the bite of a little ant would be the trigger for a catastrophe. Well, let's continue with descriptions from those who know the most about this matter... Dr. Lee Merritt, who studied Biological Weapons, believes that the Covid-19 injection is Biological Warfare, as expressed by Phillip Schneider, in Waking Times:

An award-winning spine surgeon and former president of the Association of American Physicians and Surgeons believes the current coronavirus "vaccines" are dangerous biological weapons being deployed against the population. Dr. Lee Merritt, who previously studied biological weapons while serving as an orthopedic surgeon in the United States Navy for 9 years, served on the board of the Arizona Medical Association, and has published numerous peer-reviewed articles, believes that The mRNA-altering coronavirus shots currently being distributed in the United States are rewriting our genetic code to make us vulnerable to a second virus down the road: "Back in February I believed it was a manipulated bioweapon because at the time that someone came forward with data that suggested it was censored," he said in an interview last month with The New America. Moderna admits: mRNA injections are an "operating system" designed to program humans. Based on her time spent researching biological weapons, Dr. Merritt believes we live in an era of "fifth generation warfare" in which, instead of using weapons on the battlefield, covert biological agents, economic warfare and propaganda are more effective in turning the tables of power between nations.

"We have had many biological weapons over the years and the one that worried me the most was smallpox. But most of these biological weapons were difficult to distribute or there was treatment for them," he said. "I think there is a lot of evidence showing that coronavirus is a very benign natural virus that doesn't even give most people a cold, but at most gives you a common cold." Vaccines are most effective when used against an untreatable and deadly virus, he says. While diseases like smallpox and polio were effectively treated with immunizations, scientists have discovered promising treatments for the coronavirus since the pandemic began, such as hydroxychloroquine and intravenous vitamin C. "If we are in biological warfare right now as part of this multidimensional war, if you have a treatment in your pocket they cannot terrorize you with viruses and that is important because... [the vaccine] does not prevent transmission by its own admission." Even though prevention and treatment reduce the need for a vaccine, such information is routinely censored by social media companies and demonized by the mainstream media. Even Sharyl Attkisson, a former CBS journalist, had one of her reports removed from YouTube for transmitting information that went against the official position of the World Health Organization (WHO).

"We have vaccines because we had no treatment for smallpox and it was a very deadly disease. It made sense to have a vaccine. We had no treatment for polio, so it made sense to have a vaccine, but this? Even without doing anything, this disease has a 99.991% chance of survival... as opposed to a standard viral flu season which is 99.992%." – Lee Merritt. Coronavirus numbers are widely disputed, yet dozens of doctors and scientists have been speaking out for the better part of a year about the disproportionate amount of harm done by lockdowns and forced mask-wearing. A Canadian researcher estimates that the long-term cost of lockdowns will far exceed that of the virus itself by up to ten times. Merritt explains the difference between coronavirus vaccines and regular immunizations: "[Coronavirus vaccines] don't give you a pathogen... what they do is program the mRNA. mRNA is like DNA but it is messenger RNA. It is what produces proteins in the body. It's like a computer chip that you put in a 3D printer and then you tell it what you want it to do and it prints it. We have this in engineering and this is the biological equivalent. Well, in this case they have made a piece of this mRNA to create, in every cell in your body, that spike protein (or at least part of it) and you are actually creating the pathogen in your body."

When you go to get vaccinated against the coronavirus, you are not actually receiving a vaccine like the ones we have always known. Instead, messenger RNA is injected into your body that then alters your genetic code to begin producing its own modified version of the coronavirus, which your immune system theoretically learns to fight off. Lee Merritt: In animal studies, after being injected with MRNA technology, all animals died upon reinfection. Also read: A genetics professor predicts horrible latent deaths among the elderly after immunization with RNA vaccines. According to Dr. Merritt, there have been no long-term studies to verify the safety of this form of vaccination in humans, and animal studies have led to what she calls "antibody-dependent enhancement," in which the Virus enters the body undetected because the immune system now considers it as its own, which ends up causing almost immediate death. "We have never been able to carry out a successful animal study for this type of virus. We have never done it per se. humans," he says. "The longest they have followed people after the vaccine is two months. "It is not enough time to know that we will not have that problem of increased antibodies." – Dr. Lee Merritt.

Merritt speculates that this type of procedure is exactly what a foreign adversary would use if they wanted to wage clandestine biological warfare without the process being traced back to them. "It is a perfect binary weapon. There is no way for me to know exactly what that mRNA is programmed to do and neither do you or most doctors. Doctors cannot access that data. That's for those at the top of this project... "If I were China and I wanted to take down our military, I would just make an mRNA that I know doesn't exist in nature, so no one is going to die from one vaccine and then two "Years later I release something...and it causes this immune-boosting death." – Dr. Lee Merritt. Although Dr. Merritt does not recommend whether or not one should take the vaccine, she does give some edifying advice. "If you want to get out of the pandemic right now it is very easy. "Turn off the TV, take off your mask, reopen your business and live your life." Sources: https://ejercitoremanente.com/2021/ 02/05/dra-merritt-que-estudio-armas-biologicas-cree-que-la- inyeccion-covid-19-es-una-forma-de-medicina- armada/ [4]and https://humansarefree.com/author/ascanu [5].

In another report, from Derek Knauss (January 9, 2021): I have a PhD in virology and immunology. I am a clinical laboratory scientist and have analyzed 1500 "presumed" positive Covid 19 samples collected here in Southern California. When my lab team and I tested through Koch's postulates and observation under an SEM (scanning electron microscope), we

---

4.   https://ejercitoremanente.com/2021/02/05/dra-merritt-que-estudio-armas-biologicas-cree-que-la-inyeccion-covid-19-es-una-forma-de-medicina-armada/

5.   https://humansarefree.com/author/ascanu

found NO Covid in any of the 1500 samples. What we found was that all 1500 samples were mostly influenza A and some were influenza B, but not a single case of Covid, and we did not use the BS PCR test. We then sent the rest of the samples to Stanford, Cornell and some of the University of California labs and they found the same results as us, NO COVID. They found influenza A and B. Then we all talked to the CDC and asked for viable COVID samples, which the CDC said they couldn't provide because they didn't have any samples. We have now come to the firm conclusion through all our research and laboratory work, that COVID 19 was imaginary and fictitious.

The flu was called Covid and most of the 225,000 deaths died from concomitant diseases such as heart disease, cancer, diabetes, emphysema, etc. and then they contracted the flu which further weakened their immune system and they died. I have yet to find a single viable Covid 19 sample to work with. We, at the 7 universities that did the lab testing on these 1500 samples, are now suing the CDC for Covid 19 fraud. The CDC has yet to send us a single viable, isolated and purified Covid 19 sample. If they cannot or they don't want to send us a viable sample, I say there is no Covid 19, it is fictitious. The four research articles describing the genomic extracts of the Covid 19 virus never managed to isolate and purify the samples. The four articles written on Covid 19 only describe small fragments of RNA that were only 37 to 40 base pairs long, which is NOT A VIRUS. A viral genome is typically 30,000 to 40,000 base pairs.

With how bad Covid is supposed to be everywhere, how come no one in any laboratory in the world has isolated and purified this virus in its entirety? That's because they never actually found the virus, all they found were little bits of RNA that were never identified as the virus anyway. So what we are dealing with is another strain of flu like every year, COVID 19 does not exist and is fictitious. I believe China and the globalists orchestrated this COVID hoax (the flu disguised as a new virus) to bring about global tyranny and a totalitarian global police surveillance state, and this plot included massive election fraud to overthrow Trump. Source: https://thetruedefender.com/explosive-if-true-im-a-clinical-lab-scientist-c19-is-fake-wake-up-america/ [6].

In another article, from June 29, 2015, we see, as an example of the hundreds reported in the last decade, virologists, bacteriologists, influential anti-vaccines, scientists and specialized doctors found dead in suspicious conditions, all of them being direct enemies against of the interests of vaccine manufacturing companies and their collaborators: Jeff Bradstreet, one of the main anti-vaccine activists in the United States, dies. Chimney Rock (North Carolina). (AP): A fisherman found the lifeless body of Dr. Jeff Bradstreet, a doctor who dedicated his life to fighting against vaccines. The discovery occurred on the 19th in the Broad River Rocky River in Chimney Rock (North Carolina). The Rutherford County Sheriff's Office, which is investigating the case, believes that Bradstreet, 60, committed suicide by shooting himself in the chest, according to a statement. Bradstreet was a native of Braselton, Georgia. The firearm was also found in the river and the doctor's family is raising funds to investigate his death. Bradstreet ran a clinic in Buford, Georgia, and published research on autism based on claims that some vaccines cause the disease. His son is autistic and the doctor attributed it to a vaccine that was administered when the little one was 15 months old... source: https://www.lavanguardia.com/vida/20150629/

---

6.   https://thetruedefender.com/explosive-if-true-im-a-clinical-lab-scientist-c19-is-fake-wake-up-america/

54432590074/muere-jeff-bradstreet   -anti-vaccines-united-states.html[7].

On July 11, 2013, the website of the US Center for Disease Control (CDC) published an article in which it confessed that between 1955 and 1963, about 98 million Americans received one or more doses of the vaccine "against" polio, which contained the cancer virus, called SV40 (Simian Vacuolatin 40). Evidently the CDC quickly removed the article and deleted all traces of it from Google, although someone previously noticed and took a screenshot of the post. SV40 is a virus found in certain types of apes and was discovered in 1960, and was found in the polio vaccine shortly after. This virus is believed to have reached about 10 to 30 Americans. What is understood is that SV40 has been found in certain types of cancer in humans, although it is not entirely clear that it itself is the cause of cancer, according to the majority of official scientific evidence. It is said that since 1963 SV40 was removed from polio vaccines. Additionally, in the 1950s rhesus monkey kidney cells containing the animal's SV40 were infected and used for the polio vaccine. It is said that since "no one knew" of the existence of SV40 until the 1960s, "they did not imagine" that the vaccines would be contaminated.

Interestingly, SV40 was found in the IPV (injected dose) not in the OPV (oral) version, because the injection carries the contents directly into the blood. Adds the article: <<To further confirm this incredible admission, assistant professor of pathology at Loyola University Chicago, Dr. Michele Carbone, has been able to independently verify the presence of the SV40 virus in tissue and bone samples of patients who died during that time. He found that 33% of samples with osteosarcoma bone

---

7.   https://www.lavanguardia.com/vida/20150629/54432590074/muere-jeff-bradstreet-antivacunas-estados-unidos.html

cancers, 40% of other bone cancers and 60% of mesothelioma lung cancers contained this unknown virus. This leaves the postulation that more than 10 to 30 million actually contracted and were negatively affected by this virus, to be deadly accurate.>> Source: https://breaking-news.ca/cdc-admits-98-million -americans-were-given-cancer-virus-via-the-polio-shot/[8]

The Argentine doctor Luis Marcelo Martínez explains in an interview for the program 'Contra Cara', with Juan Manuel Soaje Pino, that the protein of the supposed coronavirus is identical to syncytin (found in the ERVW-1 gene on chromosome 7), which is key for pregnancy to take place in humans. So the population is not being immunized against a virus but against its own ability to reproduce. Quoting his words verbatim, <<the placenta and the embryo depend on a protein called synsitin-1, and another called synsitin-2. These proteins are critical in early placental development. Yeah? And on the other hand, the theoretical support of the SArs-Cov-2 virus, in that the genetic sequence of the 'S' protein, of the "virus", is homologous to the genetic sequence of syncytin.>> And he adds that The supposed Sars-Cov-2 genome is a computer construct, and that the said "immunity" of the "vaccine" would be against female reproduction, but also, also against male reproduction, <<because it is enzymed by ACE2>> (enzyme Angiotensin 2 converter, or ANG2) <<which has a very strong relationship with male fertility, is also at stake in this whole network>> And he later adds, <<the "virus" is not similar to human proteins, that is a design>> <<the theoretical framework of the SArs-Cov-2 virus is a trap. The genetic design of the virus, from a bioinformatics point of view, is a design equivalent to human proteins related to reproduction. The differences between

---

8.   https://breaking-news.ca/cdc-admits-98-million-americans-were-given-cancer-virus-via-the-polio-shot/

vectorized or gene vaccines are technical differences. The public must understand that these components of genetic design will have an effect on the epigenetics and genetics of the human being.>>

Second, < < what do you intend to test? Tolerability. Test that there are not a large number of sequelae and/or deaths, because the real effects intended with these components will be observed in the long term. When you test a vaccine and want to evaluate its impact on reproduction, you have to wait years. That is why vaccines take so many years of development and testing. The confidentiality [of the vaccine component] is not for a formula to be stolen. Don't be innocent, please. Confidentiality and immunity is because there are going to be many more cases of multiple sclerosis, amyotrophic lateral sclerosis, transverse myelitis. Because? This protein syncytin-1 – against which the immune response will be mounted – is related to the onset of pregnancy and the health of the central nervous system. When syncytin-1 is canceled the patient has neurological symptoms. That's why these paintings appear. And there will be many more. Syncytin is in the brain and is in pregnancy.>> <<The intention to analyze these vaccines is blocked with the trap of the storage temperature and that it is of immediate application. In other words, if we wanted to analyze one of these vaccines, it would be quite difficult for us to access a sample to sequence it and analyze the adjuvants, the sequences of the vectors and the sequences of the fragments that are intended to be introduced into human cells.>>

<<It is possible to modulate the expression of our genes. There are genes that carry out certain specific functions.>> Genes such as male fertility can be blocked <<through epigenetic modulation. I can silence the expression of this gene, and I can achieve a specific effect, which in the short and

medium term you will not realize. Why are volunteers required, and made to sign, a "no pregnancy for two years" document? Think about that.>> What does that have to do with a "respiratory virus"? and not only will these genes be modulated on reproduction but also on behavior. So, when we talk about modifying DNA we talk about the potential of these components to generate incersional mutations. That is, the little piece of DNA particles carried by vectorized vaccines can be inserted anywhere. They are potentially risks that exist>> <<And when inserted into any site of the genome, the initial risk is cancer, and then, autoimmune diseases. Yeah? And for one to see these effects, a certain amount of time must pass. And doing this type of thing is <<acting on human behavior and discernment. Because this has [already] been done [in the past]. I can deactivate genes related to neuromodulation. There are going to be more cases of neurological sequelae>> You can see the content here: https://rumble.com/ved7xn-vacunas-covid-son-plan-de-esterilizacin-mundial.html [9].

In an interview, the Argentine doctor Chinda Brandolino gives an explanation of abortion and in her hand she holds a small-scale design of a baby to refer to the topic we are delving into, while clarifying one of the interests behind abortion, both corporate and use for vaccines. Chinda Brandolino: "This is 12 weeks old, Viviana, not even 14. Then you, with a pair of tweezers, grab a little leg and cut it off, while the child cries, you can see how the baby opens his mouth and desperately runs away with his little arms. the inside of the uterus as if seeking his mother to protect him." "In the second-third trimester, it is taken out in little pieces, it is pulled, to a certain extent you take out a little leg, a little piece, another little foot." "Suction

---

9.   https://rumble.com/ved7xn-vacunas-covid-son-plan-de-esterilizacin-
    mundial.html

abortion: a forceps is inserted, the little head is crushed, when you feel the noise (if it is big) of the broken bones, then a cane is applied, you connect it with a vacuum cleaner and like garbage it is thrown into a container." "When the child is of childbearing age, 7, 8 or 9 months to generate, breech birth is induced, that is, he is born breech and when the child's bone is in the birth canal with scissors it is cut, like "when they cut the throat of a chicken." "And this government, Fernández, is saying: I can't give you work or money, I'll keep it." "So you have to kill your child, crush the baby's head without damaging the organs so as not to reduce the price. So between 80 and 100 dollars for each children's organ."

Journalist Viviana: And what is this for?

Chinda Brandolino: for organ transplants, my love, the sale of organs is between 80 and 100 dollars. I have filmed a doctor while she eats, director of a branch, who says that they ask her for lower organs from the aborted child, probably for skin tissues, with this indifference and that she charged 120, 150 dollars. Well, organ remains are sold to very important cosmetics companies in the world...

Journalist Viviana: cosmetics?

Chinda Brandolino: Yes, and some live children are used to make vaccines, in MR-5, (I don't remember the exact acronym), in all viral vaccines, triple viral means that acronym: Lung tissue of a Caucasian male fetus with 14 weeks of gestation. That autism is produced for this reason because the deoxyribonucleic acid of the murdered child follows the brain of the child receiving the vaccine and is modified and causes autoimmune and oncological diseases. Using human DNA has entered the DNA of the child who receives it. Just look at the statistics: In 1970 there was 1 child in 10,000 with autism, in 1975 it was 1 in 5,000, in 1985 it was 1 in 2,500, in 1995 it was 1 in 500, in 2000 it was 1 in 150, in 2004 it was 1 in 125, in 2008 it was 1 in 88, in

2012 it was 1 in 68, and in 2017 it was 1 in 38. I haven't looked at the data in the last 4 years, and I don't know if I want to. Just think what the rate will be for the next 10 years.

Let's go to another case, addressing the question of how vaccines play the role of sterilization (eugenics): in the *paper* titled "A human homolog of angiotensin-converting Enzyme. Cloning and functional expression as a captopril-insensitive carboxypeptidase", whose main author is Dr. Sarah R. Tipnis, from the School of Biochemistry and Molecular Biology at the University of Leeds (UK), published on 08/2/2000 in the Journal of Biological Chemistry announces that "a new human zinc metalloprotease with considerable homology to angiotensin-converting enzyme (ACE) (40% identity and 61% similarity) has been identified." The researchers call it "angiotensin-converting enzyme homolog (ACEH)", and through an impeccable, complete and well-described experimental procedure they explain how they obtain its sequence and what tissue expression it manifests, knowing in advance that it is a non-inhibitable carboxypeptidase. by classical ACE inhibitors, and that it has a simple zinc-binding domain HEXXZ and other conserved critical residues typical of the ACE family. They demonstrate its expression and enzymatic activity using an ACEH construct, and expression of ACE mRNA and ACEH mRNA using Northern Blot in numerous human tissues, fully demonstrating a strong expression of ACEH in the testis (hypothesizing "possible reproductive functions and its relationship with fertility") and secondarily in heart, kidney, ovary, small intestine and colon, and practically no expression in lung. On the other hand, ACE is expressed uniformly in practically all tissues analyzed, with marked expression in kidney.

It is necessary to clarify that four of the six authors are deceased, Dr. Tipnis among them, and the relationship between the Pfizer laboratory and their work. In 2002, Harmer and collaborators found high expression of ACE2 by quantitative RTPCR in testis, kidney and heart, and low expression in CNS and lymphoid tissue. On November 27, 2003, a work titled "Angiotensin-converting enzyme 2 is a functional receptor for the SARS coronavirus" was published in the journal Nature, the first author of which is Wenhui Li, from the Department of Medicine (Microbiology and Molecular Genetics), Center for AIDS research, Bringham and Women's Hospital, in which they claim to have discovered that the S1 subdomain of the S protein of SARS-CoV "efficiently binds" with the metallopeptidase ACE2, thus constituting the ACE2 enzyme as its cellular receptor mediating infection in target cells. In the development of the hypothesis, they establish a "suggestive" comparison of the protein cleavage experienced by the viral proteins of HIV, Influenza and the S protein of many coronaviruses (in anticipation of the 2009 Influenza H1N1 pandemic, and the current Covid pandemic. -19)

"...Similar to the analogous human immunodeficiency virus (HIV) and influenza proteins, the S proteins of some coronaviruses—including MHV and the group III coronavirus infectious bronchitis virus—are cleaved into two subunits (S1 and S2) by a cellular protease in viruses -producing cells..." They explain how they investigated the possible "union" between the (hypothetical) S protein of SARS-CoV and its possible natural receptor in a Vero E6 cell culture using a "fusion protein" that would express residues of the S protein of SARS-CoV. Finally, after analyzing the mass of the fragments obtained after digestion with trypsin ("tryptic fragments") by mass spectrometry, they identified three human proteins, and they focused only on "one" from eight fragments with a sequence homology of 17%. with the amino acid sequence of the ACE2 protein (according to comparison of the possible tryptic fragments with protein fragments in the GeneBank database, using the Sequest software), stating that it is the best candidate protein due to "its cellular and tissue distribution" (... except that the virus enters the host through the testicle...). Given this insufficient evidence of having identified a candidate protein for a viral receptor, and taking as a descriptive model of how the nucleotide and amino acid sequence of an unknown protein with high homology and similarity to another previously known protein (ACE2-ACE) is obtained, led to carried out completely and adequately described in the work of Dr. Tipnis.

- cDNA Sequence Analysis of ACEH

- Expression of ACE mRNA and ACEH mRNA in Human Tissues

- Expression and Enzymic Activity of an ACEH Construct

- Genomic Sequence Analysis of the ACEH Gene

Suffice it to say that the description of the protocol carried out to immunoprecipitate and identify the ACE2 enzyme in the work of Dr Wenhui Li is absolutely incomplete and proves nothing. From here, in chronological sequence, there are many works in which the "broad tissue distribution for the expression of ACE2" is proposed, none with the level and weight of scientific evidence reached by Dr. Tipnis. Theoretical preparation for the next 2009-2010 Influenza A (H1N1) "pandemic": "An effort to recreate the 1918 influenza strain (a subtype of H1N1 avian strain) was a collaboration between the US Army Institute of Pathology Armadas, the USDA Southeastern Poultry Research Laboratory and the Mount Sinai School of Medicine in New York City. The effort resulted in the announcement (on October 5, 2005) that the group had successfully determined the genetic sequence of the virus, using historical tissue samples recovered by pathologist Johan Hultin from an Inuit flu victim buried in the permafrost of Alaska and preserved specimens of American soldiers Roscoe Vaughan and James Downs" (Wikipedia).

The document "The elusive definition of pandemic influenza" (Peter Doshi of MIT), published in the WHO Bulletin in 2011 Bull World Health Organ (2011; 89:532–538 / doi:10.2471/BLT.11.086173) explains clearly how the WHO changed the definition of a pandemic on May 4, 2009 (one month before the H1N1 pandemic was declared), removing the item "enormous number of deaths and illnesses." On August 12, 2009, The Journal Infectius Diseases received an article titled "What is a Pandemic?", prepared by David Morens, Gregory Folkers and Anthony Fauci, in which the authors relativize all the epidemiological aspects necessary for the declaration of a pandemic, except for the "widespread geographic extension", claiming that this is the only common denominator. In May 2010, the Rockefeller Foundation and the Global Business Network issued a report titled "Scenarios for the future of technology and International development" proposing and foreseeing a future scenario of pandemics (among others), with the need to implement consequent actions (population control).

On January 24, 2020, the article titled "A NOVEL CORONAVIRUS FROM PATIENTS WITH PNEUMONIA IN CHINA, 2019" was published (according to the editor's note) in The New England Journal of Medicine, with Dr. NA Zhu as first author. , which tells how a new coronavirus was "identified and cultured" from respiratory fluid samples of patients with pneumonia of unknown cause identified in Wuhan since December 21, 2019, describing a process of "viral culture and isolation " incomplete (the article itself states that it does not comply with Koch's postulates), and without having autopsy data on any of the patients studied. This article begins to be referenced by numerous subsequent ones and by the WHO itself as proof of the first isolation of a "new virus." It only remains to mention that from the moment the cases were identified until the publication of the work (document in the hands of the editor) a record time of 34 days passed! MARCH 11, 2020 WHO DECLARES A PANDEMIC DUE TO THE EXTENSION OF A NEW VIRAL VARIANT, WHICH DUE TO ITS ZOONOTIC ORIGIN AND MULTIPLE INTERMEDIATE HOSTS (WHICH WOULD ASSOCIATE GREATER MUTABILITY... AND INFECTIVE POWER), AS WELL AS DUE TO ITS BIOLOGICAL TARGET WITH "WIDE TISSUE DISTRIBUTION" with POTENTIALLY FATAL clinical evolution.... Conclusions:

- The industry is ALWAYS attentive to the reliable discovery of a new "actionable" gene/enzyme in accordance with the interests of power through vaccines and/or drugs.

- Dr. Tipnis discovers and reliably describes the ACE2 enzyme and the sequence of its gene (located on the short arm of the (and to a lesser extent ovary), and whose main function is most likely related to fertility and reproduction, under the watchful eye of Pfizer.

- Viruses (probably ALL) are a smokescreen to keep the scientific community distracted, establish population control strategies through fear, confinement and quarantines, and on the other hand, they are FALSELY linked to certain enzymes as a receptor in target cells , and then act on them with vaccines: Since the work of Dr. Wenhui Li (Nature 2003) is fraudulent, the existence of the S protein and by extension the virus itself is also false (there is not a single viral isolation work for batSARS-CoV, SARS and SARS-CoV2 that fully satisfies the classical Koch postulates and/or in their molecular version).

Finally, any diagnosis using new methodologies requires confirmation with previous technologies (e.g., CNV screening using NGS is confirmed with MLPA).

- The bases and strategies for declaring pandemics are sequentially established.

- The final objective: The creation of an ORWELIAN global state through the "design" of a pandemic (by theoretical definition, not by real objectification of a catastrophic situation) and in the second instance the global implementation of a vaccine to STERILIZE the total population (target of the vaccine: ACE2). [End of post]

In another study, the possible cause of the coronavirus plandemic is discussed as part of the immunological interference between POLYSORBATE 80 of the adjuvanted influenza vaccine and SARS-CoV-2. This study was carried out by Juan F. Gastón Añaños, Ana Martínez Giménez and Elisa Mª Sahún García, from the Pharmacy Service and Preventive Medicine Service of the Barbastro Hospital. The objective of this study is to analyze the coronavirus pandemic from the double point of view of Pharmacoepidemiology and Pharmacovigilance. Based on an epidemiological analysis of deaths from COVID-19 in the Health Sector served by the Barbastro Hospital, and the study of the pharmacotherapeutic history of the affected patients, it was found that the drug most common to all those who died was Chiromas®. This led to the hypothesis that the flu vaccination of the 2019-2020 campaign could be associated with a higher risk of death from COVID-19 in people over 65 years of age, that is, to the suspicion of possible iatrogenesis, a suspicion that is confirmed by accessing data from another sector.

The current situation of the Pharmacovigilance of vaccines in Spain is reviewed, seeking a means of communication of the aforementioned suspicion that is agile and dynamic. There is an apparent excess of confidence in the safety of vaccines, far removed from the principle of prudence. A possible mechanism of action is proposed for the hypothesis of immunological interference with parenteral POLYSORBATE 80, and the degree of agreement of the expected data with those observed is compared, reaching the conclusion that the hypothesis could be valid, therefore that it is decided to publish it. Keywords: COVID-19, adjuvanted influenza vaccine, POLYSORBATE 80, immunological interference, cytokine storm. The Health Sector served by the Barbastro Hospital geographically occupies the eastern half of the province of Huesca, with a highly dispersed, eminently rural population of 100,000 inhabitants. Pharmacovigilance is part of the daily work of the hospital pharmacist, who must be attentive to prevent and, where appropriate, detect and resolve possible cases of iatrogenesis in the patients they care for. Within this Pharmacovigilance work, the registration of confirmed cases of death from COVID-19 in the hospital itself as of 04/30/2020 was carried out, and the analysis of their previous treatments. Subsequently, on 05/05/2020, the study was expanded to the entire Healthcare Sector, in order to expand the sample, using the Electronic Health Record (EHR) as a data source.

Results: The first relevant data found is the fact that the 20 deaths in the Sector were all over 65 years of age. Of them, 17 had the administration of the vaccine and its batch recorded by Primary Care, and there is no record of the other 3. Those vaccinated against the flu would therefore represent at least 85% of the total deaths. This figure was higher than expected according to the vaccination rate in the Barbastro Health Sector, which, according to the Weekly Epidemiological Bulletin of Aragon, had been 63.1% in that age segment. According to these results, flu vaccination not only would not have improved the prognosis of the vaccinated elderly with respect to COVID-19, but would have worsened it. The inconsistency of data on the effectiveness of influenza vaccination in preventing complications such as pneumonia, hospitalization and general mortality in institutionalized elderly people with comorbidities has already been highlighted by previous studies with a much higher number of cases.

The data found led to the hypothesis that the flu vaccination in the 2019-2020 campaign could be associated with a higher risk of death from COVID-19 in people over 65 years of age. To test the hypothesis, a comparison of these 20 deaths/100,000 inhabitants was sought with other data from the environment, in an attempt to expand the sample. The deaths in the other Sector of the province of Huesca were analyzed, finding certain difficulties in accessing the vaccination record in the EHR. Data is accessed from a nursing home that had 94 inmates as of 11/08/2019, of which 25 have died from COVID-19, which reveals the finding that more people have died in that nursing home. with 94 inmates (25 deaths) than in our health sector of 100,000 (20 deaths), in a proportion 1000 times higher. Once the lack of registration in the EHR was solved, due to a computer problem, access was obtained to the manual Primary Care record of the vaccination in the residence, with the following results:

- Of the 80 vaccinated, 24 have died, 30%.

- Of the 14 unvaccinated, 13 are still alive today, and 1 has died. That is, 7% have died.

- Therefore, the death rate in the registered vaccinated quadruples that of the unvaccinated, for an already important sample of 94 individuals.

Confirmation of the initial suspicion is thus obtained, and a geographic-social-health component is observed that can be investigated in more depth.

Discussion: As an initial step to rule out possible contamination of the vaccine itself with SARS-CoV-2, the Microbiology Service of our center was requested to perform the PCR test on the contents of a syringe left over from the campaign, from the administered batch. to more deaths. The test result was negative. Subsequently, the composition of the adjuvanted vaccine administered to those over 65 years of age within the Public Health campaign in the Community of Aragon, Chiromas®, was studied, whose technical sheet reports on the following components: Surface antigens of viruses influenza (hemagglutinin and neuraminidase) cultured in embryonated chicken eggs from healthy chickens and with MF59C.1 adjuvant, of the strains:

- Strain similar to A/Brisbane/02/2018 (H1N1) pdm09 (A/Brisbane/02/2018, IVR-190) 15 micrograms HA (hemagglutinin).

- A/Kansas/14/2017 (H3N2)-like strain (A/Kansas/14/2017, NYMC X-327) 15 micrograms HA (hemagglutinin).

- Strain similar to B/Colorado/06/2017 (B/Maryland/15/2016, wild type) 15 micrograms HA zhemaglutinin).

Adjuvant: MF59C.1 is a unique adjuvant: 9.75 mg squalene; 1.175 mg of POLYSORBATE 80; 1.175 mg sorbitol trioleate; 0.66 sodium citrate; 0.04 mg of citric acid and water for injection. The adjuvant component is what differentiates the Chiromas® vaccine from the Chiroflu® vaccine (4), which is the one that has been administered to healthcare workers. Adjuvants (from Latin, "adyuvare", literally "to help") are substances used in combination with a specific antigen that produce a more robust immune response than the antigen alone (5). Squalene is a hydrophobic natural hydrocarbon originally obtained for commercial purposes from shark liver oil, but is produced by all complex organisms, including humans, as it is a precursor to cholesterol. It is therefore not a foreign product for our body. For the rest of the components of the adjuvant, an initial bibliographic search was carried out that led to focusing the study on POLYSORBATE 80, a cosmetic ingredient also known as TWEEN-80, Polyoxyethylene 20 sorbitan monooleate, Sorbimacrogol oleate 300, and with the acronym E-433. In the INCI list (International Nomenclature of Cosmetic Ingredients) it is called POLYSORBATE – 80.

Chemically, POLYSORBATE 80 has a hydrophilic and a lipophilic part, which allows it to improve the water solubility of hydrophobic molecules such as squalene, stabilizing emulsions. The effectiveness of POLYSORBATE 80 as a surfactant agent is confirmed by the importance of the medications that include it to enable the parenteral administration of macromolecules of the size and complexity of monoclonal antibodies (adalimumab, infliximab, tocilizumab, secukinumab...), epoetin alfa, anakinra, amiodarone...injectable solution, or triamcinolone acetonide suspension. POLISORBATE 80 is very well tolerated and is not irritating to the skin and mucous membranes topically, but the Acofarma information sheet reports that "polysorbates have been associated with serious adverse effects, including death, in low birth weight neonates." who administered parenteral preparations with polysorbates". Warnings regarding POLYSORBATE 80 are included in several drug technical sheets: Thus, the Torisel® technical sheet warns that polyvinyl chloride (PVC) bags and medical devices should not be used for the administration of preparations containing POLYSORBATE 80, since that POLYSORBATE 80 leaches di-(2-ethylhexyl) phthalate (DEHP) from PVC (7); The technical information sheet for Trangorex® warns that cases of hepatotoxicity have been reported with amiodarone after its IV administration that could be due to the solvent (POLYSORBATE 80) that carries it, instead of the medication itself.

The technical information for Chiromas® was studied, which reports "Immune system disorders: Allergic reactions, including anaphylactic shock (rarely), anaphylaxis and angioedema". We searched the literature on immunological adverse effects described for other parenterally administered vaccines that also contain POLYSORBATE 80. The following were found:

- Pandemrix®: After the flu vaccination campaign in Sweden in 2009-2010, an association between the use of the Pandemrix® vaccine and an increase in cases of narcolepsy was demonstrated, especially in children under 20 years of age who carried the HLA-DQB1*06 allele. :02, by multiplying their risk of suffering from this disorder by twelve.

- Gardasil®: Among the adverse effects detected for this vaccine against Human Papillomavirus in post-marketing, are "Immune system disorders (frequency not known): Hypersensitivity reactions including anaphylactic/ anaphylactoid reactions."

- Prevenar®: Among the adverse effects detected for this pneumococcal vaccine in post-marketing, are: "Immune system disorders: Rare: Hypersensitivity reaction, including facial edema, dyspnea, bronchospasm."

The current state of vaccine pharmacovigilance in Spain was analyzed, with the following relevant findings:

- Flu vaccines are medications whose composition changes every year, but strangely they do not carry an additional black triangle for monitoring.

- The flu vaccine is considered a prescription drug, but in the vaccination campaign there is no medical prescription, nor are individualized prescriptions issued per patient, nor are the vaccines dispensed in a pharmacy. The vaccine is administered "per protocol."

- Vaccines are frequently served on pallets from the pharmaceutical laboratory to the administration centers, without basic pharmaceutical controls or delivery notes or distributed batches.

- The document on the Pharmacovigilance Plan for Pandemic Vaccines of the AEMPS is dated October 14, 2009 (12), that is, nothing less than prior to the date on which the association of the use of the Pandemrix® influenza vaccine was demonstrated. with an increased risk of narcolepsy of 4 to 9 times higher in vaccinated children and adolescents compared to unvaccinated ones. This seems to indicate that there is widespread confidence in our healthcare environment about the safety of vaccines, and specifically the flu vaccine. Given this situation, it is decided to directly notify each of the aforementioned deaths that occur within the Hospital as a suspicion of possible ALVa (adverse event linked to vaccination) to the Aragon Pharmacovigilance Center.

Conclusions: Although the notification of suspicion of a possible adverse effect of a medication does not oblige the declarant to propose a mechanism of action for it, the hospital experience and the documentation consulted allow us to propose a hypothetical mechanism for the possible immunological interference, which requires of the concurrence of 3 elements:

- Previous exposure of the subject to the administration of POLISORBATE 80 parenterally, either through the adjuvanted vaccine or other parenteral drugs that contain it.

- Non-optimal immunological status of the subject: advanced age, concomitant autoimmune pathologies, immunosuppressive treatments...

- Subsequent infection with a strain of the SARS-CoV-2 coronavirus.

That is, by themselves, neither polysorbate nor the coronavirus would be capable of triggering the hypersensitivity reaction. The possible interference between acquired immunity against POLYSORBATE 80 and coronavirus infection would occur at the time of viral replication inside infected cells, and in subjects with a not 100% efficient immune status. But another variable must come into play: The contradictory results of the PCR tests obtained for patients at our center, with alternative results (+) and (-), seem to suggest the idea that at least two strains of SARS-CoV- could coexist. 2, one would give the PCR positive and the other would give it negative. During the replication process in the infected cell, a mutation could occur that would give rise to coronaviruses of the other strain. The (+) strain of the coronavirus, when replicating in a cell of the lung mucosa or vascular epithelium, would cause it to express some antigen similar to polysorbate on its surface, and would be responsible for the immunological interference, by confusing the immune system, not 100% efficient, making it use the acquired immunity against polysorbate against the cells in which that strain (+) is replicating, attacking and destroying them, considering them foreign cells.

The double strain would explain the fact that there are certain individuals with an immune system that is not 100% efficient and who in November-December 2019 were administered POLYSORBATE 80 parenterally as part of the adjuvanted vaccine, who only suffer the initial infectious syndrome of a mild nature due to SARS-CoV-2, and they would be those infected by the (-) strain that would generate antibodies against it and defeat it. On the other hand, in those others infected by the (+) strain, or in those in which the (-) strain mutated in the replication process to the (+) strain, the immunological interference described could take place, triggering a reaction of severe hypersensitivity, the inflammatory process known as "cytokine storm" (14), which is what would ultimately cause death. The clinical complications of this process can manifest as acute respiratory distress syndrome (ARDS), disseminated vascular coagulation, acute pancreatitis..., depending on the cells in which the coronaviruses are replicating, which are attacked by the patient's autoimmune reaction, with the very serious known consequences. The hypothesis would explain facts observed in the pandemic, such as the following:

- Geographic differences in COVID-19 cases worldwide, focusing on the northern hemisphere (Europe, United States, Mexico...), where the flu vaccination was carried out prior to winter, while in the southern hemisphere it was autumn.

- Late appearance of COVID-19 in Brazil, where the flu vaccination campaign began on March 23, 2020 (17), and has been followed by an exponential increase in the number of affected people.

- Geographic differences in COVID-19 cases at the European level, where there are very low flu vaccination rates in people over 65 years of age in Eastern European countries, such as Estonia, which does not even reach 5%, compared to Spain, United Kingdom, France or Italy, with rates of 50-60% (19). There are also differences in access to vaccines. Thus, in Estonia, the flu vaccine is paid.

- Geographic and social differences at the national level, with higher rates in elderly residences and rural areas, where the vaccination rate is higher than in residents in their own homes and urban areas. Aragon would be an emblematic case of rural and residential damage, with a higher number of cases than would be the case due to its low population density. [I will share the sources at the end of the book]. Below, in the words of Manuel Elkin Patarroyo, the scientist who developed the vaccine against Malaria, an excerpt from an interview on S TV, which was conducted with him and after which the public no longer wanted to invite him to give his opinion:

That a person allows the vaccine to be administered at a certain time really means nothing to me, I tell you. What is happening when they apply it to the person? Looking to see if it is safe, that is, if it does not harm the kidneys, the lungs, the blood, etc., etc. What we scientists call "security" the other is immunogenicity, that is, the ability to induce defenses that are capable of killing the virus in the test tube or how we do it at the level of experimental models. In this case, in the case of the Aotus Monitos, then, that is what is called immunogenicity, and the other thing is the capacity for protection, that is, protectivity, which is that both after you have been vaccinated, you have found that the vaccine does not has caused you any harm, that produced the antibodies or the white blood cell response, how much does it protect people? That is what has not been done in absolutely any of these vaccines that are being tested today. The only thing they tell you is that, look, that Glaxo vaccine, the Pfizer vaccine, the Moderna vaccine, is safe, because among the 100 to 1,000 people they vaccinated, it did not induce any kidney or liver damage. nor pulmonary, safe, safe, safe.

And the other thing is that it induces antibodies or induces defenses, but, let me make an observation, that for all my compatriots, let's not be fooled by that, the most they are telling us is that they produce antibodies that last 26 days and The one who has taken it the longest has taken it to 40 days. So, if we know well, among other things, that the molecules of this coronavirus that are here induce defenses, but they are very short-lived, they do not last more than 60 days, and, usually in an infection for an individual who has had the disease and you go and detect the antibodies, the antibodies begin to disappear after 4 weeks, that is, after a month and then by 4 to 6 months you do not have a single one of those antibodies, and that is one of the fundamental problems today in day. It is not only safety, immunogenicity, protectiveness, but also duration of the immune response. How about vaccinating people against these vaccines every 2 or 3 months? That is absolutely impossible. So, please, let my compatriots understand that, if they are selling us that the one is safe, it induces antibodies that go into Phase 3, yes, Phase 3 is, you know what? increase the number of individuals who are receiving the vaccine and find that it has not harmed them and that they are producing antibodies, but how long they last and whether they protect or not, that is what is not being said today.

Q: I want to delve into this, about the durability of these vaccines, what you say is that at the moment the vaccines that are on the horizon (40 days) yes, I would have to get vaccinated after 40 days (Laughter) that is, until the at the moment they have followed up for 40 days. And how much for the vaccine, for you, for the scientists so that it is absolutely viable for how many days, how long.

At least it lasts a year, old lady, like a kitten, usually what we ask, the scientists, is that it lasts from 5 to 10 years, that is what we scientists, those of us who are dedicated to the development of vaccines, ask for. That a vaccine protects, not that it induces antibodies because it can have them, yes, but, well, we have spent the last 45 years dedicated only to vaccines. We can produce antibodies against anything, as I say, even against cuchuco, now! But protecting that is something else! What is expected is that the vaccine will protect, protect for 5 to 10 years, but in an exceptional issue like the one now, well, man, at least 1 year and it is known that the antibodies they induce in recovered individuals, recovered from The infection does not last more than 6 months, so that is what we have to see, to see how that is induced, and none of the vaccine producers are telling the world, the people, look, we have been monitoring those vaccinated for 6 months first of all because the period of time has not elapsed and secondly they do not tell you how fast the immune response is decaying because that can be calculated, so, well, that is the issue. [End of extract]. Below, 'From strokes, TO DEATH: all the SIDE EFFECTS of the CCP Virus vaccine', is the statement of another article, translated from Life site News by TierraPura.org on December 9, 2020:

A slide presentation compiled by the FDA in October contains an extensive list of possible side effects that should be monitored along with the administration of the COVID-19 vaccine. A document prepared by the United States Food and Drug Administration (FDA), which lists possible side effects of the COVID-19 vaccine, includes among the possible side effects stroke, encephalitis, autoimmune diseases, birth deformities and Kawasaki disease. A slide presentation compiled by the FDA in October contains an extensive list of possible side effects that should be monitored along with the administration of the COVID-19 vaccine. There should be both passive and active surveillance for vaccine-related side effects. Under the previous system, the FDA will partner with the Centers for Disease Control (CDC) to manage the Vaccine Adverse Event Reporting System (VAERS), by which individuals report adverse side effects to their vaccine provider. health.

And because of a little-known federal law from the 1980s, drug companies can't be sued in court if their vaccines injure or kill someone. Instead, people affected or killed by vaccines (or their family members) should use the National Vaccine Injury Compensation Program, which was created in 1986. This program protects pharmaceutical companies from lawsuits related to injuries or deaths from vaccines. vaccines (you can see here that on Spanish television they reported on how with the Influenza A the Strasbourg Parliamentary Assembly of the Council of Europe investigated the extent to which the pharmaceutical lobby went and its setup with vaccines and they add that just before that "epidemic" The WHO had changed the definition of a pandemic to increase the "alert" level (until May 2009, for a pandemic to be declared it was necessary for a virus to spread rapidly and for the number of fatal cases to be much higher than the seasonal averages, but then it was changed, it was no longer necessary to resort to mortality, it was enough that it was appearing in different countries, and then, in June the definition was changed again): https://rumble.com/ved5yj-montaje -from-the-flu-to-repeats-with-the-coronavirus.html [10]). "It was created after lawsuits against vaccine companies and healthcare providers threatened to cause vaccine shortages and reduce vaccination rates in the United States, which they believed could cause a resurgence of vaccine-preventable diseases." , explained Children's Health Defense.

Children's Health Defense reported: "According to those affected by the vaccines and their loved ones, the program has failed miserably as a litigious and broken system in which those affected face a government vaccine program, government-owned vaccine patents, to government health officials who administer the program, and to government-paid Justice Department lawyers. There is no judge, no jury of your peers and no discovery. "Claimants feel the system is set up for their claims to fail."

---

10.   https://rumble.com/ved5yj-montaje-de-la-gripe-a-se-repite-con-el-

coronavirus.html

With active surveillance, the FDA plans to use the "Biologics Effectiveness and Safety System (BEST)" with numerous partners. MarketScan, the largest number of member companies, has more than 250 million patients. Together with the Center for Medicare and Medicaid Services (CMS), the FDA says its data may cover "approximately 55 million elderly U.S. beneficiaries over 65 years of age." It is through the use of CMS data that the FDA plans to monitor the side effects of COVID vaccines, based on rapid cycle analysis. The FDA admits a long list of possible negative side effects. The list presented has 22 records of "possible outcomes of adverse events." First on the list is "Guillain-Barré Syndrome," described as "a rare disorder in which your body's immune system attacks your nerves." The syndrome "has no known cure" and its mortality rate is "4% to 7%." In contrast, John Hopkins University estimates that the current percentage of reported deaths due to COVID-19 cases in the US is only 1.9%. "Acute disseminated encephalomyelitis," a "rare inflammatory condition that affects the brain and spinal cord," is second on the FDA's list. The third is "Transverse Myelitis", a neurological disorder that inflames the spinal cord, causing "pain, muscle weakness, paralysis, sensory problems or bladder and bowel dysfunction."

Also listed as a possible adverse effect of the vaccine is "anaphylaxis", the severe allergic reaction that can lead to anaphylactic shock (https://rumble.com/ved86l-censuran-a-los-profesionales-para-evitar-debate -covid.html [11]). A "stroke" and "seizures/fits" are other possible side effects, along with "acute myocardial infarction" or heart attacks, inflammation of the muscles around the heart, and even death. The UK government has warned that the Pfizer vaccine should not be

---

11.   https://rumble.com/ved86l-censuran-a-los-profesionales-para-evitar-debate%20-
covid.html%20

used by women who are pregnant or breastfeeding. The document adds that the effect the vaccine will have on fertility is still unknown. It also says that "women of childbearing potential should be advised to avoid pregnancy for at least 2 months after their second dose." The FDA also suggested that Kawasaki disease is a possibility after the vaccine. The disease "mainly affects children under 5 years of age" and "is always treated in hospital." Sources: https://tierrapura.org/2020/12/09/ desde-derrames-cerebrales-hasta-la-muerte-todos-los-efectos-secundarios-de-la-vacuna-contra-el-virus-pcch/ [12]. Going to another article, we read 'NO WORK: Doctor on TV admitted that the VACCINE WILL NOT STOP the contagion, and we will have to continue wearing a mask', from December 19, 2020, translated from Natural News by TierraPura.org:

Do those of the 'Deep State' believe that Americans are so naive that with their operations with lying professionals they can deceive people? Vin Gupta no longer has a conscience, everyone is positioning themselves. MSNBC medical analyst Vin Gupta is pushing so hard for you to get the Wuhan coronavirus (COVID-19) vaccine that he pretended to get one himself during a recent fake news broadcast on cable TV. If you decide to get vaccinated, we warn you that you will still have to wear a mask and avoid traveling. This is Gupta's message to Americans who are under the impression that getting vaccinated against COVID-19 will mean freedom and a normal life. Not only will nothing really change, he says, but the vaccine won't stop infection or the spread of the virus.

"Just because you get vaccinated after the second dose doesn't mean you should travel," Gupta told Meet the Press, as well as his followers on Twitter. "You could become infected and infect

---

12.   https://tierrapura.org/2020/12/09/desde-derrames-cerebrales-hasta-la-muerte-todos-los-efectos-secundarios-de-la-vacuna-contra-el-virus-pcch/

others." In other words, COVID-19 vaccines do nothing except increase the risk of death and serious side effects. In the meantime, you'll still have to carry an ID card, treat other human beings like the walking plague, and go through the motions of pandemic compliance just as if you hadn't been vaccinated—pretty compelling, right? According to Gupta, we are still "in the middle of an out-of-control pandemic," which means no one is "freeing themselves from masks." "Everything remains valid until we all receive the two-dose treatment," he added, setting the stage for the next phase of the pandemic narrative that will inevitably blame those who refuse the vaccine for things not returning to normal. "We don't think that's going to happen until June, July. "We don't know if just getting vaccinated prevents serious illness, or if it also completely prevents infection." "Don't let your guard down just because you've been vaccinated," Gupta urged people who follow the advice of TV doctors.

If COVID-19 vaccines do nothing but increase the risk of death, why would anyone get the shot? Gupta must have overlooked the report that asymptomatic spread of COVID-19 is not real, because he is also touting the idea that vaccinated people without any symptoms can somehow spread the virus to others. While so-called "experts" say they have "reason to be hopeful" that COVID-19 vaccines will prevent people from spreading the virus, Gupta and others admit this is just speculation. No one knows for sure what the vaccine will do, Gupta admits, but everyone should go out and get it, he says. Commenting on Gupta's "recommendations," writer Noah Rothman wrote that telling vaccinated people to stay indoors and masked despite being jabbed is likely to turn into a "cold soufflé." "Almost no one, at least those without diseases or loved ones at risk, is going to get two shots of the vaccine and behave as if it were still 2020," Rothman notes. "If your public messaging strategy is to insist that people who have received two doses should stay distanced, wear masks, and avoid social engagements, your messaging strategy is stupid." Department of Health and Human Services (HHS) Head Alex Azar agrees with Gupta.

He explains that people should remain "vigilant" in obeying all the suggestions made by people like Bill Gates and Anthony Fauci so that "everyone who is here now [will be] here next year for the holiday season." Source: https://tierrapura.org/2020/12/19/no-sirve-medico-en-tv-admitio-que-la-vacuna-no-detendra-el-contagio-y-habra-que- seguir- wearing-mask/ [13]. The Austrian philosopher, literary scholar, educator, artist, playwright, social thinker and occultist, Rudolph Steiner, had foreseen in 1917 a vaccine that would deprive man of his soul. In a publication from February 2021 we can read about his lyrics:

More than 100 years ago, in a series of 14 essays published under the title The Fall of the Spirits of Darkness, Steiner warned future generations of a possible measure of crowd control, much like the visions presented by Orwell and Huxley. Steiner imagined a future in which vaccines could strip us of our spiritual nature. First, a little context: "In these fourteen lectures, delivered at the end of 1917 after four years of war in Europe, Steiner speaks of the complex spiritual forces that developed during the First World War, of humanity's attempts for building theoretically perfect social orders and for the numerous divisions and disturbances that would continue on Earth to this day. Humanity in general did not wake up to the fact that, expelled from the spiritual worlds, the fallen Spirits were now intensely active on Earth. This manifested itself primarily in human

---

13.   https://tierrapura.org/2020/12/19/no-sirve-medico-en-tv-admitio-que-la-vacuna-no-detendra-el-contagio-y-habra-que-seguir-usando-mascarilla/

thinking and perception of the surrounding world." (rsarchive). According to Steiner, the fall into such destructive torpor will be marked by an era of materialism and centralization of power, in which the influences of the "Spirits of Darkness" will drive humans to devise new technologies and new means of oppression.

Excerpts from the fall of the spirits of darkness: In the past, at the Council of Constantinople, the spirit has been eliminated, a dogma has been instituted: man is only made up of a soul and a body; To speak of spirit is a heresy. They will aspire in another way to eliminate the soul, the life of the soul. And the time will come, perhaps in the not too distant future, when, in a Congress like the one held in 1912, we will see something very different develop, in which other trends will appear, in which it will be said: talking about spirit and soul is pathological; Only people who only talk about the body are healthy. The fact that a human being develops in such a way that he comes to believe that a spirit or a soul exists is a pathological symptom. These people will be sick people, and a cure will be found, rest assured, the remedy that will act on this evil. In the past, the spirit has been removed. The soul will be eliminated through the medicine. Starting from a "healthy vision of things", a vaccine will be found, through which the body will be treated from the earliest youth, if possible from birth, so that the body does not come to think that there is a soul and a spirit.

The two currents, the two conceptions of the world will be radically opposed. One will reflect on how to develop concepts and representations that are in line with true reality, the reality of the soul and spirit. The others, the successors of the current materialists, will look for the vaccine that will make the bodies "healthy", that is, constituted in such a way that there will no longer be talk of the nonsense that is the soul and the spirit, but, because they will be "healthy", from the mechanical and chemical forces that, from the cosmic nebula, have constituted the planets and the sun. This will be achieved through the manipulation of bodies. Materialistic doctors will be entrusted with the task of ridding humanity of souls. Yes, those who believe that the future can be predicted with the help of ideas that play with reality are very wrong. We must look at the future using seriously thought-out, well-founded and profound concepts. Spiritual Science is not a game, it is not just a theory. It is, in the face of evolution, a duty that must be fulfilled. [Reference to pages 104-105] I have explained to you that the spirits of darkness will blow on their guests, on the men who will inhabit them, to discover a vaccine that can, from early youth, through the body, eradicate the tendency to spirituality. Today we vaccinate against this or that disease: in the future, children will be vaccinated with a product that may be very well composed, and that will prevent children from developing in them the "follies" of the spiritual life – "follies" in perspective. materialistic, of course. [Reference page 255]

As I said before, these are innocent literary beginnings. But the purpose of all this is to find a way to inoculate the bodies so that the tendency to spiritual ideas does not develop in them, and so that during their lives men believe only in the existence of matter as perceived by the senses. Just as you are vaccinated against physiopathy, you will be vaccinated against the tendency towards spirituality. This as an indication among many things that will appear in the near future and beyond in this field, to the end that confusion is created in the forces that, through the victory of the spirits of light, wish to descend from the spiritual worlds to the earth. For this, of course, it is necessary that the conceptions of the world, the way of seeing of men, be confused, that their concepts, their representations be distorted. This is a serious situation in which we must be very attentive. Because it is one of the most important antecedents of the events that are currently taking place. I purposely choose my words precisely. I say "prepare" and I am very aware that when someone talks about preparation after what has happened in the last three years, they are saying something important. Because he who sees things in depth knows that, in effect, it is a preparation.

Only a superficial mind can believe that tomorrow or the day after tomorrow, which is not a war in the traditional sense, will end with peace, as were the wars of yesteryear. Only those who judge events superficially can believe it. Without a doubt, many will believe it when something happens outwardly that is close to what one imagines; and you will not think about everything that lies beneath the surface. [Reference to pages 255 and 256]. What Steiner advanced is a reality. And here is the evidence: Vaccine against the God Gene. Source: http://www. Verdadypaciencia.com/2021/02/la-caida-de-los-espiritus-de-la-oscuridad.rudolph-steiner-habia-previsto-en-1917-una-vacuna-que- would deprive-the-man-of-his-soul.vaccine [14]. In another report we can read that France would pay a premium of €5.4 to doctors for each vaccine they give. In addition, he will pay for giving the vaccine, he will do so for registering the person in the special health surveillance file, now operational. The remuneration is a consequence of the resistance of the French to being vaccinated, whose rates are among the highest in Europe: https://mpr21.info/francia-pagara-una-prima-de-54-euros-a-los-medicos -for-every-vaccine-they-give/ [15]. This control is

---

14.   http://www.verdadypaciencia.com/2021/02/la-caida-de-los-espiritus-de-la-oscuridad.rudolph-steiner-habia-previsto-en-1917-una-vacuna-que-privaria-al-hombre-de-su-alma.vacuna

15.   https://mpr21.info/francia-pagara-una-prima-de-54-euros-a-los-medicos-por-cada-vacuna-que-pongan/

already being carried out in many places (in Israel, for example, you can practically no longer go to work, the gym, school activities, a restaurant or the supermarket, without the vaccine certificate) and it has begun to be digitalized, promoting a virtual certificate that will later be applied as a chip implanted in the right hand. The elite's strategy on the so-called "vaccination priority order" is based on the primary interests of these technocrats, oligarchs and banksters.

The elderly, of course, are in the lead to carry out euthanasia on a large scale, since they have little chance of resisting this deadly cocktail, added to the toxic components that were sprayed on them in nursing homes, the brutal treatments to which they were subjected. with killer drugs and how they were forced to use respirators to lead them to death. As the Spanish biologist Fernando López explains in the following video, the doctors continue to make them sick and have to ask for sick leave, thus achieving a reduction in functional health personnel, and thus producing a collapse in the public care system (https://rumble.com/ved90t-quieren-acabar-con-los-mdicos-para-colapsar-el-sistema.html [16]). Then they bring in the politicians, who don't even get the real injection (https://rumble.com/ved9d9-los-polticos-no-se-vacunan.html [17]and https://rumble.com/ved7dx-hoax-vaccine -politicians-politicians-pretend-vacunarse.html [18]), to give the appearance of transparency and security. They bring in the armed and police forces, which are the ones that could prevent governments from insulting the people. Later, people with limited resources arrive,

---

16.	https://rumble.com/ved90t-quieren-acabar-con-los-mdicos-para-colapsar-el-sistema.html

17.	https://rumble.com/ved9d9-los-polticos-no-se-vacunan.html

18.	https://rumble.com/ved7dx-hoax-vaccine-politicians-polticos-fingen-vacunarse.html

because they are the scum that they want to remove from the streets and from parasitism (because governments have to be giving them aid). They continue with the rest of the people and end with the children, why, because they want that new generation for their "personal interests." On the other hand, they sell the story that they give you the vaccine "whichever is your turn," but in reality these vaccines among the different companies, and depending on the type of person, have variables. These variables are based on the premise that depending on the ethnic group, they will introduce certain compounds. This is because white racial supremacists should not be in the eye of the storm. Instead, the Israelis will go first, then the blacks, then the Asians, then the Muslims, then the Latinos and also the Orthodox Jews. The worst effects will be on these racial groups.

Why Israelis and Orthodox Jews? Just as in Nazi Germany, the population that would oppose the Zionist model had to be controlled. Israel is the scapegoat of the Jesuit power for the establishment of the government of the Antichrist. Why Latinos? Because of their Christian beliefs (starting with the most "underdeveloped" countries in Latin America, with Argentina and Spain first being the countries chosen as pilots). Why Muslims? They will be the number one instigators of terrorist attacks during World War III. They will carry out terrorist attacks, especially on American, Israeli and European soil, according to prophecies and classified information. They have been brainwashed to kill Christians, Jews and gringos in the name of jihad. The elite knows that before Christians or conspiracy theorists, the main enemies of the Antichrist are the Islamic people. That is why they destroy their morals, divide them, destroy their countries and use covert agents to incite their tribal chiefs to promote hatred towards the West. They want to take away their lands from Africans so that they can be exploited by Europeans and China. They don't want to let them become industrialized or cultured. And the Chinese? The CCP doesn't need Chinese that much. That country is full of people. They already have enough, and those who are left over – along with Tibetans, Christians and opponents of the Communist Party (CCP) – are put in labor camps, where in due course they are taken to an operating room and their organs are removed to be sold. That's enough for them. They want them to remain mostly "white", but docile, and the rest, children, biologically and mentally controlled by the Deep State, in a world of free "child trade" for their pleasure, the pleasure of some satanist pedophile psychopaths, the mother of the harlots of the Earth.

Two components of this vaccine are classified as 'Secret Defense', and they must inject 7 worse vaccines until they achieve their goal. Dr. Carrie Madej, a specialist in internal medicine, has explained clearly and simply the consequences that we would face as a human race if we introduce vaccines like those being developed by Moderna and other laboratories for the alleged Sars-Cov2. According to her, and many others who support her words, these vaccines are experimenting with RNA and DNA mutations that have never been tested in humans. There are not even large studies on them in animals. More info at: https://elinvestigador.org/vacunas-covid19-transgenicas-transhumanismo/ [19]and https://lbry.tv/@elinvestigador:0/Carrie-Madej—-Vacuna-transgencia-de-ModeRNA-—Transhumanism-2.0:3 [20]. Juan Manuel Soaje Pinto interviews the geneticist doctor Luis Marcelo Martínez, regarding the mandatory nature of the genocidal policy that the misgovernment of Alberto Fernández, and his minister of

---

19.   https://elinvestigador.org/vacunas-covid19-transgenicas-transhumanismo/

20.   https://lbry.tv/@elinvestigador:0/Carrie-Madej---Vacuna-transgénica-de-ModeRNA---Transhumanismo-2.0:3

health, the businessman Ginés Gonzáles García, intends to impose. "We are going to vaccinate 28 million people with two doses: A complete vaccination is a brutal number. The priority will be placed not only on "lowering mortality" but also "to eliminate people who can transmit the virus," said the minister. in a lapse that left him completely exposed. As we all suspected, vaccines are intended to "eliminate people", in the businessman Ginés' own words. Source: https://ugetube.com/watch/contracara-n-96-   the-vaccine-seeks-to-sterilize-the-population_Z3w266Ya8mk2aut.html [21].

Dr. María José Martínez Albarracín, the PhD in Immunology Roxana Bruno together with the Argentine geneticist, Dr. Luis Marcelo Martínez, Dr. Wolfgang Wodarg, doctor, president of the Parliamentary Assembly of the Health Committee of the Council of Europe, and Dr. Michael Yeadon, former vice president and scientist at Pfizer laboratories, an allergy and respiratory expert, is warning that the SARS-CoV-2 vaccine may trigger an immune reaction against syncytin-1 and could result in indefinite infertility in women. vaccinated. See more   at   https://cienciaysaludnatural.com [22], https://www.bitchute.com/video/6W1tDHhF3MBx/ [23]and https://cienciaysaludnatural.com/la...-afectar-el-desarrollo-normal-de-la -placenta/ [24]. Albert Bourla himself, Chairman and CEO of Pfizer, does not want to be vaccinated: https://www.brighteon.com/f3ba9c37-eb20-4ef5-8bd3-578309921d92 [25].

---

21.   https://ugetube.com/watch/contracara-n-96-la-vacuna-busca-esterilizar-a-la-población_Z3w266Ya8mk2aut.html

22.   https://cienciaysaludnatural.com

23.   https://www.bitchute.com/video/6W1tDHhF3MBx/

24.   https://cienciaysaludnatural.com/la...-afectar-el-desarrollo-normal-de-la-placenta/

On December 1, 2020, Pfizer's former Director of Pulmonology Research, Dr. Michael Yeadon [of England], and Pulmonologist and former Director of Public Health, Dr. Wolfgang Wodarg [of Germany], have filed a petition with the European Medicines Agency - responsible for the approval of medicines at the European Union level - for the immediate suspension of all studies on the Sars-CoV-2 vaccine, and in particular the BioNtech/Pfizer study on BNT162b (EudraCT number 2020-002641-42). Drs Wodarg and Yeadon ask that studies - to protect the life and health of those tested - not proceed until a study protocol is available that addresses the serious safety concerns expressed by a growing number of scientists. highlights regarding the vaccine and the study protocol. The petitioners ask, on the one hand, for so-called Sanger sequencing to be used due to the evident lack of serious studies on the PCR test. This is the only way to make reliable statements about the effectiveness of the Covid-19 vaccine. On the basis of numerous PCR tests of widely varying quality, neither the risk of the disease nor the possible benefit of a vaccine can be determined with sufficient certainty, and therefore testing the vaccine in humans is in itself contrary to ethics.

Furthermore, they demand that, for example, through animal experiments, risks already known from previous studies, which partly derive from the nature of coronaviruses, may materialize. The concerns concern in particular the following points:

*The formation of so-called "non-neutralizing" antibodies can lead to an exaggerated immune reaction, especially when the person tested is faced with the real "natural" virus after vaccination. This so-called aggravation-dependent amplification of antibodies, ADE, has been known for a long time thanks to

---

25.	https://www.brighteon.com/f3ba9c37-eb20-4ef5-8bd3-578309921d92

experiments with anti-coronavirus vaccines in cats, for example. Throughout these studies, all cats that had initially tolerated the vaccination well died after contracting the "natural" virus.

*The vaccines are expected to produce antibodies against the Spike proteins of Sars-CoV-2. However, these Spike proteins also contain syncytin-like proteins, which are essential for the formation of the placenta in mammals such as humans, and are toxic (demonstrated in 2020 by many studies that they were the main culprit in the poisoning of millions of people who were vaccinated against the supposed bug, leading hundreds of thousands to death from internal damage caused by myocarditis and blood clots). It must be absolutely ruled out that a vaccine against Sars-CoV-2 could trigger an immune reaction against syncytin-1, otherwise it could cause indefinite sterility in vaccinated women.

*BioNTech/Pfizer mRNA vaccines contain polyethylene glycol (PEG). It turns out that 70% of people develop antibodies against this substance, which means that many people can develop life-threatening allergic reactions after this vaccine.

*The very short duration of the study does not allow a realistic estimate of long-term effects. As in the case of narcolepsy following vaccination against swine flu, millions of healthy people would be exposed to unacceptable risk if an emergency authorization were granted and the possibility of observing the long-term effects of vaccination would only come after. However, BioNTech/Pfizer apparently submitted an application for emergency approval on December 1, 2020. Sources: https://2020news.de/en/dr-wodarg-an...studies-and-call-for-co-signing-the-petition/ [26]and http://www.

---

26.   https://2020news.de/en/dr-wodarg-an...studies-and-call-for-co-signing-the-

petition/

Verdadypaciencia.com/202..　　　　　　.ichael-yeadon-and-the-pulmonologist-and-former-director-of[27].

For their part, a Connecticut pathologist, Dr. Sin Hang Lee, and the Informed Consent Action Network (ICAN), have asked the US Food and Drug Administration (FDA) to require accurate counts of COVID cases -19 in the Pfizer/BioNTech COVID-19 mRNA vaccine trial. "Until an accurate count of COVID-19 cases in the vaccinated and placebo groups has been determined for evaluation of vaccine efficacy, we ask the FDA to suspend its decision regarding emergency use authorization." for this vaccine," said Dr. Lee, director of the Milford Molecular Diagnostic Laboratory. The main reason for asking the FDA for a suspension of action is that the Phase 2/3 clinical trial of the Pfizer vaccine used a presumptive RT-qPCR diagnostic test. This test is recognized by the medical scientific community for generating high rates of false positive results among qualified trial participants in the placebo group with minor symptoms such as sore throat or new cough.

The Pfizer/BioNTech vaccine trial primarily uses an RT-qPCR test that employs cycle thresholds possibly as high as 44.9 to identify COVID-19 "cases." Samples considered positive that require high levels of amplification (cycle thresholds above 30 to 35) are often false positives, Dr. Lee said. A recent review of a COVID-19 PCR test, which was signed by 22 international scientists, emphatically stated: "To determine whether the amplified products are indeed SARS-CoV-2 genes, biomolecular validation of the amplified PCR products is essential. For a diagnostic test, this validation is an absolute necessity. Validation of PCR products should be performed by running the PCR product on a 1% EtBr-agarose gel along with a size indicator

---

27.　　http://www.verdadypaciencia.com/202...ichael-yeadon-y-el-neumologo-y-ex-director-de

(DNA ruler or DNA ladder) in order to estimate the size of the product. The size must correspond to the calculated size of the amplification product. But it is even better to sequence the amplification product. The latter will give 100% certainty about the identity of the amplification product. Without molecular validation, one cannot be sure of the identity of the amplified PCR products..." A recent petition to the European Medicines Agency to suspend COVID-19 vaccine trials used similar arguments regarding the inaccuracy of the tests. of PCR that are used and the need for confirmatory sequencing.

On Dec. 1, Switzerland's medical regulator, Swissmedic, said it lacks the information needed to approve three different government-mandated coronavirus vaccines, including the Pfizer vaccine. "In a recent interview about the pending review of the Pfizer COVID-19 vaccine, FDA Commissioner Stephen Hahn promised, "We will make a determination regarding safety and effectiveness based on our strict criteria." Stephen Hahn, FDA Commissioner As stated in the petition, if Pfizer is unable to perform the necessary sequencing tests on the 180 RNA samples to confirm the vaccine's claimed 95% efficacy rate, Dr. Lee has offered to reanalyze the residue from these samples in your laboratory.

Dr. Lee said his lab is located just an hour's drive from Connecticut-based Pfizer Inc. and will submit all testing data to the FDA to support evaluation of the vaccine based on "criteria." very strict," as the FDA promised. Notary. Dr. Lee's Sanger sequencing-based method for the molecular diagnosis of SARS-CoV-2 was published in the International Journal of Geriatrics and Rehabilitation. Regarding fertility: It is unknown if the COVID-19 mRNA vaccine BNT162b2 has an impact on fertility, no studies have been performed: https://assets.publishing.service.g...onals_on_Pfizer_BioNTech_COVI

. (Page 6). Those vaccinated against COVID - 19 are at greater risk than those who are not vaccinated, this is how another investigation carried out by various experts defines this situation. COVID - 19 vaccines designed to elicit neutralizing antibodies may sensitize vaccine recipients to more severe disease than if they were not vaccinated. There is a significant risk for subjects who receive the vaccines that they may experience severe disease once vaccinated, while they may have only experienced mild, self-limited disease if unvaccinated.

Phase 1 and 2 clinical trials of vaccine candidates have only been designed around immunogenicity as an efficacy endpoint and have not been designed to capture subjects' exposure to circulating virus after vaccination, which is when it is designed for antibody-dependent enhancement (ADE)/immunopathology to occur. Therefore, the absence of evidence of ADE in the COVID - 19 vaccine data so far does not exempt researchers from disclosing the risk of increased disease to vaccine trial participants, and remains a realistic risk, not theoretical for the subjects. Given the strong evidence that ADE is a compelling, nontheoretical risk for COVID-19 vaccines, disclosure of the specific risk of worsening COVID-19 disease due to vaccination requires specific treatment, separated in a consent form. informed for easy understanding by the patient to comply with medical ethics standards. The informed consent process for ongoing COVID-19 vaccine trials does not appear to meet this standard.

While the COVID-19 global health emergency justifies accelerated vaccine trials of candidates with known liabilities, such acceleration is not incompatible with additional attention paid to informed consent procedures specific to COVID-19 vaccine risks. Food and Drug Administration Safety

Monitoring: Worklist of Potential Outcomes of Adverse Events from COVID-19 Vaccines. Subject to change:

- Guillain Barre syndrome
- Acute disseminated encephalomyelitis
- Transverse myelitis
- Encephalitis / myelitis / encephalomyelitis / meningoencephalitis / meningitis / encephalopathy
- Seizures
- Stroke
- Narcolepsy and cataplexy
- Anaphylaxis
- Acute myocardial infarction
- Myocarditis/pericarditis
- Autoimmune disease
- Deaths
- Pregnancy and birth results
- Other acute demyelinating diseases
- Non-anaphylactic allergic reactions
- Thrombocytopenia
- Disseminated intravascular coagulation
- Venous thromboembolism
- Arthritis and arthralgia/joint pain
- Kawasaki disease
- Multisystem inflammatory syndrome in children
- Disease enhanced by the vaccine

Source: Vaccines and Related Biological Products Advisory Committee October 22, 2020 Meeting and Informed consent disclosure to vaccine trial subjects of risk of COVID - 19 vaccines worsening clinical disease https://doi.org/10.1111/ijcp.13795 – Department of Biochemistry and Molecular Pharmacology, NYU Langone Health, New York, NY, USA – Division of Comparative Pathology, Department of Pathology and Laboratory Medicine, Tulane University School of Medicine, Tulane National Primate Research Center, Covington, LA, USA. Presentation: https://www.fda.gov/media/143557/download

the specific risk that COVID - 19 vaccines may worsen disease following exposure to the circulating challenge virus. Published literature was reviewed to identify preclinical and clinical evidence that COVID-19 vaccines could worsen disease following exposure to the challenge or circulating virus. Clinical trial protocols for COVID - 19 vaccines were reviewed to determine whether risks were adequately reported. COVID - 19 vaccines designed to elicit neutralizing antibodies may sensitize vaccine recipients to more severe disease than if they were not vaccinated. Vaccines for SARS, MERS, and RSV (Respiratory syncytial virus) have never been approved, and the data generated in the development and testing of these vaccines suggest a serious mechanistic concern: that vaccines designed empirically using the traditional approach (which consists of the unmodified or minimally modified coronavirus viral spike to elicit neutralizing antibodies), whether composed of protein, viral vector, DNA or RNA and regardless of the method of administration, may worsen COVID-19 disease through amelioration antibody -dependent (ADE). This risk is sufficiently hidden in clinical trial protocols and consent forms for ongoing COVID-19 vaccine trials that adequate patient understanding of this risk is unlikely to occur.

The specific and significant risk of ADE from being vaccinated against COVID-19 should have been and should be disclosed prominently and independently to research subjects currently in vaccine trials, as well as those who are being recruited for the trials. trials and future patients after vaccine approval, to meet ethical standards of patient understanding for informed consent.

Vaccine-induced disease enhancement was previously observed in human subjects with vaccines for respiratory syncytial virus (RSV), dengue virus, and measles. 1 An intensification of the disease caused by the vaccine was also observed with the SARS and MERS viruses and with the feline coronavirus, which are closely related to SARS - CoV - 2, the pathogen that causes the COVID - 19 disease. Immune mechanisms of this enhancement have invariably involved antibodies, from direct antibody-dependent enhancement, to the formation of immune complexes by antibodies, although accompanied by various coordinated cellular responses, such as the distortion of Th2 T cells. 2 – 7 In particular, both neutralizing and nonneutralizing antibodies have been implicated. A recent study revealed an in vivo IgG-mediated acute lung injury in SARS-infected macaques that correlated with a vaccine-elicited neutralizing antibody response. 8 Inflammation and tissue damage in the lung in this animal model recapitulated inflammation and tissue damage in the lungs of SARS-infected patients who succumbed to the disease. Over time, the worst damage occurred in a delayed manner in synchrony with the increase in the immune response.

Surprisingly, the neutralizing antibodies controlled the virus in the animal, but then precipitated a severe inflammatory response that damaged tissues in the lung. This is a similar profile to the immune complex-mediated disease seen with RSV (Respiratory syncytial virus) vaccines in the past, in which vaccinees succumbed to fatal RSV disease due to immune complex formation. antibody-viruses that precipitated harmful inflammatory immune responses. It is also similar to the clinical course of COVID-19 patients, with titers directly correlating with disease severity. In contrast, subjects who recover quickly may have low or no serum anti-SARS-CoV-2 antibodies. Obtaining antibodies, specifically neutralizing antibodies, is the goal of almost all current SARS-CoV-2 vaccine candidates. Previous evidence that vaccine-induced antibody-dependent enhancement of disease is likely to occur to some degree with COVID-19 vaccines is vertically consistent from controlled studies of SARS in primates to clinical observations in SARS and COVID-19.

Therefore, a finite, not theoretical, risk is evident in the medical literature that vaccine candidates composed of the SARS- CoV - 2 viral spike and eliciting anti - SARS - CoV - 2 antibodies, whether neutralizing or not, place those vaccinated at greater risk, for more severe COVID-19 disease when they encounter circulating viruses. In fact, mouse studies of previous SARS vaccines revealed this exact phenotype. Regardless, SARS/MERS vaccine candidates commonly exhibited ADE associated with high inflammatory morbidity in preclinical models, obstructing their advancement to the clinic. The ADE of SARS from both non-human primate disease and viral infection of cells in vitro clearly mapped to SARS viral spike epitopes targeting specific antibodies. This phenomenon was consistent across a variety of vaccine platforms, including DNA, vector primers, and virus-like particles (VLPs), regardless of the inoculation method (oral, intramuscular, subcutaneous, etc.). An unknown variable is how long this tissue damage lasts, possibly resulting in permanent morbidity (eg, diabetes from pancreatic damage).

Current data on COVID - 19 vaccines is limited, but so far does not reveal evidence of ADE of the disease. Nonhuman primate studies of Moderna's mRNA - 1273 vaccine showed protection without detectable immunopathology . Phase 1 trials of several vaccines have not reported any immunopathology in subjects administered the candidate vaccines. However, it was unlikely that these subjects had yet encountered circulating viruses. However, all preclinical studies to date have been conducted with the Wuhan or closely related strains of the virus, while a mutant D614G virus is now the most prevalent circulating form. Several observations suggest that this alternative form may be antigenically distinct from the Wuhan-derived strain, not so much in composition, but in the conformation of the viral spike and the exposure of neutralization epitopes. Similarly, phase 1 and 2 clinical trials of vaccine candidates have only been designed around immunogenicity as an efficacy endpoint and have not been designed to capture subjects' exposure to circulating virus after vaccination, which is when ADE/immunopathology is designed to occur. Therefore, the absence of evidence of ADE in the COVID - 19 vaccine data so far does not exempt researchers from disclosing the risk of increased disease to vaccine trial participants, and remains a realistic risk, it was not rich for the subjects.

Informed consent procedures for vaccine trials commonly include disclosure of very minor risks, such as injection site reactions, rare past risks, unrelated vaccines/viruses, such as Guillain-Barré syndrome for swine flu (the recent vaccine transverse myelitis event) and generic statements about the risk of idiosyncratic systemic adverse events and death. Specific risks to research participants arising from the biological mechanism are rarely included, often due to ambiguity about their applicability. Signed consent forms from COVID - 19 vaccine trials are not publicly available due to privacy concerns. They also vary from clinical site to clinical site, and the sample consent forms on which they are based should not be released until after the trial ends, if at all. However, these consent forms are typically very similar in content to the "Risks to Participants" section of the trial protocols, which Pfizer, Moderna, and Johnson & Johnson have publicly released for their COVID-19 vaccine trials (20 & Supplement).

Since these three vaccines are representative of the diversity of vaccines being tested, it is very likely that the consent form inferred from these protocols will be similar or identical to those of each and every vaccine trial currently being conducted. All three protocols mention the risk of disease improvement from the vaccine, but all three list this risk last or second to last on the list of risks, after the risks of the Ad26-Cov2 vector, adenovirus vectors in general , risks of vaccination in general, risks of pregnancy and birth control (which are said to be " unknown "), risks of blood collection , and risks of collecting nasal swab samples (for Johnson and Johnson vaccine), after allergy, fainting, local injection reaction, general systemic adverse reactions, and laboratory abnormalities for the Moderna vaccine and after local injection reactions and general systemic adverse events for the Pfizer vaccine. Furthermore, both Moderna and Johnson and Johnson call the risk of disease improvement caused by the vaccine "theoretical."

Finally, in citing risk, Pfizer and Moderna point to prior evidence of vaccine-caused disease improvement with Respiratory syncytial virus and dengue, as well as feline coronavirus (Pfizer) and measles (Moderna); however, SARS and MERS are not mentioned. Johnson and Johnson discuss SARS and MERS, but present an unusual scientific argument that vaccine-induced disease improvement is due to non-neutralizing antibodies and Th2-biased cellular responses and that Ad26 vaccination does not exhibit this profile. Blank consent forms for AstraZeneca and Johnson and Johnson are

also available online at https://restoringtrials.org/2020/09/18/
covid19trialprotocolandstudydocs/ [28]and although the
AstraZeneca form clearly discloses the specific risk of ADE, the
disclosure It appears last among risks only in the attached
information sheet. This company is one of the first to have been
banned in several European countries throughout March 2021
due to the side effects of its vaccines. It may seem like a mere
coincidence of the universe, but 'Astra ze Neca' means in
Romanian, "that is, killing stars." Who are we stars whose
purpose is to kill? Well, let's not be superstitious. Let's think that
it is mere chance, a coincidence...

In total, the evidence from Pfizer, Moderna and Johnson
& Johnson's protocols for their COVID-19 vaccine trials and
sample consent forms, when contrasted with the evidence of
antibody-dependent disease improvement presented in this
report and widely available to any medical expert in the field,
states that the patient's understanding of the specific risk that
receiving the COVID-19 vaccine could convert a subject from
someone experiencing mild illness to someone experiencing
severe illness. Medical ethics standards required that, given the
extent of evidence in the medical literature reviewed above, the
risk of ADEs must be clearly and emphatically distinguished in
informed consent from rarely observed risks, as well as the more
obvious risk of lack of efficacy, which is not related to the specific
risk of ADE. Based on the published literature, it should have
been obvious to any trained clinician that there is a significant
risk to vaccine research subjects that they may experience severe
disease once vaccinated, while they may only have experienced
mild, self-limiting disease if is not vaccinated. Consent must
also clearly distinguish the specific risk of worsening COVID-19

---

28.   https://restoringtrials.org/2020/09/18/covid19trialprotocolandstudydocs/

disease from generic statements about the risk of death and the generic risk of vaccine lack of efficacy.

Given the strong evidence that ADE is a compelling, nontheoretical risk for COVID-19 vaccines, disclosure of the specific risk of worsening COVID-19 disease due to vaccination requires a separate, targeted, informed consent form. and demonstration of patient understanding to comply with medical ethics standards. The informed consent process for ongoing COVID-19 vaccine trials does not appear to meet this standard. While the COVID-19 global health emergency justifies accelerated vaccine trials of candidates with known liabilities, such acceleration is not incompatible with additional attention paid to heightened informed consent procedures specific to COVID-19 vaccine risks. 19. Topic supported by NIH award R21AI157604 (to TC).

Journalist Nicolas Moras interviews Dr. Roxana Bruno about negative effects of the Astra Zeneca vaccine, alternatives in the treatment of the virus not covered in the misinformation media, and the Argentine vaccine by Argentine biochemist Hugo Luján. The day after the interview, and after tens of thousands of likes and views in less than 24 hours, the interview as well as Nicolás Morás' entire YouTube channel disappeared from YouTube, apparently due to a hack of his account. Source: https://www.bitchute.com/video/0d984DoEkeE9/ [29]Many Spanish-speaking doctors and virologists have been talking about this, as you can see in this content: https://rumble.com/ved9kj-mdicos-aunados- contra-el-engao-covid.html [30].

Brandy Vaughan, a former sales executive at pharmaceutical company Merck and founder of learntherisk.org, a website dedicated to educating people about the risks associated with

---

29.   https://www.bitchute.com/video/0d984DoEkeE9/

30.   https://rumble.com/ved9kj-mdicos-aunados-contra-el-engao-covid.html

vaccines, was reportedly found dead by her nine-year-old son last week. December 8th. According to Children's Health Defense, Vaughan reportedly died of "gallbladder complications," although the source of the report was not cited nor was the specific cause of the complications (e.g., gallbladder rupture) communicated. Shortly after learning of her death, Vaughan's friend, Erin Elizabeth, shared screenshots of a Facebook post Vaughan had written in December 2019, in which she assured readers that she was not suicidal and did not drink. no medication that would cause sudden death. «The post I wish I didn't have to write.... But given certain tragedies in recent years, I feel it is absolutely necessary to publish these ten facts... please photograph this for the record," Vaughan wrote. «I have a great mission in this life. Even when they make it very difficult and scary, I would NEVER take my own life. Period," he continued.

Referring to her son, Vaughan wrote, "Bastien means everything to me and I would NEVER leave him. Spot. He added that he had not taken medication for ten years. "In other words, I am not taking anything that could kill me unexpectedly or suddenly," he wrote. "If something were to happen to me, it's foul play and you know exactly who and why, given my job and mission in this life," he continued. Vaccine safety has come under scrutiny during the coronavirus outbreak, and pro-lifers have raised concerns about the vaccines' connection to abortion, among other concerns. Elizabeth also shared a screenshot of a text she received from Vaughan in which she expressed concern about being poisoned and was apparently referring to the death of Dr. Ben Johnson, MD, DO, NMD in January 2019. "How strange! Sometimes I worry about poisoning. Was Dr. Ben ever married? Did you live alone? Sorry for all the questions. "I am so upset by this, especially since it wasn't even about the vaccine issue but rather mammograms, which you would think is a 'safer' issue."

Vaughan, who worked as a pharmaceutical sales representative for Merck, explained how he got his start as an activist exposing the dangers of vaccines and the pharmaceutical industry in a video shared in 2015. He begins by revealing that he used to represent Merck's drug Vioxx. "When it came out that Merck had falsified safety data and that Vioxx actually had a double increase in heart attacks and strokes [for] people taking it, it really made me realize that there was a lot of corruption going on behind the scenes and "That just because a drug is on the market doesn't mean it's safe," Vaughan said in the video. She explained that later, during a well-child visit for her son, a doctor "stormed out of the room" when she asked to see a package insert for the vaccine. "That was a big red flag for me, knowing what I knew from being a pharmaceutical sales rep before. "And I started researching vaccines, ingredients, and flawed safety data." Part of what she discovered is that aluminum is an important adjuvant in vaccines, which was another big "red flag" for her. When her grandmother was diagnosed with breast cancer, the doctor found high levels of aluminum in her tissues. He told her that the aluminum found in traditional deodorant was linked to breast cancer.

«The more I looked into this, the more I realized that vaccines are not for public health. It's actually about the profits of the pharmaceutical companies. "It's basically playing Russian roulette with our kids," Vaughan continued. "I was motivated to get more involved in this fight when I became aware of the mandatory vaccination bills that were sweeping the country[.]" Vaughan founded Learn The Risk, a nonprofit organization, "in response to one of the first mandatory vaccination laws for education in the country, California's SB277," according to its website. SB277, which became law in 2015, "prohibited parents from citing their personal beliefs as a reason for not vaccinating their children" to attend school. It was when Vaughan returned from a protest rally against SB277 in Sacramento that he began to experience acts of intimidation, he explained in a video shared in 2015. He described how he came home from Sacramento to find a key to his house, which he had previously hidden in the bushes, placed in the lock of the door of his house. "I had my locks changed that day and installed a $3,000 alarm system two days later," Vaughan said.

Her alarm company later informed her that someone had set off her alarm at 3:45 a.m. and she immediately disarmed it with the master code, which Vaughan said no one but her had. Whoever entered proceeded to walk down his hallway, activating the monitor's sensor, and opened and closed the dining room window before leaving the house at 3:49 in the morning. "After the incident I spoke to some security experts who have worked on business intimidations, and they said they were probably bugging their house." Vaughan described how just a few days later, he found his computer moved from its hiding place above his microwave, to the center of his kitchen floor. After leaving the city for a couple of weeks, she returned with a friend to find a ladder, which she had stored in her garage, right outside a bedroom window in her house – the only window with the blinds open. A neighbor informed him that he had not seen the ladder there the day before.

Just days after what happened, he found a duck figurine on one of his outdoor tables. «When I spoke to the security experts, I said, I don't understand the duck. And then I realized that I had been using my phone and having a lot of conversations [with] people asking me, are you staying at home? What are you going to do? And I use the term repeatedly: I'm not going to stay in my house. "I feel like an easy target, because they can come in at any time." "So it was quite disturbing coming home. "It's just a clear message that, again, I was being watched." «It's quite scary. After all these intimidation tactics it is very difficult to feel safe and protected, but I am not going to disappear – I mean I am not going to be silenced, because these are important issues, and we have to expose what is really happening behind the projects of mandatory vaccination law."

«I hope we can continue this fight. "We may have lost the battle, but we still have a war to win," Vaughan concluded. In his 2019 Facebook post, Vaughan wrote: "If something were to happen to me, I have arranged for a close group of my friends to start a GoFundMe to hire a team of private investigators to find out all the details." "There have been many on this mission or a similar one who have been killed and it is time for this b———- to stop. "Darkness cannot win." Source: https://tierrapura.org/2020/12/17/muerte-bajo-sospeccha-hallaron-muerta-a-ex-ejecutiva-farmaceutica-que-denunciaba-el-negocio-de-las-vacunas/ [31]. I myself saw a video of Brandy Vaughan talking about how they had been scaring her, breaking into her house, moving things, deactivating the alarm systems and threatening her shortly before she was murdered. This business of going after anti-vaxxers is just the beginning of the Purge (https://rumble.com/ved7sn-threat-to-brandy-vaughan-before-killing-her.html [32]). Spain will create a registry of people who refuse to be vaccinated against the coronavirus, according to a report dated December 29, 2020. It will share the document with the rest of European countries, although maximum respect for the protection of personal data will supposedly be

---

31.   https://tierrapura.org/2020/12/17/muerte-bajo-sospecha-hallaron-muerta-a-ex-ejecutiva-farmaceutica-que-denunciaba-el-negocio-de-las-vacunas/

32.   https://rumble.com/ved7sn-threat-to-brandy-vaughan-before-killing-her.html

maintained. as stated by the Minister of Health. Source: https://actualidad.rt.com/actualidad/378400-espana-crear-registro-negar-vacuna-coronavirus [33].

In short, we are not talking about a vaccine but about an experimental gene therapy, officially, and unofficially about a killer cocktail. Not all injections have the same content, some are trick syringes, for politicians and celebrities, others are saline solution or serum, but in general, altered or not, they should generically have a portion of the virus in question so that the body recognizes it and acquire immunity. The first problem here is that if there is no virus, what are they inoculating it? In essence there is a mixture of things that are not related to any antidote but to a babel of products, from graphene, luciferase, aluminum, mercury, copper, kidney particles from aborted fetuses, polysorbate 80, messenger RNA, protein S, nano particles and more things. To make matters worse, there are more and more cases where injected individuals are synchronized via Bluetooth. Yes, it sounds like a joke and even I took it with some skepticism the first time I saw it. After a few months I began to check it out for myself and with colleagues. Vaccinated people appeared on the phone's Bluetooth tracking devices.

It does not surprise me, since I have been hearing about this type of nano technologies since I was a teenager, and since the beginning of 2020 I had already heard student doctors talk about how they were told to design chips coated with synthetic material measuring microns in diameter, which can generate radiofrequency. I don't know if the morguellons are also involved here, but studies in this regard also show that the morguellons also transmit data via Wireless. This information was even provided by journalists who talked about DARPA studies and

---

33.   https://actualidad.rt.com/actualidad/378400-espana-crear-registro-negar-vacuna-coronavirus

their interest in putting nano robots in vaccines. It sounds cool to talk about transhumanism, bionic people, but the reality is becoming a cyborg, an android, a half-robot. It is not the fact that they can make you live longer with nano robots inside your body, or with a new experimental drug, or that they give you mechanical or bionic parts, or that they reconstruct parts mutilated or damaged by cloned or laboratory-grown ones. in accelerated growth. That all sounds nice. It is the question of the control they will have over you through those same devices. In August 2021, there were already close to 11 million people dead in the last 8 months after the vaccination campaigns, as adverse effects that they try to hide. In itself 33 million people have suffered from this experiment. Partly because they are testing how much graphene the body can handle, and it doesn't matter if people die, because they will say through their purchased media that it is a mutation of the virus, a variant, which, ironically, only affects vaccinated.

Before moving on to the following, I will leave you with some details from a document leaked in August 2021 from the Colombian Ministry of Health. This confirms what other documents from Pfizer and Moderna had exchanged with the CDC and the WHO, such as the fact that it is not known if the vaccines will be effective, it is not known what effects they will have, it is not known what they will produce in the long term, and on the contrary, they provide a long list of adverse effects, from mild to serious, although they omit death, which is reported in hundreds of thousands of people worldwide. These documents, from between January 5 and March 25, 2021, include some of the compounds that - at least, officially, although hidden from the public - these pseudo-vaccines possess. If you have been vaccinated, you will have heard that depending on your age and race (although they say "country") you are given one vaccine or another. You can't choose the company. They must give placebos, to later know if there was a difference between some groups or others, and thus determine long-term effects. This is also being done suspiciously. Anyway, they evaluated the injections from AstraZeneca, Moderna, Jansen and Pfizer-Biontech.

The AstraZeneca is recombinant ChAdOx1-S. What is this? It is essentially a recombinant, replication-deficient chimpanzee adenovirus vector that encodes the putative SARS-CoV-2 Spike glycoprotein. This is produced in genetically modified human embryonic kidney (HEK) 293 cells. This Spike protein is identical to synsitin, which is responsible for sexual reproduction and fertility, so in reality what is being attacked is not It is a virus but synsitin, to produce sterility in those who undergo this injection. That is, the AstraZeneca injection has as its main purpose eugenics, apart from, like all the others, introducing graphene, luciferase and other nanobots into the body. A vaccine, supposedly, is an attenuated portion of a virus that is injected so that your body adapts and the next time it comes strong you are immune to it. Why is an adenovirus taken from a chimpanzee? Because there are no human samples, because it was never actually isolated. Coronaviruses are a type of flu that infects certain animals and does not spread to humans, but now it is injected into humans. Since it cannot be passed through air or saliva droplets, they are injected intravenously. Besides, do you say that that chimpanzee contained SARS, or MERS, or some coronavirus? No. They introduce you to a chimpanzee adenovirus, which is not even SARS-CoV.

Moderna is a dose of 100 micrograms of mRNA, encapsulated in SM-102 lipid nanoparticles. This RNA is messenger, a single-stranded capped at the 5' end, produced by acellular in vitro transcription from corresponding DNA templates, which codes for the viral spike protein (Spike, or 'S') of the SARS-CoV-2 virus. CoV-2. As with AstraZeneca, Moderna is also responsible for sterilization. Apart from that, this specifically modifies human DNA, because it adds messenger RNA to the codes of our own chromosomes. However, they make you a genetically modified organism, apart from the fact that, in all cases, you are the property of the company that owns the compound that was injected into you, as an experimental subject. With this they inject you with messenger RNA and a pattern that will affect syinsitin, they do not inject you with an attenuated virus.

The Jansen contains a dose of adenovirus type 26 that encodes the SARS-CoV-2 protein no less than 8.92 log(19) infectious units (IU). Here again they inoculate you with an adenovirus that supposedly does have the code for this SARS-CoV-2 in a certain proportion. In other words, this is supposed to be a vaccine. That does not mean that it is necessary or effective, or does not produce adverse effects.

The worst of all, as far as I know, Pfizer-Biontech, is outrageous. After dilution, each 0.3 mL contains 30 mcg of modified nucleoside messenger RNA (modRNA) encoding the spike (S) glycoprotein of the putative SARS-CoV-2 virus. Likewise, each dose contains lipids ((0.43 mg (4-hydroxybutyl) azanediyl), (hexane-6, 1-diyl), (2-hexyldecanoate), 0.05 mg 2 ((polyethylene glycol)-2000)-N, N-ditetradecylacetamide, 0.09 mg 1,2-distearoyl-sn-glycero-3-phosphocholine and 0.2 mg cholesterol), 0.01 mg potassium chloride, 0.01 mg potassium phosphate monobasic , 0.36 mg of sodium chloride, 0.07 mg of dibasic sodium phosphate dihydrate and 6 md of sucrose. Why all these things? Many of these components are toxic. Both hexadecane and hexane are hydrocarbons. Do we need blood fuel to kill a bug? Polyethylene glycol is a polymer used in industry, and certain laxatives are produced from it. In general, these products cause kidney failure, but they are harmful to the body. More than an antiviral, it seems like a cocktail to poison.

XI. MUZZLES ARE FOR SLAVES

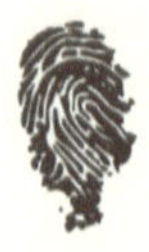

What does a muzzle and air reduction have to do with any health? The use of a mask has been a psychological measure taken by governments to permanently remind the subconscious that it is in a state of alarm and that it is censored, apart from harming its body. The initial reaction of the governments before the bug crisis was to order the population to wear a muzzle, without providing any scientific evidence of this measure, as with the rest of the measures. Many months before, various governments had already purchased supplies of this nature from China, as well as gels, gloves, thermometers, syringes and hygienic suits. Did someone "prophesy" to them what was coming? Or could it be that they already knew it because it was an agenda? What does a muzzle have to do with a protection system? The manufacturers' own boxes clearly indicate that these masks "do not provide any type of protection against coronavirus covid-19, or other viruses or contaminants." That is, they wash their hands. And they do it at a coherent level, of logic and common sense, that is, based on pure science. These masks are merely hygienic in nature. Why then so much madness with people wearing it no matter what? It is a symbol for the subconscious mind: "obey." If you've ever seen the movie 'They Live' (1988) you'll find all of this quite memorable, starting with how forces "above" use the airwaves, propaganda and subliminal messages to instill in people the idea that they obey and obey, submit.

We see that several terms have been given to the use of the muzzle since the beginning of the quarantine, such as chinstrap, mask, covers, tapabocas, or mask, among others. In biblical Hebrew we have the word Sapam (Leviticus 13,45, Ezekiel 24, 17 and 22, Micah 3,7 and 2 Samuel 19,25) it is a mustache or mustache, in the context of something that covers the face from below the nose. In the book of the jewish priest Ezekiel it is used in the phrase 'jaateh al sapam' (rolling up the beard), as in covering the lower part of the face. The RVA translated this as 'rebozo', which is a type of shawl, or garment used to cover the upper part of the body. The Hebrew term Jasam (Deuteronomy 25:4) is also used as a muzzle. This has two archetypal meanings: to put the brakes on and to silence. Bozal is an adjective referred to in Spanish as a black person who has recently left the country. In colloquial use it refers to someone who is inexperienced, novice, apprentice and unskilled in performing some art or performance. Silly person, of little understanding and stupid. It is said of horses and mares that are not yet trained. This word in its etymology is composed of the noun "bozo" from the Latin "bucc ĕ us", mouth and the suffix "al", which indicates relationship or belonging. Notice, the word Jasam appears in Ezekiel 39:11 in the context of the meaning of 'obstruct', hinder, cover up, plug up or stop.

Apart from telling the mind that the person should keep quiet and not give an opinion, it also incapacitates him, telling him that his hands are tied. However, there is another element also embedded in the symbolism that a muzzle represents for the mind, which is the 'loss of identity', since we identify ourselves through the face, and our expressions are first reflected with the features of the mouth. and the cheeks, apart from the eyes. In the Middle Ages, slaves – usually black – wore a muzzle. Hence the combination of the concept between black, slave and muzzle.

This was given to the subject to make it clear to him that he was 'inferior' to his masters, and that he should 'keep quiet' with his master. To this we must add the component of educating the person in the belief that they are 'stupid' and 'inexperienced', so their "masters" are the ones who think and decide for them. In itself, considering that the "most lethal virus in history" can be prevented by wearing a cloth in the mouth does not coincide with the suits and equipment always used in the face of biological or viral threats, which include waterproof suits and safety masks. Here we have, through a key symbol of psychological and non-verbal communication, an unmistakable graphic idea: censorship.

Just last night I shared a fragment of a Netflix movie with my students, from before the pandemic, where they expressed the use of vaccines to introduce pathogens. Well, in the morning my post was censored from the public, arguing that it was "false information", verified by Facebook "independent reviewers". If it's a clip from a movie, including the trailer, what exactly is the false information...? There is no such thing as Facebook "independent reviewers." These are algorithms that, through artificial intelligence, put together definitions, images and words that pass through the networks and configure elements that they subsequently censor. Phrases such as "dangerous vaccine" will never be reviewed, but the program automatically identifies it and marks the publication or comments as "false", without you having the option of a discussion, refutation or justification under documentation. Next we even see advertisements and posters where the "normality" is to see models that come out with a muzzle on: psychological adaptation. They tell the person's mind, "shut up, for your health," "don't give your opinion, the government is in charge," "obey, everything will normalize," "follow the rules, for everyone's safety." Just as an

Illuminati said decades ago, <<we will have a totalitarian and dictatorial global government, whether by consent or by imposition.>> We see the combination of both: public consent and imposition, repressing dissidents.

When one reviews the passages of the New Testament that were written in the common Greek language - or Koine - one comes across the repetition of the muzzle issue, specifically on two occasions. Both argue "not to muzzle the ox that threshes." The apostle Paul explains that this passage that evokes Deut. 25.4 argues not to hinder those who are doing their work, or not to make the work of those who are doing their work difficult. In his case, this verse was intended to make people understand that they should not act as a "stumbling block" to those who were in charge of God's work, and that they should remember that everyone's contribution is what allows the minister of God to be able to comfortably dedicate yourself to what you do, without worrying about how to get money for rent, services, food, transportation, etc. So we find that a commandment of God is not to prevent people from carrying out their functions, and this is exemplified by the use of the muzzle (1 Cor. 9:9 and 1 Tim. 5:18). The word that the apostle Paul used in Greek in his letters was 'Fimosei', which is also translated as 'to command silence'. In the Vulgate translation it refers to "putting a tie on the snout" or "tying the snout." Animals that are muzzled are primarily so that they do not bite. Do we bite? We are not angry beasts, the subconscious mind understands that, we unconsciously begin to "see each other as a danger": every human being, your neighbor, is a threat.

There are two other aspects that should be mentioned in this section, which are of a medical nature: Masks are a source of oral bacteria and an impediment to breathing oxygen (inhaling the expired CO_2 itself for a long time). First of all, can you see light through a mask? Then a virus can pass. Any virus that is smaller than 200 nanometers in diameter can clearly pass through pores that filter out 100-micron particles. What then are the muzzles preventing or filtering? The passage of pure air, oxygen. First, the mouth has a multitude of bacteria, hence the "pleasant" smell when we smell our breath when we wake up. Now let's put our head in a bucket or bucket and spend a couple of minutes breathing our own air. Some breathe through their nose, but most people use their mouth. And even if they didn't use it, when they talk, they are scattering those particles into the muzzle. Then you breathe in those bacteria. It's pure mathematics, if your breath smells bad, it's because those bacteria are not from rose or lily cells. Why does garbage, fish, rotting food smell bad? They are bacteria. That's why bad breath exists. With that muzzle you breathe in your own oral bacteria, mites that stick to the muzzle fabric, and CO2 from expiration. Is it good to breathe mites? What are mites? Tiny ticks that eat the dead skin and defecate all around. Much of what is attributed to respiratory allergies is both mites and primarily the feces of these tiny ticks.

But let's go to the aspect of the cells, which is the one that personally seems angular to me when it comes to people's health. There are aerobic and anaerobic organisms in this plane. What's that? Those that exist through the air and those that do not. If you like the Bible you can find various passages where it is described that "the life of organisms is in the air." In the Vedanta culture of India, there is this philosophy of Prana, which maintains that life is sustained by an invisible energy that is in everything, called by the Chinese the 'Ki', or 'Chi' (the Ka of the ancients). Egyptians). This Prana/Ki is the invisible energy or spirit that gives life to all things. That energy is in the air and moves within the atmosphere thanks to wind currents. In universal perfection, the existence of algae and trees participate in the renewal of this energy. Why can't an organism live without air? To begin with, if it were not like that, why the lungs, or the gills? Aerobic organisms transform Prana, Ki, Chi, as leaves do with photons. It is worth saying that in Hebrew culture we also talk about this Prana/Ki, which is called Jai, about the deformation of the sound Khai, which came from Ki, which is the same one that gives shape to the sound Gai ('mother earth', provider of life). The Hebrew Chai is translated as 'life', but it is an invisible energy, the Ruach (spirit, wind) that gives life to everything.

That life exists because there is an atmosphere, and because there are oceans, and because there are trees. It is a set, it is a whole, it is an "ecosystem", a perfectly elaborate mechanism. We breathe Prana/Ki/Jai and the alveoli of the lungs push it to the heart and from there to the bloodstream thanks to the erythrocytes (blood cells or red cells). They transport that air throughout the body, oxygenating it. Oxygen - whose symbol we know as 'O' - enters the body in molecules grouped with two atoms per structure (O2), which is the amount necessary for its essential function. This consists of reaching the various types of leukocytes (blood cells or white cells) and entering through their membrane to go to the mitochondria. Oxygen first accesses the internal state of the cell, where, as in everything, there is a symbiotic synaptic communication (let's say, something like "wireless"). Thus, the structures in proteins and amino acids of the bases that structure the chromosomes in the nucleus of the cell are reassembled. That means that what goes in maintains human DNA, who we are, and what our health depends on. The function of life is here, but mostly in the fact that when oxygen enters the cellular mitochondria it produces a "combustion", a chemical reaction that generates ATP (adenosine triphosphate), the cellular fuel. That is the key to organic life. However, we live, number one, by the air, by the oxygen that we breathe.

Now, the largest volume of oxygen on the planet per cubic centimeter is concentrated in the troposphere (the lower layer of the atmosphere). This ranges from 17% to 29%. White cells require, at least, a percentage of 15% for survival. By "subsistence," I mean, to live, the limit. I mean, I can "subsist" on one coconut a day, but is that life? Is that balanced nutrition? Is it about subsistence or living? Being at the limit of capabilities the system is at risk. I can survive on a coconut a day, but I better not get bitten by a mosquito or bitten by a crab. Or God forbid that I don't get cold, because if I get the flu, I get the flu, and once I get the flu, I have little chance of beating the flu. Now let's do a simple mathematical exercise: if the amount of oxygen between cities and mountains is between 17% and 29%, where is there the highest and lowest concentration of pure air? In the cities? In the mountains? The higher the altitude, the higher the pressure. The more trees, the more pure oxygen. The closer to the sea, the more pure oxygen. In cities, less pure oxygen. Inside your house, even less pure oxygen. And by "pure", I mean "clean", because another thing is the actual amount of oxygen per cubic centimeter. The equation would give us something like 17% in the worst conditions, and 29% in the best conditions. The worst conditions are near the subsistence limit of white cells. But we add a component: a filter. The amount of oxygen that now enters per cubic centimeter in each inhalation is reduced. Strictly speaking, every second with a muzzle is time that is shortened on your body's life chronometer.

Thanks to the algae in the ocean, and the trees – secondly – the air remains purified. We inhale 'O2', and it reaches the cell and energizes it (oxygenates it, maintains life), but there is an exchange. All organisms produce waste. The "poop" of the cell is a composition – in essence – of atoms with 6 protons, 6 electrons and 6 neutrons (666), called carbon (whose symbol we know as 'C'). Yes, and the atomic number of carbon is also 6, curious? Translate '6' as waste. But this waste returns through the bloodstream and returns from the heart (symbol of life and emotions) to the lungs (symbol of the desire to live and the possibility of living), and from there it is expired. That molecular structure comes out as CO_2 (one carbon atom and two oxygen atoms per molecule) and goes with the air towards the currents that take it to the trees and algae, which absorb it and feed on it. That's right, the food of trees and algae is carbon. Oxygen only acts as transporter, as a connector, as a companion, as a catalyst. Ergo, the tree and the algae take the carbon and release clean, new oxygen, which returns to us. Between the photons they receive from the Sun and transform into energy (photosynthesis) thanks to the structure of the leaves, trees and plants maintain their existence. In themselves, plant cell organisms transform energy through structures that we call green (due to the frequency range).

But we have a problem. The CO_2 that we expel does not go away when we have a muzzle on, like the type of mask that people have put on since 2020. On the contrary, it stays in the muzzle and that is what we breathe in again. Not only does clean oxygen not enter, but the cellular waste itself is aspirated: the cells absorb their own feces. And that happens hour after hour and day after day in a large part of the population. What results do these actions give after a few weeks and a few months? Mathematics... the immune system is weakened and cells die. In addition to this, oxygen does not reach the brain properly. The brain can only last 4 to 5 minutes without oxygen, but what would happen if instead of doing it all at once I dosed it with oxygen? What is the difference between smoking 100 cigarettes in 2 minutes and smoking 7,000 in a year? When is it considered suicide or murder, if you kill in slow motion or fast motion? If someone smokes, they are not fined - although they are killing themselves and poisoning those around them - nor are they imprisoned, but if a person is not wearing a muzzle they are fined. What is the difference? I would say, what do they have in common? That masks are sold by China, and they have a global business, like gels, gloves, gowns, temperature sensors, etc., and cigarettes are sold by tobacco companies. The common one is BUSINESS. The more people get sick, the more customers for pharmaceutical drugs and the more patients for expensive medical treatments.

Do you know what cerebral hypoxia is? It occurs when not enough oxygen reaches the brain. The brain needs a constant supply of oxygen and nutrients to function. Cerebral hypoxia affects the largest parts of the brain, called the cerebral hemispheres. However, the term is frequently used to refer to a lack of oxygen supply to the entire brain. It is no longer just that a person becomes idiotic in the long term due to lack of oxygen (you become stupid, literally), but it can even kill you. In cerebral hypoxia, sometimes only the oxygen supply is interrupted. This can be caused by: Inhaling smoke (smoke inhalation), such as would happen during a fire, Carbon monoxide poisoning, Asphyxiation, Diseases that prevent movement (paralysis) of the breathing muscles - such as amyotrophic lateral sclerosis (ALS) -, High altitudes, Pressure (compression) on the trachea, Suffocation. In other cases, both the supply of oxygen and nutrients are stopped. Brain cells are extremely sensitive to lack of oxygen. Some of these begin to die less than five minutes after the oxygen supply is interrupted. As a result, brain hypoxia can quickly cause death or serious brain damage.

There is a lot of talk about carbon monoxide as the cause of these problems. Then we have, lack of oxygen to the brain, and the inhalation of carbon monoxide. Although in its known state it is popularized as a chemical produced from the incomplete combustion of natural gas, the truth is that it is generally formed from other products that contain carbon. For example, carbon monoxide is an odorless gas that causes thousands of deaths each year in North America. Inhaling carbon monoxide is very dangerous, in fact, it is the leading cause of poisoning death in the United States. Now think about whether wearing a muzzle saves you from a bug or kills you. To begin with, there is no evidence that "coconut" is transmitted through the air. Fauci's staunch enemy already said it at the time, and that cost her 5 years in prison. Judy Mikovits, who once worked alongside Anthony Fauci, already said from the beginning of the pandemic that coronaviruses ARE NOT TRANSMITTED THROUGH THE AIR. That the only way to get infected is through an injection, and I was convinced that SARS-Cov-2 had not inoculated the population in the flu vaccination campaign of December 2019. It saddens me to see people exercising, on the beach, outdoors or in the countryside with a mask. Being told to use it in a closed space with many people has a scientific part, but wearing it in open spaces shows where brainwashing and the lack of knowledge and common sense have reached.

The Facebook channel Cima TV Perú recently interviewed a health professional. She expresses that she has a degree in Physiotherapy and that we must seek information on our own, not stick with just one type of information. She says that this is the pandemic of fear because from the moment you wake up, instead of breathing oxygen, you see, in Television news of death, you cannot go to work, you cannot visit your relatives, comments that in Peru they have been locked up since March 16, you cannot go to work. How do you pay for electricity, water, how do you feed your children, if now you have to take care of your health? What is really killing is fear since it is related to the stress hormone, she explains that cortisol, say international professionals, in high quantities in the blood decreases the Immune System, lymphocytes cannot reproduce as they always do, So no matter how much you are eating healthy, drinking water, doing exercises locked up at home, if your Cortisol hormone is elevated, any virus, any bacteria, TB (Tuberculosis), hepatitis, pneumonia can arrive and the consequence will be having to go to a Hospital Center.

If you arrive with a cough because you got a simple flu, what are they going to tell you? Possible covid, while they are doing your test, then you already live in fear and now you arrive at an emergency. If you are in fear, the Immune System begins to collapse, but how can I not live in fear if there is no food, if there is no work, how can I not live in fear if I have all the bills every month. She reflects and asks: Has the government cared about us? If you are from the Province, you know it better than me. In 2018 there was cold weather (the cold air is a mass of cold air coming from Antarctica that contributes to the sudden drop in temperature in the jungle. It occurs every year in Peru with a frequency of 6 to 10 times, reported the National Service of Meteorology and Hydrology (Senamhi)), in 2017, 2019 and, surely, in 2020 as well, and no press said anything. How many animals die from the cold? How many geriatric people die from the cold? Did the government do something? Every year in the cold comes chikunguya, cholera, etc.

Another question for reflection is the following: how many hours do you use a mask? And it explains the amount of fungi that people have in their respiratory cavity, the amount of bacteria, we have always had them since it is part of our body, having enzymes that degrade them, the fungi, the bacteria, because oxygen enters and begins to work. the metabolism correctly, but now nowadays those bacteria that have been there all our lives, but the oxygen does not enter correctly and when we speak, those saliva particles stay on the masks, we keep them anywhere, we do not expose them to the sun and put it back on. If this mask is exposed to a microscope, we will observe a large number of bacteria, mites and fungi. That is what we inhale every day. We are taking recycled oxygen. When oxygen does not arrive adequate to the brain, it is the case that the person may suffer from hypoxia (Hypoxia is a situation that occurs when the amount of oxygen transported to the body's tissues is insufficient, causing symptoms such as headache, drowsiness, cold sweating, fingers and purple lips and even fainting.) your brain does not work at 100%.

The health professional emphasizes: This is chronic, it is not going to be in 2 or 3 months, so they need you to be with this for 1 year, 2 years, even 3 years, so that slowly more and more people continue inhaling their own mushrooms. and mites. The Sun kills viruses and bacteria through ultraviolet rays, now they force you to be inside your house because sunlight does not enter. It is necessary to breathe the viruses and bacteria found in the environment naturally so that the macrophages start working every day and fight them. [End of his presentation]. The Spanish researcher, Rafael Palacios, shared the rates of psychological reactions in children due to the use of masks, which is clearly not taken into account, because these are the results that globalists seek: 53% of children suffer headaches, 49% are less happy, 44% no longer want to go to school, 38% suffer from learning problems, 25% develop new fears, 15% play less... what is this drama doing in homes and on the physical and mental health of children? The famous novelist, George Orwell, wrote at the end of his work '1984': <<the important thing is to keep the population in a continuous state of fear, for which the news contradicts itself from one day to the next, thus maintaining a state of endless national emergency, justifying... any abuse by the authorities.>>

[UPDATE 03/30/21: I've considered adding an addendum on another point I didn't get to, which is about morgelons. NASA and the UN have worked together for decades in the development of technologies that serve the Great Deception project, from which the core of the Blue Beam is outlined. The core of this well-elaborated plot lies in the recreation of an atmospheric film that makes the world believe that a messiah has appeared to save humanity. This "great messiah", or substitute for Jesus Christ, is the so-called Antichrist, as defined by Christianity (or the Al-Dajjal (or simply 'Dajjal'), of Islam, Armilius for Judaism, or Maitreya for Buddhism). The strategy of creating a holographic space show is the real work of NASA, which in collaboration with DARPA develops the so-called Future Strategic Warfare technologies for the year 2025. What is this? The infrastructure and mechanisms designed for the "future war", where the objective would not be other nations but the civilian POPULATION. That's right, as stated in the 114-page document by NASA Langley Research Center Chief Scientist Dr. Dennis M. Bushnell, entitled 'Future Strategic Issues/Future Warfare [Circa 2025]'. According to this document, the use of Smart Dust, morgelons, nanobots, transhumanism, nanometer tracking devices, artificial insects, wave weapons and explosive dust would be used to reach anywhere and attack people.

What is Smart Dust? The "Smart Dust" is a group of intelligent nano drones that interact with each other like flocks of birds. They can function remotely or respond to a generalized program of response and action. This Smart Dust is even explosive and can charge morgelons. Its use has been intended, among other things, to infiltrate bunkers, remote or almost inaccessible places where insurgents or groups of dissident individuals may be hiding. Hunting humans would be easier with the use of this Smart Dust. Nanotechnology, we see, is the number one tool in this anti-population combat strategy. Introducing nano devices into the body, whether nano particles, morgelons, chelates (heavy metals), micro chips, viruses or nanobots (tiny robots) is the cornerstone of this Illuminati masterstroke. This would lead to complete control over our body by the "masters of the world", and the transformation of our organism into a "transgenic" and "transhuman" creature, thus losing our pristine nature, and turning towards cybernetics, or the post-human. Morgelons – or "morgellons" – are officially a "dermatozoic parasitic delirium", since we do not want to accept the real version of their origin: extraterrestrial.

Morgelons look like tiny fibers of different colors like worms or worms that glow in a certain light, which in essence would be more like self-replicating holographic fibers that would read people's DNA and transform into an electromagnetic wave that can be tracked by satellite, as an antenna to send signals), according to various researchers and experts in new technologies. Accompanied with these morgelons are the "Co-Opted Insects", or false flying insects, used for years in military and secret service operations of the US, Israel, England or Russia. These robotic insects could listen to communications or carry a pathogen that they would inject into a subject, causing, for example, a president or leader of a nation that refuses to follow the Illuminati's guidelines, or stops cooperating with them, to appear, SURPRISELY, dead or terminally ill due to a sudden pathology or attack to the brain or heart. The ability for nano drones to replicate and expand like a halo of smoke has been mentioned in various exhibitions of new technologies, but its existence has not been officially recognized due to its implications. This science, as recognized by a senior government official to a German researcher and technology developer, is of "extraterrestrial" origin and "cannot be controlled." This leads us to discover how the film 'The Day the Earth Stood Still' revealed them to us in 2008, although due to negative primacy few would suspect that said alien development exists, or is even used by NASA, DARPA and the US Armed Forces.

The most terrible thing about this, and the reason for commenting on it in this chapter, is that recently (March 2021) more and more reports, photographs and video recordings have emerged showing morgelons in the masks that China has been marketing throughout the world. The balloon. In 2012, the CDC presented a justification for the appearance of morgelons due to the debate that began with the initial cases investigated in 2002, but they stated that it was not a disease – as some maintained – but merely "cellulose and cotton", which does not coincide with the evidence seen in zoom on these ORGANISMS, where they are observed moving, and even interacting through physical contact with human skin. The closest to discredit were previous studies carried out between 2006 and 2007, burying the idea in bacteria or plant pathogens. All in all, what are these morgelons doing in masks that are SUPPOSEDLY sterilized for "hygienic" use? It is no longer merely the fact that morgelons can send information abroad, but it has been witnessed how they produce serious adverse and horrible dermatological and organic reactions in human beings.]

Sorry, I wouldn't want to move on to the next thing without sharing an anecdote. I call it "the sneezeman debate." To my surprise, it is something that practically no one talks about, despite its obviousness. In a debate I was shocked to see how my detractor nullified his ability to reason when faced with elementary issues. They scold you in public places if you take your nose out of the mask, almost as if you were a risk, as you can shoot a laser beam at them with your nose and destroy them all. It sounds like a joke, but it's how people act robotically, apart from not seeing the dictatorship behind this simple exercise. It's as if most people have stopped thinking. The reasoning is that the bug is supposedly transmitted by saliva droplets. First of all, no bacteria resists solar radiation, so if you expose it to the outside it dies. However, it borders on absurd to be cleaning the exterior surfaces. The Sun is the greatest purifier that exists. Secondly, the anatomy of the nose means that what you breathe in and out points downward, not forward, if you are not one of those who breathe through your mouth. And no, we are not dragons, we do not breathe powerful breath through our noses. So if someone is just half a meter away from us, the worst thing that can happen to them is our breath. Thirdly, it is stated that the problem is the drops when speaking, so why do they tell us to cover our nose inside a muzzle? Ah, because of the sneeze. Of course, because when we feel like sneezing we do it from the rooftops, ensuring that our bacteria reach as far as possible and are lovingly shared with those around us. I don't know what it will be like on your planet, but on mine, wherever you go, when people sneeze they lower their faces and point towards the ground, and they almost always cover themselves with their hands. Apart from that, out of mere politeness we would never do it in front of us when there are other people, and even less so when we are all enthralled with the story of the murderous sneezes.

Now let's do numbers. If 0.07% of the planet has supposedly been infected. By what method was it infected? Those millions of supposedly infected people have never, in all the time I have been collecting information, testified that someone spat in their face before knowing that they were sick. Some talk about having been infected at a party, but do you share your glass with others? And if you know they are sick, all the more reason? And if you feel bad, don't you isolate yourself? I see people exercising, in a car, on the street, METERS away from any human being, with a muzzle on. What does this mean psychologically? It is notorious what the official media has achieved. In one of the demonstrations that were held in Santa Cruz de Tenerife, in the Canary Islands – against all this outrage – I heard the testimony of a lawyer, who said that when the measures to be taken on the people began, what the politicians of the island was, FIRST OF ALL, to allocate an initial fund, not to health measures, or even isolation, or security, but to give it to the media, so that they could follow a script that they were going to give them. Yes, the same script that all the news shows repeat for almost everyone.

The saddest thing about all this is seeing children, not only in schools, but in the parks themselves and on the street, with a mask - and I say this as the father of a little girl -, being that in that phase of growth This is when your brain needs the most oxygen. They are damaging their brain, apart from the other organs in formation. People damage their brains, hearts, lungs, and immune systems by obeying the fallacies of the intoxicating media, especially those who spend hours in front of a television and believe everything they are told. And I can't help but say that we forgot basic biology classes. We have two main types of cells: leukocytes and erythrocytes. Leukocytes have a half-dozen groups, but they all contain a nucleus, in which the DNA chains, the chromosomes, are found. These white cells have mitochondria. Having been created as aerobic organisms, WE LIVE BY AIR. Hold your breath for at least 3 minutes to see what happens. There are those who have spent their entire lives without seeing sunlight, or without getting into a river, a lake, a pool or a beach. We can go days without drinking water and even weeks without eating. There are those who even barely make any type of movement for decades. But what we cannot under any circumstances avoid is breathing.

That air brings oxygen to the white cells thanks to the work of the red cells. Our body is made up of millions of all these cells. Are you aware of what you do to your body by not breathing well? It's not just breathing, it's how you breathe, the patterns of taking in air, holding it, releasing it, the depth of the breathing force, the quality of that air and its quantity. What do you think happens to your body in the long term if you deprive it, with each breath of air, of 20% of that oxygen? Our body's energy comes from how that oxygen is converted into energy by the mitochondria. They are draining your energy by telling you to breathe through a mask for hours every day, even in adverse circumstances where it is difficult to breathe well. But that's not all, your cellular waste, which is carbon, you breathe it again, because it stays in that mask, and you swallow it with your own oral bacteria and the mites that stay there, plus the morguellons that the Chinese give us. they put on the masks. What a deadly mix.

We are the resistance. The prophet Mashah (Moses) wrote in Dbarim (Deuteronomy) 25:4 that <<You shall not muzzle the threshing ox>>. A muzzle is being put on the world to prevent it from "threshing", from doing its job, from working. Progressively we will see ourselves more and more bound, we, who are currently stopping the manifestation of <<that wicked one, whom the Lord will kill with the spirit of his mouth, and will destroy with the brightness of his coming; wicked one, whose coming is by the work of Satan, with great power and signs and

lying wonders, and with all deception of wickedness for those who are perishing, because they did not receive the love of the truth to be saved.>> (2 Thess. 2 :8-10) Meanwhile, this is the call that Ihoshua (Jesus) makes is for you to listen to the Truth, share it with your fellow human beings and prepare yourself with those who the Holy Spirit puts you on the path to live for a few years , while evil on Earth unleashes its fury. <<The only thing that is asked of you is that you make room for the truth. You are not asked to invent or do what is beyond your understanding. The only thing that is asked of you is that you let the truth in, that you stop interfering in what is to happen in itself and that you recognize again the presence of what you thought you had rejected.>> (A Course in Miracles 21, II ,7:2)

XII. THE ERA OF SURVIVALISM

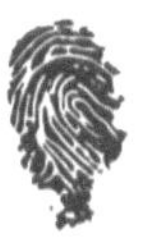

Iremember hearing Dr. Alberto de La Torre, a pharmaceutical chemist at the Universidad del Valle (Colombia), speak frustratedly about not being allowed to test the benefits of chlorine dioxide. You already know how to boost your immune system, teach it to others (get fresh air, walk, make love, stretch, go to the gym, swim, eat fresh fruit, fresh vegetables, sunbathe, interact with others, laugh, enjoy your hobbies). You already know the deception that is being perpetuated, do not fear, do what you must and tell others. You already know what is going to happen, do not start fighting with the system, nor put your hope in it, go, rather, and prepare yourself, you will be helped along the way. You already know how to avoid electromagnetic fields (look, I myself have everything made of wood in my office, I walk barefoot, I have vulcanized stones and plants to reduce the waves, and I keep the phone away (and I don't put it to my ear when talking). I myself have thought about putting a pseudonym in this book, to evade the attack on me, so that I do not become the center of attention when it comes to persecuting another contributor of light. There are many, many of us - although you may not believe it or see it at first glance - who are telling the truth, although, unfortunately at the moment, not many are preparing for survivalism for these years of Orwellian tyranny that are coming. Don't wait until it's too late. My grandfather's family waited until the last minute to leave Germany when the Nazi Party came to power. Almost none survived, few were seen again after WWII. Let's learn from history.

I would like to start this last chapter of the book by adding an article about our great friend Bill Gates and his master plan to hide the Sun. The plan seems strangely similar to the plot of "The Immortals II", but it could be a reality within a decade. Every day, more than 800 giant planes would lift millions of tons of "chalk dust" to a height of 19 kilometers above the Earth's surface and then spread it around the stratosphere. In theory, dust in the air would create a gigantic umbrella, reflecting some of the Sun's rays and heat back into space, thus protecting Earth from the devastating effects of climate warming. The project is being funded by billionaire and Microsoft founder Bill Gates and supported by scientists at Harvard University. In fact, plans are so advanced that initial 'cloud cover' experiments were due to begin months ago. This initial test, known as the Stratospheric Controlled Perturbation Experiment (SCoPEx), would use a high-altitude scientific balloon to lift about 2 kg of calcium carbonate dust, the size of a bag of flour, into the atmosphere, at about 20 kilometers over the New Mexico desert.

This would seed a tube-shaped area of sky half a kilometer long and 90 meters in diameter. Over the next 24 hours, the balloon would be steered by propellers back through this artificial cloud, its sensors monitoring both the sun-reflecting abilities of the dust and its effects on the thin surrounding air. However, SCoPEx is on hold as it could trigger a disastrous series of chain reactions, creating climate changes in the form of severe droughts and hurricanes, killing millions of people around the world. "Our idea is terrifying," said Lizzie Burns, one of the leaders of the Harvard team. "But so is climate change." But creating "a gigantic umbrella" for Earth could have devastating consequences. One of the problems we face is that spreading dust into the stratosphere can seriously damage the ozone layer that protects us from dangerous ultraviolet radiation. Climatologists are also concerned that such modifications could inadvertently disrupt the circulation of ocean currents that regulate our climate. This in itself could trigger a global outbreak of extreme weather events that could devastate crop areas, wipe out entire species and fuel disease epidemics. The potential for disaster doesn't even end there. Trying to dim the Sun's rays would likely create climate winners and losers.

Scientists may be able to establish the perfect climate conditions for farmers in the American Midwest, but at the same time, this environment could lead to devastation in Africa. Because it is not possible to change the temperature in one part of the world and have nothing happen to the rest. Everything in the world's climate is interconnected. Additionally, any change in global average temperature would change the way heat is distributed around the world, with some places getting warmer than others. This, in turn, would affect rainfall levels. Heat drives the water cycle, in which water evaporates, forms clouds, and falls as rain. Any change in heat would cause a change in rainfall patterns. And worst of all, there is no way to predict how the global climate will respond in the future to having a giant chemical umbrella placed overhead. Even this terrifying technology could provoke wars between countries, which would accuse each other of causing the catastrophes. However, Harvard scientists defend their project by ensuring that it is completely safe. David Keith, one of the SCoPEx members, said uniformly seeding the entire global atmosphere with low levels of reflective dust should not be a risk. Professor Keith also suggested that the world's richest nations should create a global insurance fund to compensate poorer countries for any damage unintentionally caused by their sun protection experiment.

The truth is that we are left with Keith's last statement: creating a global insurance fund to compensate poorer countries for any damage caused by the project. How can we compensate for the deaths of millions of people due to scientific madness? Even if we accept this crazy plan, how do you shut down such a global cooling system? And what unforeseen consequences would arise if they suddenly did so? Well, in the following report from October 16, 2009, from the magazine 'Biodiversidad', you will be able to read Silvia Ribeiro talk about geoengineering and the use of these weapons for psychic-mental work on humans. "With honorable exceptions like Bolivia, almost no government or industry proposes going to the true causes of climate change and transforming them. The proposals on the table are market measures (such as carbon trading) that will not serve to reduce greenhouse gas emissions, or technological measures that, without remedying the situation, entail strong social, environmental and economic impacts, and will increase the injustices caused by global warming. Geoengineering is the new card of the oil lobby to negotiate in Copenhagen.

The governments of great powers show growing enthusiasm with the prospect of not having to change anything or reduce emissions at their sources and have already begun to divert public resources for research and experimentation in this new technology, which with its drastic climate manipulations occupies more and more spaces in media, conferences and meetings. They are expensive proposals (with a very risky approach) to manipulate entire ecosystems or large portions of the planet with the aim of combating (so they say) global warming. From the proposals of some scientists (which seemed like science fiction, far from being taken seriously and put into practice), we quickly moved on to the pressure to experiment in the real world. Today the campaign to prove the "necessity" and viability of geoengineering is carried out by the most influential private institutions that want to maintain the world system based on oil." "Geoengineers, armies and oil magnates. A century of industrialism based on fossil fuels that produced oil "civilization" caused climate chaos of dramatic proportions: extreme warming of the planet, more violent and frequent hurricanes, more droughts and floods, melting of the poles and glaciers, rise in sea level with risk for island and coastal populations, disruption of agricultural cycles, greater desertification. Harsh conditions on the most dispossessed populations. For decades, intentional manipulation of the climate became a military objective.

From now declassified documents we know that the United States government caused rains in the Vietnam War that lasted months to destroy roads and crops for the Vietnamese. "Weather as a Force Multiplier: Owning the Weather in 2025" is a classic US Air Force document from 1996, which outlines ways to manipulate the climate for war purposes. Recent proposals come from scientists like Paul Crutzen, Nobel Prize winner in Chemistry, who proposes launching sulfur nanoparticles into the sky to block out the sun and cool the earth. Their logic is that governments are not going to make the necessary decisions to stop greenhouse gas emissions and that the only way out is large-scale technological manipulation that reduces solar radiation that reaches the earth or artificially increases absorption. of CO_2."

You should know that this covering up the sky is precisely an initiative promoted by Bill Gates. Let's continue with the article: "His speech converges with the high-profile institutions and organizations that make up the so-called "international coal lobby." Heavily financed by big oil companies like Exxon and Chevron, and by transnational auto and energy companies, they have insisted for thirty years that climate change is "natural" and that any measure that cuts the use of fossil fuels — especially oil and coal — would be an unjustified attack on "development," sources of employment, and the "right" to consume more and preserve the "American way of life." Geoengineering is a perfect fit for these institutions and the governments of the countries that have caused the most climate alterations, such as the United States, to continue arguing that there is no need to change energy production and consumption patterns based on fossil fuels, because "geoengineering will restore any collateral impacts that these have had or may have in the future."

"The transnational agribusiness and agrofuel companies, forestry monoculture companies, synthetic biology companies, the new biochar capitalists and philanthrocapitalists like Bill and Melinda Gates, among others, finance and converge in this discourse and these strategies. Gates, by the way, has already applied for a patent to control hurricanes. Now everyone "recognizes" that it is urgent to take measures against climate change, but with technological remedies and geoengineering megaprojects. Thanks to their powerful lobbying and financing, they have gotten the United States Academy of Sciences and the Royal Society of the United Kingdom to prepare reports endorsing the need for more research and experimentation in geoengineering, subsidized with public resources. Facets, impacts, controls, calculations. The technological fixes promoted by geoengineering have serious problems."

"Some propose fertilizing the oceans with iron or urea nanoparticles (which supposedly cause plankton to grow that absorb CO2 and take it to the bottom of the sea), others use transgenic algae or algae processed with synthetic microbes that, dumped in the sea, are said to absorb CO2; pumping the deep layers of the ocean to the surface with immense tubes to cool the surface temperature and increase the absorption of CO2; shoot the so-called "stratospheric sulfate" atomized from cannons or balloons to form a layer of aerosols that imitates the effect of a volcanic eruption that blocks the sun's rays and lowers the temperature; place millions of mirrors made of ultra-thin aluminum fabric in the space between the sun and the earth to reflect the sun's rays, preventing them from reaching the earth; throwing salt water into the clouds so that they reflect more of the sun's rays; burning large amounts of organic matter – crops, trees, plant residues – to produce charcoal, burying it in the soil as fertilizer and thus "sequestering carbon", planting transgenic trees and crops with Terminator technology (resistant to drought, floods, saline soils and others), or finally seed clouds to cause rain, dissolve or redirect hurricanes."

"In the case of ocean fertilization, the experiments and published studies show that it does not work — CO2 is released again — and would produce impacts on the food chains of the sea, lack of oxygen in the deep layers of the ocean, toxic over-fertilization with nitrogen, temperature change in marine currents, impact on fish populations and coastal climate regulation. It is the only climate manipulation on which a moratorium has been achieved by the Convention on Biological Diversity since 2008. The other manipulations have strong impacts on the acidification of seas and land, on the ozone layer, on the balance of rainfall, on the trophic, in the balance of ecosystems, depending on the technological patch in question. Any remedy that involves monocultures (and GMOs worse) entails more use of agrochemicals that release greenhouse gases, multiple social, economic and environmental impacts, serious long-term contamination in forests and crops, greater soil erosion and larger eroded areas. There are common problems. To have an effect on the planet's climate, manipulation must involve

megascale violence. This means that while some countries and/
or companies define what is altered, how and when, many or all
of us suffer the consequences."

"Proponents argue that "experimentation" must be allowed,
because it does not harm anyone and then it will be decided
whether to expand it. But there are no mathematical models
or speculations that can predict what will really happen in the
multiple interactions of ecosystems, plant, animal and human
populations: the planetary climate is a complex and
interconnected system with infinite dynamic variables. But the
geoengineers are pushing for the "tests" to be on a megascale,
which would subject us to planetary engineering and the climate
dictatorship of those who control it. These proposals involve
large investments and sophistication and are proposed directly
by the most powerful transnationals on the planet. Even if they
are proposed by governments, they depend on technologies
patented by companies. For them it means new big profits and
that the impacts are assumed by society. Almost all of the
proposals (biochar, ocean fertilization, monoculture of trees and
transgenic crops, agrofuels, transgenic algae, synthetic trees,
ocean mixing, cloud seeding) aim to sell their projects as carbon
credits on the public or private market."

"Geoengineering is proposed by some countries and
companies, which, not by chance, are the most extreme causes
of climate change. They argue that the climate crisis cannot wait
for a global consensus process in the United Nations, because
multilateralism is too slow and bureaucratic a method for
responding to climate emergencies. What will happen if the
United States wants a couple of degrees colder and Russia wants
a couple of degrees warmer? Will the countries of the global
South have to endure whatever they get in the tug-of-war?
Geoengineering will be a trigger for upcoming "climate wars."

If we are all threatened along with the planet, the poorest and most vulnerable countries will suffer 90 percent of the impacts. Peasants, indigenous people, artisanal fishermen, forest dwellers and nomadic shepherds are those who will suffer the greatest impacts from the collateral damage of geoengineering. If one of the first remedies that was intended to be implemented in the real world (ocean fertilization with urea in the Philippines) had been carried out, it would have ended the livelihoods of 10,000 artisanal fishermen. Bjorn Lomborg, famous "researcher" who denies climate change, assures that geoengineering is very cheap. According to him: "We could counteract global warming if 1,900 unmanned ships shoot seawater into the air to thicken the clouds. The total cost would be about $9 billion, and the benefits of preventing temperature rise would total about $20 trillion. This is equivalent to a benefit of 2 thousand dollars for every dollar spent."

"Lomborg's calculations are speculative, arbitrary and false. They exemplify what the oil lobby institutions disseminate to demonstrate that geoengineering is not only a solution but a good investment for governments. None of them "counts" the immense environmental, social and even economic costs that would entail trying to repair or minimally "adapt" to the new impacts. Conclusions. It may seem like a discussion far removed from our daily lives, from the serious and urgent concerns of social organizations and movements, but it is essential that we know these new scenarios and the risks they entail. Geoengineering will be presented by powerful lobbyists and governments as the only "politically viable" solution at the climate change negotiations in Copenhagen. The Group, etc., has concluded that geoengineering is a wrong and highly dangerous response and that its experimentation and development in the field should be prohibited internationally.

Any government or company should be prohibited from making any decision about it unilaterally, since the consequences will necessarily affect us all. [End of publication].

<u>PREPARATIONISM</u>

Concepts such as preparationism, survivalism, or bushcraft are no longer a trend exclusive to Americans. In the last two decades, more and more people from different countries are aware that some serious event can occur that puts the lifestyle we socially have in check. I am talking about measures to survive, whether in the short, medium or even long term, in the face of a disaster of great proportions, such as the collapse of markets, a war, a natural disaster, an epidemic or the sum of two or more of the previous ones, or all of them. Preparationism is the discipline, art or ideology of preparing places, resources and knowledge for an apocalyptic future, even if it were not immediate. Survivalism is the art of studying various ways to survive in a hostile environment, outside the comforts that a city or home provides. Bushcraft is the ability to create shelter and conditions to be outside the city or home.

As the years go by we see that the phases of development of the Apocalypse seem to be on our heels. I believe that in 3 phases the elite has planned to impose its dictatorship, a Police State. The first phase was the era of "terror", where cuts to freedoms began with the excuse of invisible jihadist enemies; The second was from 2020, with the story of the supposed pandemic of a new mutant coronavirus; The third, designed to reinforce the previous two and ensure that no more loose ends are left, is with the use of scalar wave weapons. The powers that be must make sure they achieve their goals as soon as possible, because the longer it takes, the more people will learn the truth and the greater the protests will be. Graphene is also part of this plan, so that once demonstrations are banned, Martial Law will be declared, and since people who are hungry and tired of so much manipulation will not follow orders, they will control the crowds with microwave weapons. Those that contain graphene within the body, or other heavy metals such as aluminum or mercury, will be the worst off.

This phase 3 of deprivation of rights and civil liberties is at the same time phase one of the Blue Beam project. On the one hand, it has the purpose of causing landslides in certain locations where they know that there are archaeological sites of ancient civilizations, and whose content will be publicly known, confirming the existence of extraterrestrials, to launch the other phases of the Blue Beam. The other part of this maneuver is to produce all kinds of environmental disasters in the sky, the desert, the sea, the forests, the coasts and the cities to establish the definitive State of World Emergency, State of Siege and Martial Law under the pretext of take control of the situation. From then on, the military and police forces will be permanently patrolling the streets and the restrictive measures will be increased, with constant Curfews and limitations on movement. In this way they will also distract the army, so that it does not act in favor of the people in the face of the arbitrariness of the state, and, as if that were not enough, to avoid a possible military-civilian coup d'état, nations will enter into wars with other nations, commanding the armed forces abroad.

Then we will see civil war, because reactionary humanity in the face of the deprivation of its rights and in the face of so many abuses will burst with fatigue. The world will refuse the implantable chip as a financial substitute, they will reject the dictatorship and oppose the State. Those who have allowed themselves to be injected will be seeing hallucinations, hearing voices in their heads, believing they see ghosts, they will commit mass suicide, they will believe they see alien invasions, they will go like crazy looting houses for their resources... those who knew this was going to happen, or were Opening their eyes along the way, they will abandon the cities. They will then be able, at least for a few months (hopefully a couple of years), to live off the countryside, heal themselves with plants and cleanse their body of everything that was put into them. They will be able to freely use hydroxychloroquine, chlorine dioxide (CDS), ivermectin, make vitamin and mineral cocktails, enjoy the sun, fresh air, baths (sea, river, lake, pool), the forest, the organic, and ecological vegetable food. Certainly this utopia will be interrupted for a few years, due to severe environmental disruptions, but it will finally lay the foundations for a new world.

"Blessed are those who suffer persecution for righteousness' sake, for theirs is the kingdom of heaven." (Matt. 5:10 – RVA 60) As I have explained the last 6 years, it is necessary to understand that the interpretation that various theologians have had about the chronology and terminology of the cycle of historical transition between the current era and the coming era have many shortcomings. I have been warning for years about the importance of studying how to leave the cities and go live in the countryside, the mountains or the forest. Some think that living far from cities is a "cool" alternative to connect with nature, others because they no longer want to be "slaves of money", but others have as their main motivator seeing that various apocalyptic prophecies come true. I would like us to take a few minutes to make sure if this is actually true, or on the contrary, we see ourselves, as on many other occasions in history, wanting to adjust things that do not fit with our time, either because some want Jesus Christ to return soon, or because others love the action and adrenaline of fiction described in eschatological predictions. One of the parameters to be considered unequivocally is the context of the events; The second is the order of the prophecies; the third the context of the prophecies; and the fourth is the correct interpretation of the prophecies (to which we must previously add a correct translation of the words used in the text).

I will do the work of simplifying the most significant events that concern the present. I have already done this in previous works, but this time in light of the COVID-19/COVID-21 Agenda. Thanks to these elements, the perception and understanding of various advertisements, which until now were not applicable or understandable, is more lucid. I will go in chronological order of events to avoid descriptions of individuals who announced it and the prologue of what they were talking about, since in the end they were referring to the same thing that concerns us in our present. I won't go too far back, just starting from some substantial examples that follow the context of the circumstances:

1. Isaiah 9:11 prophesied 9:11 (attack on the Twin Towers), the beginning of a series of wars in the Middle East and the awakening of the Islamic "enemy."

2. Much of the prophecies, both biblical and parabiblical, describe that there will be a time when deceit and lies will reign. The context of this is applicable to today because of how politicians lie, the media manipulates information and how all things are presented to society distorted, retouched and biased. This is a component that persists and will be the master key of the Antichrist, who will use deception to achieve his ends. This is something unique that has never before been possible to do because of the dark power over all of humanity at the same time, especially because they did

not have the technologies and resources that exist today.

3. Apostasy is also referred to, and is clearly seen. The value of religion and the principles that were maintained are degraded. Decidedly before WWII you were still a heretic if you contradicted the Catholic Church, however, the tendency to attack the figure of Jesus, for example, was more of a fashion that began to be seen in the mid-90s. It is Freemasonry that has led this trend, and the Rockefellers who have weakened religious faith due to their multiple social brainwashing campaigns.

4. Colossal advance in technology and science, mentioned by both the Jopi Indians and the prophet Daniel.

5. In line with deception is ignorance of the truth and failure to understand what is happening. Daniel also said it in this order of things, arguing that, furthermore, those who do understand would be those who would be chosen for the future kingdom.

6. Likewise, Yeshua (Jesus) and the prophet Yoel (Joel) warned that the Holy Spirit would come upon many at this time to give them courage, knowledge and impetus to warn of the things that are happening and that will happen, and this would then be the " new gospel" of this generation: warn what is coming and who is behind all this. This is the Resistance, what is increasingly persecuted, censored and silenced, and those who will be part of those chosen for the new kingdom: <<If anyone goes into captivity, he goes into captivity; If anyone kills with the sword, he must be killed with the sword. Here is the patience and faith of the saints.>> (Rev. 13,10). Yeshua referred to them saying, "He who perseveres to the end will be saved" (Mark 13:13),

knowing that only Resistance will remain firm despite the attacks, deception, persecution and tribulation: <<With your patience you will win your souls.>> (Luke 21,19).

7. Oppression and reinforcement of dictatorial imperialism, a detail especially mentioned in the prophecies of Ezra and Baruch. There were isolated dictatorships, and they have still been seen, true or not, in Cuba, Venezuela, North Korea, Russia, China, Chile, Italy, Germany, Spain, Iraq, Libya... however, none of that compares to the new communism, Nazism, Marxism, fascism, Francoism and other "isms", which has emerged globally since quarantines were announced in almost all countries in the world in March 2020.

8. People who call themselves Christ, or the return of Jesus, or the reincarnation of Jesus, or the one sent by Jesus, as savior. Definitely, if someone had come out with this story several centuries ago, it would end up in hell.

Now let's look forward to events to see, according to social behavior, the consequences of the crisis caused by the COVID-19 Agenda, added to the COVID-21 Agenda. Although I am writing these lines on Wednesday, February 17, 2021, these words and their application must be recorded at the moment you may be reading this chapter. There is a first element that is present in the prophecies that Yeshua (Jesus) provides about what they define as "signs" of the "end" of this era, to invite the return of the Lord. Revelation and Yeshua's references are, without a doubt, the most extensive and clear when it comes to reporting on these events. Yeshua begins his warnings by announcing that there will be "false Christs," that is, pseudo messiahs, false saviors, who would say they come in the name of Jesus, or they themselves are Jesus. Well, this has been seen for several years, and it would not be surprising if it were seen more frequently, especially because "in the country of the blind the one-eyed is king", and in a time of crisis, fear and uncertainty, inventing That you are a savior puts you on a pedestal and many people after you. Some think this matches the description of the White Horse of Apocalypse and the Q movement, or supporters of Donald Trump. True or not, or to some extent false or not, is something that will become evident in due course. However, it is true that we can find ourselves faced with a bad translation and misinterpretation of the biblical passage.

Let's see, the verse says, <<Take heed that no one deceives you. For many will come in my name, saying, I am the Christ; and they will deceive many.>> (Matt. 24:4-5, RVA 60). To begin with, anyone can say, "I come from Jesus," whether well-intentioned or not. You can believe what you are saying; You may be right, or lying. But if you say that you come from Jesus, it does not mean that Jesus appeared to you and said, "come from me", or it may be, it is enough that you have an ideal based on a Christian concept, for example, such as principles ethical, moral, spiritual or religious. On the other hand, saying that you are "the Christ" refers to a conception of a Greek word. He is actually saying "I am the Chosen One," "I am the Anointed One," "I am the heir to the Throne," "I am the Messiah," "I am the Deliverer," or "I am the Savior." So here the case of Donald Trump fits in like a glove, who might not be lying in his statements and intentions, but in reality he is just a man. However, people could later become disillusioned or disappointed by their trust in him. The meaning of the word used in the Greek text, Planísousin, fits here, relating to erring, making mistakes, getting confused, getting lost, being deceived, becoming disillusioned, disappointed, losing focus or failing. It would not be strange if Trump left a military legacy, to say the least, and his former generals began a series of maneuvers to "reestablish," at least, the United States. That would fit the description of the White Horse, as it also fits very well. good with Trump's victory in the 2016 elections. However, this barely receives any room in the prophecies, because the Red Horse follows directly.

Ergo, the next element that accompanies these indications is war. Here, like a funnel, all the "end-world" prophecies meet. Let's see, according to the COVID-19 Agenda, there would be about 18 months to achieve mandatory vaccination implementation. If this started with the 2020 World Quarantine, everything would be ready, according to your plans, by approximately September 2021. In the worst case scenario, few people would have time to escape such a macabre plan. At best, the White Horse "helps us out," but only to slow things down, giving us a short window of time, while simultaneously allowing more people to open their eyes. How do you achieve it? It seems the only way that is plausible under the circumstances: war. It is notorious that the scenario of the global war confrontation is the hidden agenda of the Illuminati. It is my assumption that the world leaders who are participating in this, having allowed themselves to be bought off by Soros and his henchmen and bosses, have not been informed of this move. They believe that they will receive a paradise plot somewhere in the Caribbean while their country enters the gears of the Illuminati's planetary dictatorship, and they will simply give people mandatory vaccines, let's say chips, and a strong police state. I think they were not told about the "Trojan horse" trap.

One of the reasons that lead me to this deduction are other prophecies, such as those of Baruch, Enoch, Ezra or Billy Meier, about the perplexity and bewilderment of world leaders when military tension increased and the outbreak of a thermonuclear conflagration became evident.

What ties this together perfectly – from my personal point of view – is in the description of this programming. In accordance with the COVID Agenda, in March 2020 the implementation of concentration camps was accelerated from January 2021; Labor Reform would be promoted and Universal Basic Income was presented as a solution to the economic crisis since February and March 2021, when the story of Covid-21 infections would begin; Between April and June, food would become scarce in supermarkets and there would be great economic instability; between April and July new confinements would begin; and from July riots would begin, and local governments would begin to withdraw while military controls in the cities increased. This business of "riots" and "military control" actually translates into civil unrest in the streets. This was also prophesied by Enoch, Baruch, Ezra and Yeshua, among others, and, clearly, in its context. Yeshua would have said – according to the description of the doctor Luke – that this would be the second thing to happen: <<And when you hear of wars and seditions, do not be alarmed; because it is necessary that these things happen first; but the end will not be immediately.>> (Luke 21:9, RVA 60) Social unrest would increase. This translates into what is also defined in the Greek text as riots, commotion, tumult or disorder. It is logical that many people end up getting tired of the nonsense, their economy is about to completely fall apart, they find themselves incapable of dealing with expenses and commitments, and hunger squeezes and clouds reasoning.

With the precedent of the 2020 Quarantine, this time people will take to the streets outraged, with more than compelling reasons, and in all parts of the world. This, from my point of view, is the outbreak of civil wars that will be unleashed, propagated and expanded from now on throughout the planet, until the Blue Beam Agenda has been completed, or at least, to a large extent achieved. to complete. I will include another element: covid-21 vaccine. Operation LockStep is designed to put such pressure on society to accept mandatory vaccination, and while in the first phase people were locked up, 5G antennas, which are the key to why graphene is injected into the world, were withdrawn around the world. people. It is the main part of the agenda of the 2020 and 2021 lockdowns. Weaken the minds of the people so that they crave this vaccine, and if there is resistance, also exhaust it everywhere and by all plausible means. The covid-21 vaccine would be presented in July, precisely, and the vaccination wave would already be a fact by August of this year. This would only further stress the people, especially those who refuse to be poisoned. To appease this there would be the idea of Universal Basic Income, which additionally allows the elimination of all debt, even if you must abdicate your property rights. This idea, proposed for September 2021, coincides with 50 years of the inflationary petrodollar financial system that allowed the banksters, masters of all the banks, to create money from nothing and put nations in debt. According to the prophetic scenery of 'I Pet Goat II', Barack Obama's work is followed by the fall of the Statue of Liberty, which in turn is followed by the monitor (screen) where a reptilian brainwashes the youth (while being intoxicated with drugs and injections) and finally the markets collapse to break out nuclear war.

The hour will come when all who do iniquity will receive what they have sown. We, who faithfully believe in reincarnation, are aware of the law of cause and effect, and that no one escapes it. In the last decade, doctors, virologists, scientists, and other experts in self-healing, natural medicine, and expensive treatments have been murdered all over the world. Because? At this point the answer is more than obvious. They will return in their next incarnation, and continue their path of growth. Others are now repressed, but they fight, despite everything and the high level of censorship. All of us who are speaking are the prophets of this generation, no longer with rags, beards, disheveled hair or words from a biblical vocabulary, but we prophesy, we predict, we announce, we declare the truth, we say what is necessary so that many can know the truth. TRUE. We are the voice that cries out today from the networks and the web, although they censor us, delete our posts and our videos. We talk in the street, although we are prohibited from approaching others. The level of deception and brainwashing on neutral brothers in the world is so serious that they hear us and are confused, disconcerted, misplaced, because they have been presented with a false world, and they have believed it.

I have had face-to-face discussions with state officials and doctors, and they themselves, after agreeing with me, remain silent and confused. There is no holistic knowledge, however, they do not see the image in perspective, they do not know what is behind it or imagine it (and they will not even want to know when they find out how deep the "rabbit hole" is). The mere question of pedophilia is shocking. The first time I heard about this was back in 2008. I was affected for at least 3 days. The pain I felt in my heart and soul bathed my cheeks with tears. I couldn't believe it, but something inside me told me that it was true. More of that came to me about two years later, with Abdullah Hashem's YouTube series, 'The Antichrist-Dajjal will be a Metamorphic Reptilian'. This made me understand the depth of the rabbit hole, and the very creepy, well-crafted and titanic program of mind control directed by the CIA, in turn motivated by the usual ones. It was with the quarantine of the "bug" that I saw many prophecies and words of the Bible different, in light of events, and I understood that we were already at the beginning of the Great Tribulation. The prophet David, who was king of Israel about 3,000 years ago, spoke of the beginning of this in his 91st psalm, and Yeshua did too, but neither announced this "pandemic" because it is not a pandemic. What they did say was that we would be in a time of DECEPTION.

That is the beginning of everything, <<For this reason God sends them a deceptive power, so that they believe the lie...>>> (2 Thes. 2:11, RVA 60). They said what would be true, such as the deprivation of rights and the dictatorship, such as <<a lot of oppression>> (2nd Ezra and 2nd Baruk). Likewise Daniel said in his chapter 12 that <<many would be cleansed and purified and made white>>, and <<the wicked will act wickedly, and none of the wicked will understand, but **those who understand will understand** .>> (verse 10, KJV 60) . This is the time of inner purification, of awakening, of awareness, of inner perfection, of demonstrating who we are. We understand what is happening, and we must be a light on those who do not understand, because they have fallen into the web of deception and lies. That is our mission, <<those who are wise will shine like the brightness of the firmament; and those who teach righteousness to many, like the stars forever and ever.>> (Dan. 12:3, KJV 60) We are the prophets of the present, of whom Joel said, <<I will pour out my Spirit on all flesh, and your sons and your daughters will prophesy; Your old men will dream dreams, and your young men will see visions. And also on the male and female servants I will pour out my Spirit in those days.>> (ch.

2:28-29, RVA 60). What are these visions and prophecies about? In warning what is happening and where it is headed: the New World Order.

This is what Yeshua was referring to when he stated that this gospel would be <<preached, as a testimony to all nations, and then>> is when <<the end>> would come (Matt. 24:14). Yeshua was not speaking of the kingdom of heaven at that time, but of the kingdom of Belial. He spoke of a message, or news (gospel) that would be made known everywhere so that it would remain a record, that would be a testimony to all humanity. As in this passage and in Joel 2:28, other verses remind us of this current mission, and the consequences, where many will be persecuted and killed for speaking the truth: <<Because they shed the blood of the saints and the prophets, You have also given them blood to drink; because they deserve it.>> (Rev. 16,6, RVA 60) And he points to the source of evil on our planet, as guilty of this: <<And in it was found the blood of the prophets and saints...>> (Ch. 18,24). Saints and prophets? We have to see things according to the proper prism. Whoever announces and predicts falls into the category of prophet. He who has innocence and inner purity is a saint, and that includes little children: <<See that you do not despise one of these little ones; because I tell you that his angels in heaven always see the face of my Father who is in heaven.>> (Matt. 18,10, RVA 60). And just as the murder of prophets – whether today or yesterday – will bring divine "revenge", in the same way the mortality, abuse and exploitation of the innocent will bring its retribution: <<And whoever causes any of them to stumble for these little ones who believe in me, it would be better for them if a donkey's millstone were hung around their neck and they were drowned in the depths of the sea. Woe unto the world because of offenses! for stumbling blocks must come, but woe to that man through

whom the stumbling block comes! Therefore, if your hand or your foot causes you to offend, cut it off and throw it away from you; It is better for you to enter life lame or maimed, than having two hands or two feet to be thrown into eternal fire.>> (Matt. 18,6-8, RVA 60)

Before the so-called Rapture there will be a great persecution against those who follow the truth, although it will not be as terrible as that which will come after that event. At that time those who are connected to the Light, vibrating in the Truth, guided by the Holy Spirit and his angels will be protected. However, many have been suffering from the attack of tyrants and will continue to fall before the hunt of the masters of the world: <<When he opened the fifth seal, I saw under the altar the souls of those who had been killed because of the word of God. God and for the testimony they had. And they cried with a loud voice, saying, how long, Lord, holy and true, will you not judge and avenge our blood on those who dwell on the earth? And they were given white garments, and told to rest for a little while, until the number of their fellow servants and their brothers, who also were to be killed like them, was completed.>> (Rev. 6,9- 11, RVA 60) Although some have been killed, both these and those who remain alive will be taken, as I have already explained in my other books regarding the theme of the Rapture. And in the meantime, those who are attuned to the Spirit and his messengers will be protected, as noted in Psalm 91 of David.

Many people ask me about how to manage what is to come. Well, I have written these tips to provide light and logistical and technical information on issues that you should consider. How to live in a world without money? How to stay afloat in the face of what is going to be unleashed on a global level? A self-sustaining community. Start by...

1. AWARENESS AND INFORMATION

2. SELL

3. BUY

4. MEET

5. ESTABLISH INFRASTRUCTURE

<u>1st. Awareness.</u>

Each individual must become aware of the situation and document everything as best as possible. This is my forecast for the next 10 years.

I) China will buy more land, install more biometric recognition surveillance cameras, establish more concentration camps, expand its maritime fleets in the Pacific, and together with Russia they will buy all the gold possible. They both plan to destroy the US.

II) The value of gold will go down.

III) More satellites programmed for the Blue Beam project will be taken into space and 5G – and then 6G – antennas will continue to be installed for the same purpose.

IV) The idea of new coronavirus infections and in greater numbers everywhere will be promoted.

V) Lockdowns will be extended again, this time under greater control, hygiene and police and military surveillance measures.

VI) The borders will be closed again and there will be no more tourism or travel between countries.

VII) Banks will give less and less credit and will ask for more requirements to lend money.

VIII) It will not be possible to sell anything of great value due to the social evaporation of cash.

IX) Decapitalization will reach the point where it will not be possible to pay rent or water or electricity services.

X) Mandatory vaccination will begin to be implemented in all parts of the world to damage the DNA of humanity and introduce nanoparticles that help triangulate geolocation control and mental control systems. This vaccination will be mandatory and must be certified, and without this document children will not be able to attend school or go to work or receive benefits from the state.

XI) People will be more encouraged to report their neighbors and fellow humans who do not attack the imposed rules and do not get vaccinated. Social tension between couples, families and neighbors will increase, increasing the number of conflicts between them.

XII) Access to food will be reduced since supermarkets will not have supplies, since supplies of products will be cut off because farmers are abandoning the fields to go to the cities. Food will become increasingly scarce and its price will rise greatly.

XIII) More sources of employment and types of work will disappear rapidly. The level of unemployment will exceed limits never seen before in all of history.

XIV) Drug trafficking and prostitution will increase to make some money among people.

XV) Social stress, anxiety, helplessness, hunger, frustration, anguish and anger will bring people together on the streets in demonstrations, violating the imposed quarantine regulations. There will be disturbances to businesses and public works. This will lead to protests with cases of violence and confrontations with law enforcement. This will spread throughout the planet on a large scale. Governments will not have enough prisons and will have to set up concentration camps.

XVI) The banks will become insolvent and there will be no more money in circulation. US markets will crash and the Federal Reserve Bank and Treasury will declare the end of the US dollar.

XVII) After the fall of the economy in the USA, that of the European Community will immediately follow. The treasury bonds held by all central banks in the world will lose their value, creating a collapse of the global financial system that will lead to a global structural collapse.

XVIII) The world supply of oil will be reduced rapidly, which will raise its price and slow down the commercial system.

XIX) The most powerful nations in the world will rise up in thermonuclear war against each other, air war, with transatmospheric missiles and satellite weapons, with viral and bacteriological war, and cyber war. This is to restore their economies.

XX) Social protests will rise to the level of civil war, looting, riots and homicides. The cities will be an apocalypse.

XXI) New virulent diseases will spread among the population. These have been created in laboratories in order to be spread among crowds to reduce the population.

XXII) The Deep State will use geophysical weapons to cause massive earthquakes in certain locations. This is so that evidence of extraterrestrial intervention in our past is discovered and this is announced in the news media. Likewise, these weapons will be used to alter the weather and use it against enemies. This will change the natural cycle of the seasons throughout the planet, and will cause tornadoes and hurricanes in areas where that did not exist, and will bring rain in desert areas, drought in cold areas, altering the entire biosphere and the energy fields of the globe, causing disorders. in animals and in humans.

XXIII) To stop the irrational deployment and launch of nuclear arsenals and set the stage for the new global government, the Blue Beam project will come into force.

These 23 points that I have shared are called in Jewish and Christian eschatology, 'The Birth Pains', referred to in the book of Revelation as 'The Great Tribulation', or the first phase of what is known as Revelation itself. Those who are aware of the implications of all this are going to prepare, and not wait until the last minute, when it is impossible to do anything about it to be safe.

2nd. Sell (and save).

Properties. Any property near cities will be a risk to the safety of its tenants due to looting that will spread and increase following the demonstrations and riots that will occur with the fall of the economy. There will be no water or electricity supplies or the possibility of purchasing food or any basic necessities from supermarkets.

Vehicles. At some point it will become reckless to travel on the roads. There will be no fuel available. To maintain the vehicle, a distribution of appropriate mechanics from a workshop will be necessary. It will be impossible to buy spare parts for vehicles.

Articles and objects. As long as there is money movement and the markets function, it is essential to sell everything that is not strictly a priority and that has some commercial value.

Electronics and appliances. Due to low electrical power supplies it is not advisable to take things that will not work or will draw too much voltage. Only equipment that can operate at low power, that is charged or powered by solar panels can be viable. The rest must be battery-operated devices.

3rd. Buy.

- Get land away from cities and towns.
- Perishable foods (preserved, canned) and long-lasting.
- Drinking water, which must also be neutralized from any biodevelopment with drops of bleach every couple of months.

- First aid material (hydrogen peroxide, alcohol, betadine, sodium bicarbonate, gauze, tape, band-aid, scissors, scalpel, syringe, thermometer, aspirin...)
- Personal hygiene material
- Survival material (knives, flint, matches, lighters/lighter, flashlights, batteries of various calibers, water purification tablets, water filters, compass, thermal blanket, fireproof and waterproof fabric, walkie-talkies, mountain boots, hammock, tent, watch, radio, repellents, net/mesh or mosquito net...)
- Gold and silver
- Cryptocurrency
- Seeds (short and medium cycle) and fruit trees (these are obtained in fairly grown nurseries, and which can already begin to bear fruit, or in less than a year after transplanting)
- Fuel
- large batteries
- Solar or photovoltaic panels, or wind fans
- Leisure material (balls, board games)
- Gas bottles (cylinders)

4th. Community.

Contact people who have the same awareness, decision-making capacity and commitment to working together. To warn of the importance of Eco Villages, self-sustainable communities or mini cities. Although it is true, since before 2001 I had already been talking about a large part of these "apocalyptic" topics, but it was not until 2012 that I began to be aware of the importance of considering having places of refuge and support in the face of what is happening. came. When Obama planned to retain office in the US and impose Martial

Law was the time I took this task most seriously. Thank God, 2016 was not yet the time, and thank goodness, because I could only supply my home for a maximum of 3 months, and I had no land to flee to. In 2018 I began to feel again that it was important to re-motivate these ideas of survivalism and eco villages, but it was finally mid-2019 when I felt it was time to get to work. Since then I have promoted eco villages and I myself organized what I called Neo Eden, to be developed, either in the Canary Islands, somewhere in Honduras or in Colombia. It's a lot of work, but we are making progress on all the logistics, while advising others who feel the same way.

An eco-village works as a team, cooperatively, performing the functions necessary for the maintenance of the community. They have to create an assembly and hold weekly meetings to evaluate the affairs of the village and the distribution of daily activities. Here they must explain what each of the members are good at, what specialty they have to contribute. Main work areas:

◈ Surveillance
◈ Cleaning, recycling and order
◈ Agriculture
◈ Child care
◈ Early childhood education
◈ Kitchen
◈ Social activities and cooperative and raid workshops
◈ Crafts
◈ Assembly and labor

5th. Infrastructure.

- Set up shacks or prefabricated homes if the land does

not consist of already built homes.

- Set up dry toilets, which contribute to the composting process, or if you decide to go with conventional methods, install toilets, if the land does not already have them installed. Likewise, if there are no showers, they should be installed, taking advantage of the drainage for irrigation.
- Install self-sustainable energy systems and electrical wiring, if you do not have it
- Obtain at least one water source from which collection can be made and install a water tank close to the core, where it is deposited.
- Install a dining area
- Install a kitchen area that can operate with a wood oven, barbecue, gas stove, or simply a fire
- Install a washing area
- Install a meeting area, or central area, where the first aid area is also located
- Install a children's study area
- Install a reading, library, relaxation area
- Install a children's play area
- Install a board game area
- Install an outdoor recreation, game and sports area
- Install a recycling area
- Install an exercise area
- Preferably install a refuge area under the ground, which would be the task that would require the most time and study.

So consider investing in:
- Food
- Food

- Water
- Energies
- Fuel
- Gold

Also, keep in mind that preparing for a self-sustaining system means thinking about:

- Households
- Electricity
- Water
- Feeding
- Leisure
- Trades
- Barter

How do we see ourselves then with all this, and how do we make estimates to more or less foresee how to locate ourselves in time and know how we are in time and what things the circumstances will allow us depending on what moment? Some "approximations" can be traced around what 2021 to 2030 would be like, but we already know that this cannot be taken 100%, but merely as a comparative scale and general idea. We must consider, first of all, the elements that have given rise to the current movements, prior to the Covid-21 Agenda, part of 'Agenda 21':

a. Gender ideology => destroy homes and the power of families, and degrade youth, restrict religion, reeducate children to the elite model (brainwashing... Ludovik effect)

b. Pro-abortion => reduce overpopulation... phase after the 'AIDS Agenda' (use condoms to avoid pregnancies), sicken and kill healthy people, and finance big pharma and the medical industry, restrict religion

c. Climate change => financing control over Africa and big pharma, and control over open spaces (privatization of the environment and exploitation of new natural resources)

d. Biological threat => test the power of the political establishments and transfer them to supranational organizations (WHO + big pharma), increase surveillance technology and the militarization of the streets, reduce the groups of revolution and dissidence (eliminate marches, protests and demonstrations , and keep them away so that they do not organize or conspire against the state or have human warmth (then they would have to do it digitally, but by doing so the AI will know)), frighten the population to make it docile, promote new vaccinations (reduce the population world and feed big pharma and the medical industry), eliminate the crippled and elderly (reduce government costs in public health and pensions), all cities and houses are turned into prisons (like the goat in i pet goat ii)...disarm, ridicule and demoralize Christianity.

e. Pharmaceutical and medical business

f. Ecumenism and Disarmament of the Abrahamic religions

g. Control of the media

Later we will see ourselves with the Covid-21 Agenda, which consisted of starting with isolation facilities from November 2020. That is, concentration camps. Then January with: Complete secondary block. New confinements. Third blockade. Complete flight restriction (priority flights only?). Quarantine.

Maximum restriction. New IMF meeting on the Great Reset, Promotion of Labor Reform, Global Vaccination Movement. And so on, February, start of the covid-21 phase (https://www.joblo.com/horror-movies/news/covid-21-lethal-virus-unleashes-new-trailer-online [1]), labor reforms underway: fourth industrial revolution... part of the so-called 'Great Reset' proposed in June 2020 by the World Economic Forum (WEF), which will shift capitalism to collectivism (added to the 'UBI Agenda' to take away the people's ownership and purchasing power and private capital to pass into the hands of the government). In this way, throughout 2012 they would be forced to accept the new vaccine and its certificate. If the majority of people oppose vaccination, methods will be released to kill many people (it will be survival of the fittest). This is the type of thing that was already exposed in the protocols leaked in 2020 for 2021:

April:

- Second supposed wave of the pandemic...
- Would propaganda restricting access to wild places (nature) be promoted with the excuse of contact with animals that could cause new epidemic outbreaks and the sale of wild animals for consumption? At least the forests would be privatized...

May – PHASE 2:

- Greater implementation of UBI in more countries.
- Those who accept the vaccine will be at war with those who do not. Anarchy will begin on both sides.

June:

---

1.   https://www.joblo.com/horror-movies/news/covid-21-lethal-virus-unleashes-new-trailer-online

- It has been 50 years since the government chaired by Richard Nixon announced its decision to abandon the so-called gold standard and global debt and the inflationary crisis began.
- Failures in the supply chain. Food shortage. Great economic instability. Inventory.
- Alleged third wave of the pandemic...?
- Social atomization
- Propaganda of social betrayal. Tell your neighbors.

July:

- Military deployment within cities, and controls, travel points.
- health passport and digital ID? Whoever does not accept it will be taken to concentration camps or will receive a house in prison and their belongings will be confiscated.
- Total border and flight control.
- I work from home. Strictly digital employment

August:

- Protests and demonstrations
- Abort any possible revolution
- Total submission to the authorities
- Imposition of vaccination certificate
- Mandatory vaccination
- UBI with vaccination certificate
- Proposal to eliminate debts and end individual property

September:

- Market collapse
- World War
- Civil war and riots
- Hunger and food shortage

October:

- technocratic government
- Empire of transnationals
- Tech Big Brother
- Mass surveillance
- Elimination of alternative media
- Martial law

November:

- Purge
- Elimination of dissidents
- Tyrannical immigration control
- Elimination of social and political opposition
- Closure of airports and borders.

December:

- Elimination of physical money
- Change of the economic model
- biological warfare

January 2022:

- False democracy
- Imposition of identification chips and monetization

Beyond this, I have already addressed the issue in other manuscripts, but roughly speaking, we see that it is quite likely that the systemic breakdown will be triggered by the combination of the fall in monetary stability in people, along with the pressure to get vaccinated. and want to make that become mandatory law. According to the prophetic chronology, we are already in the time of those "false prophets and false Christs", who appear on television and the networks, led by Bill Gates, Melinda Gates, George Soros, Pope Francis, Elon Musk, Kamala Harris, Hillary Clinton, Barry Soetoro (Barack Obama), Anthony Fauci, Joe Biden, Tedros Adhanom, Mitt Romney, Jared Kushner, Benjamin Netanyahu, and many others (from world leaders and politicians to spokespersons for international and supranational organizations). This would be followed by social unrest that would lead to seditions, protests and demonstrations on a global scale, which would be accompanied by several wars between certain nations until falling in a matter of weeks into a series of planetary conflicts, both internal (civil war) and external. (Third World war). This would not have to happen overnight, but the process of these events will make most minds still asleep react. In the subsequent months, earthquakes would shake the globe greatly, and chemical and bacteriological agents would be released in densely populated areas, where hunger due to food shortages would already be creating a social shock. Then, to make matters worse, the Purge will begin. When you see these things coming, it is time for them to have had every book to have carried out their exodus from the cities.

<u>PROPHETIC TIMES?</u>

With this section I do not intend to give a biblical lecture (this book is not about this topic, which has already been addressed ad nauseam by me in other works), I just want to add a couple of details as a mere retraining exercise. It is more of a curious approach than a prophecy. Twenty centuries ago Ihoshua, known to the Western world as Jesus Christ, was asked how this age of humanity would end to begin a new generation on this planet. As Jews, those who questioned him had hope for a Coming Kingdom of peace, utopia, love, immortality and happiness. Regarding this question, Ihoshua – or Ieshua, as others knew him – spoke to them about certain signs that would be a reference. These "signs" had already been described by other Jews centuries ago, from the prophet Daniel to the scribes Ezra and Baruk. Later, a disciple of Ihoshua, named Yochanan (John), added other unique details to the description, as the apostle Paul would have done a few years earlier. But it was not only Hebrews who, for whatever reason, knew what these events would be like. These statements supported the following issues that I will list, leaving the authorship of the individuals.

You must understand that the context of what they were talking about was specific, specific, not generic. I will present below my conclusion in this regard after almost two decades studying the words of these and many other people who had premonitory dreams. I will just make a summary of some of these references that they gave. All of this revolves around the theology of the Antichrist, which is defended by both monotheistic and polytheistic religions, and which is an important reference in the philosophy of Freemasonry.

1. The Wicked One will be preceded by a multitude of deceptions. By saying 'precede' it means that for its public appearance the world will mostly be under a global "deception".

2. There will be a multitude of news. This means that despite the great deception worldwide, all kinds of reports would spread tirelessly. Be it misinformation or truth, phenomena that we see comparing news media and social networks.

3. Those who understand will understand, those who do not understand will remain deceived. This aspect argues that only people dedicated to searching, who are hungry to know and in their hearts desire to understand, will find out what is really happening, and will become more informed and give that knowledge to others.

4. Those who are wise will shine into eternity. These words, allegedly spoken by the archangel Gabriel, speak of a world where the deceived will be led into slavery and destruction, and those who seek will advance at full speed. Two sides will be created, as the passage refers, creating a social bifurcation of the deceived and the knowledgeable. And those who advance towards the truth will be more and more enlightened, and will be with those who think and feel as they do.

5. The above is the antithesis of the passage from the Apocalypse of John, which describes the deceived masses as individuals who will be brought to the extreme suffering and harm of their incarnation. Your body and mind will be completely affected. As? Because of new technologies, because of the poison and the nano devices inside his body.

6. They will antagonize each other, parents and children will betray themselves to the authorities. Many will lose love because of deception and fear, and will even harm their fellow men. Because of this whole network of deception, people will be turned against each other by their beliefs and ideologies, based on fear and brainwashing in some, and the ideals of freedom in others.

7. Politicians, leaders and leaders will hesitate not knowing what to do, so there will be a change in global power, leading to a centralization of power, removing individual government structures.

8. The people will incite more and more and larger protests and demonstrations, and these will increase to produce unstoppable waves of sedition against the system and civil unrest.

9. This will explode into a worse and prolonged situation due to the collapse of the markets. The references speak of hunger,

food shortages and drought. That is, a systemic fall in the markets.

10. The deceived society will admire and adore the State for having provided them with a basic income, but it will be conditioned to a chip, its numbering or its certificate. It is obvious that this is what we are getting to. Without the implanted chip, the certificate numbering or the certificate itself, no one will be able to be part of the system: they will not be able to buy or sell.

11. The climate will be disrupted, from worse to worse, and with this pretext humanity will be deprived of its rights, justifying that a State of Emergency is necessary due to severe climatic disorders.

12. A dictatorship will be established worldwide. Finally, whoever opposes the State will be eliminated. Artificial Intelligence will be under the total control of everyone and their networks.

The prophecies announce certain radical events after which, years later, the entire system of this super state will collapse. With the collapse, all those who have nano devices in their body will suffer great pain, since the collapse comes from solar radiation, which in those days will be very high. In this way this era will end and a new one will begin without the domination of the Illuminati, and under the help of beings from the stars, but the responsibility of those who will have achieved full consciousness of the Light of which we are all part.

CONCLUSION

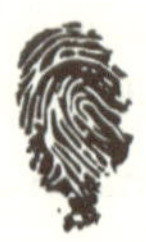

A virus was created in the genetic laboratories of Wuhan and used as a scapegoat to push the global control agenda. To prevent it from getting out of control, it was not made lethal, but rather less harmless than the flu. People thought they were sick with that virus, but few actually caught it. The symptoms were actually the effects of high-frequency waves spread throughout the planet's major cities, toxins dropped from airplanes, and pathogens injected through flu vaccines. That did the same thing as the common flu and atypical pneumonia, but the mega-rich paid their pawns to bribe the leaders of almost all nations to force medical centers to say that people had it was "covid." , and so that they would not give them anything that would alkalize them, but, on the contrary, that they would let them get worse, and when they got worse, they would intubate them so that they would die.

This is how they upset the people and the news spread panic, pushing the people to believe that a "vaccine" was their salvation. This false salvation was nothing more than a genetic component that sterilizes people, causing other types of side effects in the short and medium term. So, there they were injected with the laboratory virus, along with many more things for the Blue Beam Agenda and Agenda 2030 (World Dictatorship with the help of wave weapons and nano technology) . This is just the beginning of propaganda that motivates people to be injected with strange compounds so that microscopic technologies can be put into their bodies, in order to change our race and make it a zombie species. Then they tell them that one injection is not enough but many, and also trackers, and later identification systems and payment technologies, embedded in devices under the skin, to make payments, sales, purchases, transactions digitally from there.

The powers that be, whose philosophy is Luciferian, want to establish a world government led by a single sovereign. Under him, first 10 supreme leaders, and then 7, would be the masters and lords of the entire Earth. They would divide the planet into 10 regions and the rest of the countries would disappear as independent nations. One world government, one planetary leader, one currency, one army, one flag, one religion... one dictatorship. Artificial intelligence, supercomputers, biometric technology, satellites, 6G antenna networks, drones, surveillance cameras and the police state would serve this purpose. Covid-19 is nothing more than the name of the agenda that sets the stage for this new world that the most powerful in this world have been planning for centuries.

Every human being would have a quantum chip or tattoo on the back of their right hand, and some on their forehead, and their DNA would be changed by introducing tiny agents into their body that make man increasingly a machine without feelings or consciousness. nor spiritual reason. Progressively, anyone who opposes this imperialism will be sanctioned, imprisoned, annulled as a citizen and, finally, murdered. More and more people will escape from this insane movie created by plutocratic psychopaths lacking all love and kindness, and will see a new life in the forests or fields, at least temporarily, at least while the monopoly of those crazy tyrants remains. When your dictatorial digital system collapses, we, those who have escaped from the cities and absolutist control, will be the heirs of the new world, and we will establish the foundations of a new beginning, based on freedom, peace, union, fraternity, respect and immortality.

In 2011, when I was writing my second book, I received information from 2009 about a globalist agenda that sought to implement a digital vaccination certificate worldwide as a platform to insert nano devices into the human body and a personal control microchip. These pseudo-vaccines would be part of a eugenics program to reduce overpopulation worldwide. Although, for more than twenty years my father had been warning that the shadow power on this planet intended to insert an identification chip into each human being, and only through which economic transactions would be carried out. Without the implanted microprocessor, the certificate number, or the digital certificate itself, there will be no access to anything (the person who does not have it will be undocumented and will be completely outside the system, ending up being imprisoned).

In December 2019, the news did not stop talking about a new global epidemic, as the Pharmaceutical Industries promote/finance every year. The word "covid" appeared. Then, at the beginning of 2020, an Italian doctor repeated what I had been hearing for several weeks from other Spanish and American researchers: COVID was the acronym for CERTIFICATE OF VACCINE IDENTIFICATION DIGITALLY. This was confirmed as the months passed and I received information from the French military, and later from several colonels of Russian intelligence and the Canadian army, who spoke of COVID as an agenda for a coup d'état against humanity, to establish a dictatorship. globally, and eliminate human rights. He had already learned of this plan more than a decade ago from US Naval Intelligence officer Bill Cooper, and had written and exposed much of it since then.

We have reached the limit of the exponential growth of human beings, according to the globalists. The consumption of resources, environmental pollution, the exorbitant level of political corruption and the arrival of the Fourth Industrial Revolution represent a critical mass that the aristocracy defines as a potential danger for the planet. The new Labor Reforms are designed to eliminate the work of the worker, the physical labor force. Everything is becoming digital, becoming controlled by supercomputers, artificial intelligence and robotics. The unemployment rate will skyrocket like never before in history and governments will not have the capacity to respond to social needs. The IMV or UBI comes into force with the condition that every person abdicates their rights and freedoms, and loses possession of property, passing everything into the hands of the State. This "state" would be centralized, first by the WHO and finally by a World Government, on the basis of the UN, since all local governments will disappear.

The global economic model system will end. Instead of currencies and currencies, everything would be run by a cryptocurrency. A microprocessor on the back of the right hand or on the forehead, or a certificate or digital numbering would be the only provisions to make any type of payment or collection. Every structure of corruption would be eliminated, no drug trafficker will be able to hide his wealth nor will any personality be able to trust in tax havens. What is not digitized will be worthless, and the Super State will know how much you have, what you spend it on and where you got it, and will eliminate you if you oppose the new empire. All personal data will be digitized and all systems will have absolute control over people's mobility, activities, thoughts and emotions, using microchips, nano robots, biometric recognition cameras, satellites, drones and fingerprint and iris readers. Anyone who opposes or protests will be taken to concentration camps, without the possibility of any trial.

In November 2020, various information was leaked again from classified documents, which warned of the agenda starting in 2021 for the New World Order (called by the media 'New Normality') with the establishment of concentration camps in Canada, Spain, Australia and Germany, like those already existing throughout the US under FEMA control. The documents reflected that there would be new "waves" of alleged infections, as part of the COVID-21 agenda to collapse the economy, create social unrest, withdraw local governments, modify laws and implement a digital vaccination certificate (COVID). Spraying aerosols from airplanes and using elevated microtesla waves from high-frequency antennas would put people's health in a critical state, calling it a "viral pandemic." They would then use tests for bacteria, justifying that they detect viruses, so that they would push the use of military elements under State of Siege and Martial Law. Anyone who opposed the official version would be censored and attacked, even if they were eminent in the field of medicine, biology, virology, chemistry or science. Any public debate that refutes the use of draconian measures instead of health measures - or that presents already known natural alternatives - would be annulled: getting fresh air, swimming in the sea, eating alkaline, getting sunlight, doing physical activity and social sharing (stimulate hormones and neuropeptides).

The year 2020 began with extreme vaccination campaigns against a virus that was never isolated or purified and for which there is no evidence of its existence nor a REAL molecular photomicrograph, with fraudulent tests and categorization of healthy people (labeled according to the anti-scientific term "asymptomatic", which does not exist in the jargon of medicine).

George Soros reportedly bribed almost all world leaders to take Martial Law measures with health excuses, and those who refused were ridiculed and some of them even turned up dead. This financing would be supported by the Chinese Communist Government and the Pharmaceutical Industry. It is this industry, the most powerful in the world, owned by the Rockefellers (masters of the banking system, the education system and the majority of the oil monopoly) and Bill Gates, who finance more than 73% of the WHO funds, and also those who control and finance the main Media. In this way, throughout 2020 clinics, hospitals and doctors were paid to report every death as "death due to covid" (from €4,000 to €8,000 per person, and the clinic/hospital would receive more than €40,000), and Since then, any person sick with anything would be classified as "infected with covid", without any authentication by autopsy. This has been widely denounced by various experts, such as doctor and senator Scott Jensen on CNN, with documents in hand that exposed it. Thus other doctors in other countries showed the same protocol that they were told to follow and are still fighting against this Coup d'état against Humanity (as it has been called by Russian Military Intelligence and the French army).

The objective of injecting the population was planned since 2009 in the Rockefeller memoranda, and it clearly states that Operation LockStep (Confinement) would be carried out for this purpose. The Confinement was also used for a global distribution of 5G antennas, used as psychotronic weapons that will act on bodies invaded by the graphene of pseudo-vaccines (since they are not vaccines but experimental gene therapy for DNA modification). Companies that would normally take between 10 and 20 years to design a vaccine already knew what they were going to market, based on studies of mRNA, which, never before used in humans for 20 years, always killed the animals in which it was administered. . The US Department of Military Advanced Technology Studies working for the DoD (DARPA) had designed nano devices with graphene and luciferase (nano particle crystals) to be incorporated into the contents to be inoculated into the population. That, together with the Spike protein and the messenger RNA, would be responsible for mass sterilization, canceling the activity of synsitin 1 and 2. The side effects and deaths in the millions in the short and long term (next 2 years) would be justified as sick or deaths from a new strain or mutation of that virus, as in the case of the so-called Delta strain in the summer of 2021.

Fear has done the rest through the action of cellular stress, suggesting so many people who get sick from a mere nocebo effect mixed with cofactors (as is the case of 70% of the dead in this drama, who were really elderly people or people with previous conditions), whether the flu and other pathologies are called covid). Those who refuse to accept the new guidelines (they will soon be classified as Terrorists and taken to Concentration Camps without the right to a trial) must leave the cities or be arrested. George Orwell's words will have been fulfilled, and if Jesus Christ and others were right, dissent and resistance will push for civil war in every major city in every major country. In effect, all this is expected to lead to the systemic collapse of the world economy, and therefore, burst into a Third World War and an escalation of hunger for many years, full of violence and riots under a permanent Police State and social apathy and mistrust.

Frederick Guttmann R.

<u>SOURCES</u>

FOR THIS WORK I HAVE CONSULTED THE WORKS AND OPINIONS OF MORE THAN 250 EXPERTS WORLDWIDE. HERE ARE THE NAMES OF MOST OF THEM.

1. Aaron Russo – former American politician and film director
2. Albert Bourla – spokesperson and CEO of Pfizer
3. Albert Pike – American lawyer, soldier and writer
4. Alberto de la Torre – pharmaceutical chemist from the Universidad del Valle, Colombia
5. Alberto Martí Bosch – doctor, oncologist of Spanish origin, who has dedicated his life to research into alternative therapies for the treatment of cancer
6. Alberto M. Wulff – Venezuelan doctor residing in Miami
7. Andreas Kalcker – German biologist and promoter of the CDS
8. Aldous Huxley – British writer and philosopher
9. Alejando Sousa – graduate in medicine and surgery, specialty in urology, Regional Hospital of Monforte
10. Alexander Chuchalin – Russia's leading pulmonologist, former member of the Ethics Council of the Ministry of Health
11. Alexandria Ocasio-Cortez – activist and politician
12. Almudena Zaragoza – graduate in biology and faculty member of the General Council of Biologists of Spain
13. Anna Forbes – British medical doctor
14. Antonio Gutiérrez – Secretary General of the UN
15. Antonio Palazon Bru – bioanalyst from the Miguel Hernández University, Spain
16. Alexandra Henrion Caude – French geneticist and research director of the SimplissimA International Research Institute.
17. Alberto Sangrillo - Berlusconi's doctor and head of intensive care at the Italian San Raffaele hospital in Lombardy
18. Anthony Fauci – American doctor
19. Ana María Oliva – Spanish doctor

20. Alex Azar – head of the US Department of Health and Human Resources (HHS), politician, lawyer and former pharmaceutical executive

21. Alicia Verónica Rubio Calle – parliamentary deputy of Vox (Spain)

22. Andrew A. Marino – Health Sciences Center, University of Louisiana, USA.

23. Andrew Poland, Sir – Professor and Director of the Oxford Vaccine Group

24. Andrew Zimmerman – world-renowned pediatric neurologist

25. Amaia Foces – Spanish doctor in India

26. Alexander Lukashenko – President of Belarus

27. Ángel Luis Valdepeñas – co-founder of Doctors for Truth Spain

28. Andry Rajoelina – President of Madagascar

29. Alexander Fomin – Russian colonel general and deputy defense minister

30. Andrew Kaufman – expert in advanced thoracic microscopic invasive surgery and oncologic thoracic surgery at Mount Sinai Hospital in New York

31. Anna de Buisseret – British lawyer

32. Anthony Holland – OPEF (Oscillation Wave Field Pulse Specific Frequency) scientist

33. Antonio Aguirre - surgeon

34. Alfred Webre – former advisor to former President Jimmy Carter

35. Amy Offutt – US integrative physician

36. Arthur Firstenberg – doctor, writer and activist

37. Ana Martínez Giménez - pharmacy service and Preventive Medicine service of the Barbaso Hospital

38. Anne Fierlafijn – Belgian medical doctor

39. Antoine Béchamp – French biologist

40. Ariyana Love - Goodwill Ambassador to Palestine (ICSPR), independent journalist, human rights activist and naturopathic

doctor.

41. Angus Dalgleish – Professor at St George's Hospital

42. Bartomeu Payeras I Cifre – biologist, specialist in microbiology, graduated from the University of Barcelona

43. Birger Sorensen – Norwegian virologist

44. Ben Edwards – General Physician of the United States

45. Ben Tapper - doctor and communicator

46. Brandy Vaughan – former pharmaceutical industry representative, when she was a sales executive for the pharmaceutical company Merck

47. Bernard Rimland – American research psychologist, writer, influencer and speaker

48. Benjamin Netanyahu – former Prime Minister of Israel

49. Bob Hall – Republican senator from Edgewood, Texas

50. Bill Posey – member of the US Congress

51. Bill Gates – founder of Microsoft and one of the main financiers of the WHO

52. Barre Lando – physicist from the USA

53. Boris Dragin – graduate in acupuncture (Sweden)

54. Bruce Harold Lipton – American cell biologist, known for his belief that genes and DNA can be manipulated by a person's beliefs. He is a visiting professor at the New Zealand College of Chiropractic, and is the author of the best-selling book 'The Biology of Belief'.

55. Carl G. Jung - Swiss psychiatrist, psychologist and essayist

56. Carlo T. Motemagno – professor of biomedical engineering

57. César Carballo Cardona – coordinator and physician of emergency medicine and

58. Chinda Brandolino – prestigious Argentine doctor

59. Carlos González de la Cuesta – head of the alert service at the Ourense hospital.

60. Carlos Huamani Cueva – Peruvian researcher, writer and inventor,

studied computer science and specialized in pedagogy

61. Christiane Northrup – physician and author in obstetrics and gynecology

62. Claudia Kücherer – German molecular biologist

63. Claus Koehnlein – German doctor

64. Carrie Madej – internist and owner of Phoenix Medical Group, Georgia (USA)

65. Catherine Austin Fitts – former housing secretary under George HW Bush and director of the investment bank Dylon & Red, Swiss UBS, economist editor of the Solari Report

66. Carlos Astiz – journalist, doctor in information sciences and Spanish university professor

67. Cristina Martín Jiménez (Spain) – journalist, writer and expert in geopolitics

68. Chuck de Caro – American journalist and CNN correspondent

69. Charles Lieber – chair of the chemistry department at Harvard University, and expert in microsensor development

70. Charles Darwin – English naturist

71. Chris Sky – Canadian activist

72. Christopher Exley – English chemist and researcher, professor in bioinorganic chemistry and leader of the Bioinorganic Chemistry Laboratory at Keele University, also honorary professor at the UHI Millennium Institute

73. Christine Lagarde – former director of the International Monetary Fund

74. Daniel López Acuña - former WHO Crisis Director, graduated from the Autonomous University of Mexico and the Johns Hopkins Bloomberg School of Public Health

75. Daniel Estulin – former Russian counterespionage analyst

76. David Gracias – professor at the Whiting School of Engineering, John Hopkins University

77. Dennis M. Bushnell - NASA scientist and lecturer, head of NASA

Langley Research Center, responsible for technical oversight and formulation of advanced programs.

78. Dider Raoult – French infectologist and microbiologist, member of the French COVID-19 Scientific Council that advises the French government in the face of the pandemic. Doctor by training and then researcher at the Faculty of Medicine of the University of Aix-Marseille

79. Diego Posada – Colombian doctor, expert in biophotonics and frequencies

80. Donald Trump – former US president

81. Dan Burton – US Congressman

82. David E. Martin – professor, businessman, writer and famous inventor

83. David Weldon – physician member of the US Congress.

84. Deepak Chopra - Hindu doctor, writer and lecturer. Winner of the Ig Nobel Prize in Physics in 1998.

85. Dolores Cahill – immunologist and molecular biologist

86. Daniel Cullum – American medical chiropractor

87. David Rockefeller – owner of Rockefeller banking, the pharmaceutical industry and main financier of the WHO

88. Diego Martínez - doctor

89. Dominique Belpomme – professor of oncology at the Descartes University of Paris

90. Eduardo Yahbes - doctor

91. Elon Musk – American businessman

92. Elizabeth Evans – British medical doctor

93. Enric Corbera - industrial technical engineer, naturopath, qualified in Psychology, and also a lecturer. He is known for promoting the Bioneuroemotion method (Spain)

94. Elizabeth A. Rauscher – renowned American physician

95. Eric Schmidt – president of Microsoft and former director of Google

96. Ella Naveh – Israeli biologist and epidemiologist with a master's degree in public health
97. Edward Snowden – former US National Security Agency official
98. Elisa María Shún García - pharmacy service and Preventive Medicine service at the Barbaso Hospital
99. Elke F. de Klerk – Dutch medical doctor
100. Enrique Costa Vertcher - internist and graduate in Medicine and Surgery from the Faculty of Medicine of Valencia in 1979.
101. Eric Ménat – French doctor
102. Félix Guttmann Van Katz – flight captain and captain of the Colombian merchant navy, and former member of Intelligence in the Israeli army, and rabbi
103. Frank Suárez - Specialist in obesity and metabolism (Cuba)
104. Fernando Ferreira – Doctors for Truth of Uruguay
105. Fernando Vega – Doctors for the Truth of Uruguay
106. Florin M. Selaeu – director of the John Hopkins Inflammatory Bowel Diseases Center
107. Francoise Barre-Sinoussi – director, RRI, Pasteur Institute, and Nobel Laureate in Physiology of Medicine 2008, France
108. Fernando López Mirones – renowned Spanish biologist and scientific communicator
109. Freddy Portillo – renowned doctor, Honduran doctor
110. Fritz Springmeier – American investigative journalist, writer and historian
111. Geert Vanden Bossche – German virologist and one of the world's leading vaccine specialists
112. Galit Tzefler Naor – Israeli physician and medical district director of the Health Maintenance Organization
113. George Orwell – British journalist, essayist and critic
114. Gregory Stock – biophysicist
115. Guiseppe Mazzini – Italian politician and journalist
116. Gunter Frank - German doctor

117. Heiko Schöning – founder of Doctors for Truth

118. Hunter Lundy – American lawyer

119. Heinrich Fiechtner – doctor and member of the parliament of Baden-Württemberg, Germany

120. Hilde De Smet – Belgian medical doctor

121. Heiko Santelmann – German medical doctor

122. Helen Schucman – psychologist and clinical researcher, was a professor of medical psychology at Columbia University in New York.

123. Hippocrates of Cos – Greek physician, father of medicine

124. Iñaki Gabilondo – Spanish journalist

125. Igor Shepherd – military doctor in St. Petersburg, studied under the Strategic Rocket Force, expert in bio-weapons, anti-terrorism, chemistry, biology, radiology, nuclei, high-precision explosives and pandemic preparedness, manager and medical doctor of the department and unit Wyoming state public health preparedness on the Covid response team, worked for the Soviet Communist Government until he immigrated to the US to work with said government.

126. Irit Yankovich – Israeli lawyer

127. Jane Burgermesiter – Austrian science journalist

128. Jeff Bradstreet – one of the leading anti-vaccine activists in the US, who ran a clinic in Buford, Georgia

129. José Delgado – doctor with 30 years of experience in internal medicine

130. John McAfee – founder of McAfee antivirus

131. José Antonio Campoy – former head of information at the EFE agency and director of the magazine Discovery DSalud, Spain

132. Jon Ander Etxebarría – dean of the College of Biologists of Euskadi

133. José Ortega – lawyer specializing in legal matters

134. José Cabrera Forneiro – Spanish forensic doctor and psychiatrist,

expert in forensic medicine

135. Juanjo Martínez – Spanish doctor

136. Janci Chunn Lindsay – molecular biologist and toxicologist (USA)

137. John Hutchison – Canadian scientist

138. Jerry Mander – president of the International Forum on Globalization

139. James Giordano – head of the Bioethics Studies Program, scholar-in-residence, leader of the Military Medical Ethics subprogram and director of the O'Neill-Pellegrino Program in Brain Science and Global Health Law and Policy at the Pellegrino Center bioethics clinic, and professor from the department of neurology and biochemistry at Georgetown University Medical Center in Washington.

140. Jaume Cortés – expert in electrosensitivity

141. Javier Milei – Argentine economist

142. John Virapen – former representative of the pharmaceutical industry

143. Jesse Ventura – American politician, actor, television host, writer and retired wrestler

144. Jovenele Moïse – former president of Haiti

145. Judy Anne Mikovits – former American research scientist, director of antiviral drug mechanism laboratory at the National Cancer Institute, renowned researcher in molecular biology and virology, her 1991 doctoral thesis revolutionized HIV/AIDS treatments, has published more than 50 scientific articles

146. Jim Carrey – American actor and activist

147. Javier Villamor – Spanish journalist

148. José Luis Gettor – Argentine emergency doctor

149. Joseph B. McCormick – American epidemiologist

150. John Ioannidis – world leader in diets and big data

151. John O'Sullivan – member of Principia Scientific International

152. John L. Badalamenti – US judge

153. Javier Sciuto – doctor from Doctors for Truth of Uruguay

154. John Magufuli – former president of Tanzania

155. John Kopchinski – former Pfizer sales representative

156. Jesus of Nazareth – Jewish doctor

157. Jail Bolsonaro – president of Brazil

158. Johan Denis – Belgian medical doctor and homeopath

159. Jane M. Orient – CEO of the Association of American Physicians and Surgeons

160. Jane Roberts – American medium

161. Joe Rizoli – clinical laboratory scientist

162. José Luis Sevillano – Spanish doctor in France

163. Joseph Mercola – one of the world's most renowned doctors, proponent of alternative medicine, practicing osteopath, and Internet businessman

164. Juan Carlos Perez Olmedo - doctor

165. Juan F. Gastón Añaños – pharmacy service and Preventive Medicine service of the Barbaso Hospital

166. Karen Kingston Bombshell – former Pfizer employee

167. Kelly Brogan – American medical doctor

168. Kary Mullis – American biochemist, Nobel Prize in Chemistry for the invention of the polymerase chain reaction (PCR)

169. Konstantin Pavlidis – professor of cognitive science, biomedical researcher and holistic healthcare practitioner in London.

170. Karina Acevedo Whitehouse – academic at the Autonomous University of Querétaro, Mexico

171. Karina Sarno – hospital care physician and doctor of psychiatry

172. Klaus Schwab – director of the International Monetary Fund

173. Kate Shemirani – natural nurse from the United Kingdom

174. Katrin Korb – German medical doctor

175. Kevin P. Corbett – retired nurse and health scientist from the United Kingdom

176. Knutt Wittkowsky – former head of the epidemiology department at Rockefeller University in New York

177. Lida Obregón – doctor, Hipólito Unanue scientific award, Peru

178. Luc Antoine Montagnier – 2008 Nobel Prize in Biology

179. Leonardo González Bayona – UBA doctor, CENIC family medicine from Argentina

180. Leslie Kenderesi – Canadian officer cadet

181. Leonard Horowitz – American dentist with a postgraduate degree in his specialty and in Public Health

182. Luis Miguel Benito – area specialist at the El Escorial university hospital (Madrid), expert in the digestive system and endoscopy

183. Luis Marcelo Martínez – Argentine geneticist, master in molecular biology

184. Luis de Miguel Ortega – Spanish lawyer

185. Lawrence Palevsky – American doctor, renowned board-certified pediatrician, sought-after speaker and published author

186. Lee Merritt – renowned US doctor and orthopedist

187. Larry Pavelski – doctor

188. Liu Chuang – Chinese scientist

189. Magdalena Nevado – deputy of the Vox political party, specialist in transpersonal therapy, master's degree in Political and Business Communication, member of the ProVida association.

190. Martin Paul – professor emeritus of biochemistry and basic medical sciences at Washington State University

191. Manuel Elkin Patarroyo – immunologist, creator of the malaria vaccine (Colombia)

192. Magda Havas – graduated in biology (B.Sc) and environmental toxicology (PhD) from the University of Toronto

193. Maureen McDonnell – American nurse with 34 years working in birth education, clinical nutrition and pediatrics

194. Mark McDonald – US doctor and child psychiatrist.

195. Manolo Fernández – Peruvian researcher

196. Margareta Griesz-Brisson – German neurologist
197. Mariano Arriaga – Argentine clinician and eye surgeon, member of Doctors for Truth
198. Mariano José Ludeña – Argentine doctor
199. Moritz Von Der Borch – German medical journalist
200. María José Albarracín – graduate in medicine and surgery, professor of clinical diagnostics, and professor of biology, immunology and laboratory techniques
201. María Eugenia Barrientos – doctor from El Salvador
202. Mike Yeadon – former vice president of Pfizer Global
203. Marc Van Ranst – Belgian virologist and researcher
204. Michael Schnedlitz – parliamentarian, liberal general secretary of the Austrian Freedom Party
205. Milton William Cooper – former US Naval Intelligence officer
206. Mohammad Adil – medical doctor from UK
207. Michael Ganoe – Israeli journalist and actor
208. Mikael Nordfors – medical doctor from Sweden
209. Max Tegmark – American physicist
210. Máximo Sandín – Spanish doctor in biology
211. Marta López – researcher at the National Institute of Biotechnology (CSIC), who did her thesis in Spain with SARS, and worked in the US unraveling the flu
212. Matt Hepbun – US Army infectious diseases doctor, DARPA officer and retired colonel.
213. María Van Kerkhove – doctor, technical director of COVID-19 for the WHO
214. Martin Kulldorff – professor of medicine at Harvard Medical School, and biostatistician and epidemiologist at Brigham and Women's Hospital
215. Marty Makary – surgeon, John Hopkins professor and editor-in-chief of MedPage Today
216. Miralles Boye - doctor

217. Na Zhu – Chinese internal medicine doctor

218. Nicholas P. Mizell – US magistrate

219. Nicholas Weid – science writer

220. Nicola Tesla – American inventor, electrical engineer, mechanical engineer and physicist

221. Nils R. Fosse – Norwegian medical doctor

222. Nour De Sam – Belgian medical doctor

223. Norbert Wiener – American mathematician, founder of cybernetics

224. Natalia Prego – co-founder of Médicos por la Verdad, specialist in community medicine

225. Nayra Txako – biologist from the Canary Islands

226. Nevers Mumba – politician and former vice president of Zambia

227. Nirdosh Kohra – surgeon, graduated as a medical doctor from the Anahuac University of Mexico

228. Oriol Mitjá – specialist in infectious diseases, and researcher at the Barcelona Institute for Global Health (ISGlobal)

229. Oswaldo Restrepo – doctor and surgeon, specialist in occupational medicine, with training in epidemiology and risks (Colombia).

230. Óscar Aguilera – Cum Laude doctor in fundamental biology and Marie Curie postdoctorate of excellence in mathematics and sciences

231. Pablo Campra – doctor from the University of Almería

232. Patrick Smith – professor at John Hopkins University

233. Patricia Fernández – biochemist with a master's degree in immunology and neuroscience

234. Pinkie Feinstein – Israeli psychiatrist

235. Peter Jennings – Australian Strategic Policy Institute

236. Peter Daszak – British zoologist, president of Eco Health Alliane and WHO inspector

237. Piotr Rubas – Polish medical doctor, internist in Germany

238. Pierre Gilbert – French doctor

239. Pamela Mas – Argentine doctor

240. Peter McCullough – Doctor of Internal Medicine, renowned board-certified cardiologist and academic professor of medicine (USA)

241. Peter Gøtzsche – physician and biologist, specialist in interim medicine, director of the Nordic Cochrane Center in Copenhagen (Denmark)

242. Peter Gariaev – doctor, professor of biological sciences, nominee for the 2021 Nobel Prize in Medicine, creator of quantum genetics, wave genetics.

243. Richard Barlet – American doctor with 28 years of experience

244. Richard John Roberts – doctor who won the Nobel Prize in Medicine in 1993.

245. Richard Ebright – molecular biologist at Rutgers University in New Jersey

246. Rotem Brown – Israeli lawyer

247. Robert DeNiro – American anti-vaccine activist, actor and film director

248. Reiner Fuellmich – German lawyer

249. Ryke Geerd Hamer – German medical biologist, creator of the Germanic New Medicine

250. Robert Kennedy Jr. – nephew of former President John F. Kennedy, politician, lawyer, and founder of Childrens Health Defense

251. Richard J. Codey – President of the New Jersey Senate

252. Rashid Buttar – coach, doctor and director of medicine in the USA.

253. Roberto Petrella – Italian doctor

254. Robert Koch – German physician and microbiologist

255. Rudolf Steiner – Austrian philosopher, literary scholar, educator, theater artist, social thinker and occultist.

256. Rudolf Virchaw – father of pathology

257. Ralf ER Sundberg – medical doctor from Sweden, formerly dedicated to back treatments at the Karolinska Institute

258. R. Zac Cox – British holistic dentist and homeopath, member of the Medical Alliance of Doctors

259. Rian Cole – doctor, anatomical pathologist with studies in immunology and virology

260. Roxana Bruno – Argentine immunologist

261. Ricardo Delgado – Spanish biostatistician

262. Robert Malone – doctor who created the mRNA vaccine

263. Robert L. Brennan – distinguished scientific researcher in the Research Management and Statistics Area of the American College Testing, who postulated the Generalizability Theory

264. Robert Becker – orthopedic surgeon and researcher in electrophysiology and electromedicine. He worked as a professor at the Upstate Medical Center in New York.

265. Rand Paul – physician and US senator

266. Richard Nikolaus Graf von Coudenhove-Kalergi – Austrian politician and geopolitician

267. Richard Dearlove – former director of MI6

268. Ron Johnson – US Senator

269. Satoshi Omura – Japanese doctor, 2015 Nobel Prize winner

270. Scott Jensen – doctor and US senator

271. Sara R. Tipnis – graduate from the School of Biochemistry and Molecular Biology, University of Leeds, UK

272. Sunetra Gupta – eminence in the field of infectious diseases at the University of Oxford

273. Simone Gold – American doctor, author and activist

274. Sherri J. Tenpenny – American osteopathic physician and activist

275. Steve Forrest Hotze – Texas doctor, radio host and conservative Republican activist

276. Steven Weller – Australian Professor, BE (Hons.I.) degree in Computer Engineering, ME degree in Electrical Engineering,

Ph.D. in electrical engineering from Newcastle University, BSc from Monash University

277. Stephen Hahn – Commissioner of the US Food and Drug Administration (FDA)

278. Salvador Pané – researcher at the Institute of Robotics and Intelligent Systems at the ETH in Zurich (Switzerland)

279. Senta Depuydt – Belgian freelance journalist, representative of the organization 'Children's Health Defense' in Europe, together with Robert F. Kennedy Jr.

280. Stefan Lanka – renowned German virologist

281. Stéphane Bancel – CEO of Moderna

282. Stephanie Seneff – senior research scientist at MIT

283. Sandy Lunøe – former Norwegian pharmacist

284. Dr. Sebi – famous holistic doctor, personal health advisor to Michael Jackson (Honduras)

285. Sucharit Bhakdi – Professor and Head of Medicine

286. Tom Cowan – American doctor

287. Tony Holohan – Irish doctor

288. Teresa Morera – former pharmacist and naturopath

289. Tiffany Dover – nurse

290. Tom Renz – attorney for Ohio, USA

291. Theresa A. Deisher – founder, president, spokesperson and leading scientist of the Pharmaceutical Institute, CEO and managing member of the Georgetown Biotechnology AVM, USA, PhD in molecular and cellular physiology, holds more than 47 patents for testing discoveries clinics in the US, Europe and Japan, with more than 30 years of experience in pharmaceutical leadership, including Genentech, Repligen, ZymoGenetics, Immunex and Amgen.

292. Thierry Baudet – Dutch MP

293. Vittorio Sgarbi – Italian deputy

294. Vernon Coleman – writer qualified as a doctor in England

295. Vladimir Kvachkov – colonel of the Russian General Intelligence

> Bureau

296. Vladimir Ze'ev Zelenko – Ukrainian-American medical doctor
297. Vivian Burnett – Mexican naturopath
298. Vin Gupta – Affiliate Assistant Professor of Health Metric Sciences at the Institute for Health Metrics and Evaluation (IHME) at the University of Washington
299. Wu Zunyou – head of epidemiology at the China Center for Disease Control
300. Wolfgang Wordarg – German doctor, epidemiologist, and president of the Health Council of the European Commission
301. William Bramley – writer and researcher
302. William Ross Adey – US professor of anatomy and physiology
303. William L. Van Bise – inventor of an external electromagnetic field that, by impulse, reduced heart and brain pain. He worked in American laboratories specializing in wave magnetic superconductors.

And many more sources such as CIA agents - whose names cannot be named for obvious reasons -, Chinese and French army reports, scientific documents and works, records, law decrees and memoranda.

<u>SOME LINKS OF INTEREST</u>

- Words from Dr. Patricia Fernández about the immune system: https://www.facebook.com/permalink.php?story_fbid=106875124801086&id=100990325389566 [1].

- Movie sets with color schemes and actors in Israel where the "hospital pandemic" is filmed: https://www.facebook.com/Karalieneeee/posts/3531926520365165 [2].

- Interview with lawyer Miguel Iannolfi, by journalist Verónica Ressia, on her radio program, La Hora de Vero: https://lbry.tv/@ElCanalDeQQ:e/LA-HORA-DE-VERO!—-24- 11-20:6 [3].

- Casualties in Spain due to vaccination effects: https://okdiario.com/espana/aluvion-bajas-profesores-policias-bomberos-militares-efectos-vacuna-astrazeneca-6899405?utm_medium=Social&utm_source=Facebook#Echobox=1615103433 [4].

- Another link of interest: https://lbry.tv/@ReVelionenlagranja:e/20-11-12-ABRE-LOS-OJOS-(1):e

- National death index (Ministry of Health): https://www.mscbs.gob.es/estadEstudios/estadisticas/estadisticas/estMinisterio/IND_TipoDifusion.htm [5], https://www.mscbs.gob.es/estadEstudios/estadisticas/docs/indNacDefunciones/2020_Defunciones_8.pdf [6].

- About the PCR tests Ministry of Health: https://www.mscbs.gob.es/gabinete/notasPrensa.do?id=4824 [7].

- Creative diagnostics laboratory PCR test leaflet: https://drive.google.com/file/d/14_MB6_QDiJV_TPykIf4HsGttTRV2u4FV/view?usp=sharing [8].

- Kary Mullis, inventor of PCR tests, talks to us about whether their efficiency in detecting diseases is true:

  - https://lbry.tv/@ReVelionenlagranja:e/Kary-Mullis-(inventor-de-los-test-PCR)—'They are not useful-for-detecting-diseases':8 [9]

1. https://www.facebook.com/permalink.php?story_fbid=106875124801086&id=100990325389566

2. https://www.facebook.com/Karalieneeee/posts/3531926520365165

3. https://lbry.tv/@ElCanalDeQQ:e/LA-HORA-DE-VERO!---24-11-20:6

4. https://okdiario.com/espana/aluvion-bajas-profesores-policias-bomberos-militares-efectos-vacuna-astrazeneca-6899405?utm_medium=Social&utm_source=Facebook#Echobox_43ec3e5dee6e706af7766fffea512721_1615103433

5. https://www.mscbs.gob.es/estadEstudios/estadisticas/estadisticas/estMinisterio/IND_TipoDifusion.htm

6. https://www.mscbs.gob.es/estadEstudios/estadisticas/docs/indNacDefunciones/2020_Defunciones_8.pdf

7. https://www.mscbs.gob.es/gabinete/notasPrensa.do?id=4824

8. https://drive.google.com/file/d/14_MB6_QDiJV_TPykIf4HsGttTRV2u4FV/view?usp=sharing

    ° https://lbry.tv/@ReVelionenlagranja:e/EL-INVENTOR-DEL-TEST-PCR:0

    [10]. Flu mortality rates in the world, according to the WHO:

- https://www.who.int/es/news/item/14...ory-diseases-linked-to-seasonal-flu-each-year [11],

- Tuberculosis mortality rates in the world, according to the WHO: https://www.who.int/es/ news-room/fact-sheets/detail/tuberculosis#:~:text [12]=

- In 2018, 251,000 people with HIV fell ill with TB. Pneumonia mortality rates in the world, according to Our World in Data, in 2017: https://www.enterarse.com/20200422_0001-que-es-la-neumonia-y-cuantas-muertes-causa-en-el-mundo #:~:text [13]=.

- US   mask   leaflet: https://drive.google.com/file/d/ 1C4q4wGS1RMspghd3El3IVxlNbj8NdZv8/view?usp=sharing [14].

- What the WHO says about the use of masks regarding COVID-19: https://lbry.tv/@ReVelionenlagranja...EL-USO-DE-LAS-MASCARILLAS-QUE-NO-TE-MIENTAN:3

- Brief Spanish documentary about the great reset plot: https://lbry.tv/@thebigreset:1/movie:2

- Documentary on the effects of microwaves: https://www.youtube.com/ watch?v=wEbfKW3Sjok

- Countries with the most coronavirus deaths per 100,000 inhabitants: https://www.rtve.es/ noticias/20201107/paises-muertos-coronavirus-poblacion/2012350.shtml

- Mortality rates in the world caused by smoking, according to the WHO: https://www.who.int/ es/news-room/fact-sheets/detail/tobacco#:~:text [15]=

- Mortality rates in the world of alcoholism, according to the WHO: https://www.who.int/es/ news/item/21...-3-million-people-each-year—most-of-them-men [16]

---

9. https://lbry.tv/@ReVelionenlagranja:e/Kary-Mullis-(inventor-de-los-test-PCR)--'No-sirven-para-detectar-enfermedades':8

10. https://lbry.tv/@ReVelionenlagranja:e/EL-INVENTOR-DEL-TEST-PCR:0

11. https://www.who.int/es/news/item/14...ory-diseases-linked-to-seasonal-flu-each-year

12. https://www.who.int/es/news-room/fact-sheets/detail/

 tuberculosis#_853ae90f0351324bd73ea615e6487517__4c761f170e016836ff84498202b99827__853ae90f0351324bd73ea615e6487517_text

13. https://www.enterarse.com/20200422_0001-que-es-la-neumonia-y-cuantas-muertes-causa-en-el-

 mundo#_853ae90f0351324bd73ea615e6487517__4c761f170e016836ff84498202b99827__853ae90f0351324bd73ea615e6487517_text

14. https://drive.google.com/file/d/1C4q4wGS1RMspghd3El3IVxlNbj8NdZv8/view?usp=sharing

15. https://www.who.int/es/news-room/fact-sheets/detail/

 tobacco#_853ae90f0351324bd73ea615e6487517__4c761f170e016836ff84498202b99827__853ae90f0351324bd73ea615e6487517_text

- Mortality rates in the world due to poor diet, according to the WHO: https://www.elperiodicodearagon.com...uertes-estan-provocadas-mala-dieta_44330.html

- The lie of asymptomatic people, PCR and vaccines, dr. luis marcelo martinez geneticist. Right Direction program. exclusively the Geneticist Dr Luis Marcelo Martínez... From the team of Argentine Epidemiologists: https://www.bitchute.com/video/imUUbuzhIQiQ/

- Doctor Enric Costa: "I don't care about the term denialist, because I actually deny COVID." Interview with Doctor Enric Costa on Radio Ya in the program Seamos Francos directed by Álvaro Romero: "I don't care about the term denialist, because I actually deny COVID": https://mowplay.com/video/v-5scAgftFSXA

- Javier Navascués. Deputy Director of El Correo de España. Radio and TV presenter, speaker and scriptwriter. He has been a sports editor for El Periódico de Aragón and Canal 44. He has collaborated in media such as EWTN, Radio María, NSE, and Canal Sant Josep, Adelante la Fe, of which he was director, and Agnus Dei Prod. Actor in the Cura documentary from Ars and in another work against cultural Marxism, John Navasco. He has viral videos like El Master Plan or El Valle no setouch. He currently has a blog on the prestigious InfoCatólica portal and occasionally participates in Somatemps, Ahora Información, Español Digital and Radio Reconquista in Dallas, Texas. Collaborate with the John Paul II International Association: https://elcorreodeespana.com/politica/855364050/Dr-Enrique-Costa-La-pandemia-es-un-fraude-pues-milagrosos-ha-desaparecido-la-gripe-y -everything-is-counted-as-Covid-By-Javier-Navascues.html [17].

- According to a scientist from the Israeli army, the virus disappears on its own in less than 3 months: https://www.infobae.com/america/mundo/2020/04/22/el-fin-del-crecimiento-exponential-un-cientifico- Israeli-assures-that-the-spread-of-coronavirus-decreases-to-almost-zero-after-70-days/?fbclid=IwAR1apQD0QVaYlnX1Sqx0m_KdxoYVL-eeLWpj_oErVIVyh8kWVwlIQ7Lus7Y [18]

- The common flu kills more than covid-19: https://www.newtral.es/la-gripe-mas-letal-que-el-coronavirus-ncov-hasta-la-fecha/20200201/?fbclid=IwAR2sE-

---

16. https://www.who.int/es/news/item/21...-3-million-people-each-year--most-of-them-men

17. https://elcorreodeespana.com/politica/855364050/Dr-Enrique-Costa-La-pandemia-es-un-fraude-pues-milagrosamente-ha-desaparecido-la-gripe-y-todo-lo-cuentan-como-Covid-Por-Javier-Navascues.html

18. https://www.infobae.com/america/mundo/2020/04/22/el-fin-del-crecimiento-exponencial-un-cientifico-israeli-asegura-que-la-propagacion-del-coronavirus-disminuye-a-casi-cero-despues-de-70-dias/?fbclid=IwAR1apQD0QVaYlnX1Sqx0m_KdxoYVL-eeLWpj_oErVIVyh8kWVwlIQ7Lus7Y

3U2_z_sapm0l8hpBPkvtzZxFT1D0ReXM5zWZQRUjYQ1dZGeAhEZi0[19]

- An Argentine doctor in Brazil complains about the great montage perpetuated with the story of the bug: https://www.youtube.com/watch?v=BgK5iXOWf6s&feature=youtu.be&fbclid=IwAR0Om4bEkEbkYIVDuHUciCECrlLsyomIH

- Here is what the reality of vaccines is from a documentary directed by actor Robert De Niro: https://www.youtube.com/watch?v=P0JB0oS6yIQ&fbclid=IwAR0K_GrXkLDskl5lgfBvMLsJiWnVboHc-AbK3SrhUCa0wxiuGhrd5pq427k

- ID 2020: https://www.periodistadigital.com/politica/opinion/20200327/identificacion-digital-id-2020-terrorifico-plan-diabolico-bill-gates-controlar-humanidad-noticia-689404286249/?fbclid=IwAR2SMgXWp5BnMWC7KsMyV-tkHjCHdLPly7UyMMGv2Ol4TLEhlBHPLyVf7E4 [20].

- 5G global control and triangulation system: https://www.youtube.com/watch?v=YasR24R9bv4&fbclid=IwAR1gEjnxoE7_32BSxeVFB4V20gXYC75rM0LSCV8SGuQ-oQ1qGl9AjpL0GbY [21].

- Chips in humans: https://www.youtube.com/watch?v=RfDsn6SuSY0&feature=youtu.be&fbclid=IwAR3LhFxVkkE76spcqnlKwKo5617z4_WqVH8I [22].

- A short documentary about the current financial collapse: https://www.youtube.com/watch?v=MedO6qIDsv4&fbclid=IwAR2DLSmkVzYQQKHDYbtpln4hqe8_K0OJaeYlgCURdRTdj_IK [23].

- Electromagnetic fields and public health - Electromagnetic hypersensitivity: http://www.who.int/peh-emf/publications/facts/fs296/en/

---

19. https://www.newtral.es/la-gripe-mas-letal-que-el-coronavirus-ncov-hasta-la-fecha/20200201/?fbclid=IwAR2sE-3U2_z_sapm0l8hpBPkvtzZxFT1D0ReXM5zWZQRUjYQ1dZGeAhEZi0

20. https://www.periodistadigital.com/politica/opinion/20200327/identificacion-digital-id-2020-terrorifico-plan-diabolico-bill-gates-controlar-humanidad-noticia-689404286249/?fbclid=IwAR2SMgXWp5BnMWC7KsMyV-tkHjCHdLPly7UyMMGv2Ol4TLEhlBHPLyVf7E4

21. https://www.youtube.com/watch?v=YasR24R9bv4&fbclid=IwAR1gEjnxoE7_32BSxeVFB4V20gXYC75rM0LSCV8SGuQ-oQ1qGl9AjpL0GbY

22. https://www.youtube.com/watch?v=RfDsn6SuSY0&feature=youtu.be&fbclid=IwAR3LhFxVkkE76spcqnlKwKo5617z4_WqVH8Ix_YlrXyi_en3iKVOg18khPg

23. https://www.youtube.com/watch?v=MedO6qIDsv4&fbclid=IwAR2DLSmkVzYQQKHDYbtpln4hqe8_K0OJaeYlgCURdRTdj_IKN5kMXHarLJU

- Guideline of the Austrian Medical Association for the diagnosis and treatment of EMF-related health: http://www.scribd.com/doc/87308119/Guideline-of-the-Austrian-Medical-Association-for-the-diagnosis -and-treatment-of-EMF-related-health-problems-and-illness-[24]EMF syndrome.

- IARC Monograph volume 102 Non-ionizing radiation, Part 2: Radiofrequency electromagnetic fields http://monographs.iarc.fr/ENG/Monographs/vol102/ [25].

- European experts on disarray over EHS - electromagnetic hypersensitivity: http://communities.washingtontimes.com/neighborhood/between-rock-and-hard-place/2012/apr/1/european-experts-disarray-over-ehs-electromagnetic/

- Latest case history updates: http://www.mast-victims.org/

- Biological and Health Effects of Microwave Radio Frequency Transmissions, A Review of Research Literature - 2013 http://www.national-toxic-encephalopathy-foundation.org/wp-16content/uploads/2012/01/ Biological_and_Health_Effects_of_Microwave_Radio_Frequency_Transmissions .pdf [26].

- RPS3 - ARPANSA Radiation Protection Standard No. 3: http://www.arpansa.gov.au/publications/codes/rps3.cfm

- Radio Frequency Toolkit for Environmental Health Professionals - BC Center for Disease Control: http://www.bccdc.ca/NR/rdonlyres/9AE4404B-67FF-411E-81B1-4DB75846BF2F/0/RadiofrequencyToolkit_v4_06132013.pdf

- Electromagnetic fields modulating bioeffects in acute experiments (summary of Russian research): http://www.bemri.org/component/docman/doc_download/78-grigoriev-bioeffects07.html?Itemid=4 [27];

- The Biological Effects of Weak Electromagnetic Fields: Problems and Solutions Professor Andrew Goldsworthy: http://www.cellphonetaskforce.org/wp-content/uploads/2012/04/Biol-Effects-EMFs-2012-NZ2.pdf [28];

---

24. http://www.scribd.com/doc/87308119/Guideline-of-the-Austrian-Medical-Association-for-the-diagnosis-and-treatment-of-EMF-related-health-problems-and-illness-

25. http://monographs.iarc.fr/ENG/Monographs/vol102/

26. http://www.national-toxic-encephalopathy-foundation.org/wp-16content/uploads/2012/01/ Biological_and_Health_Effects_of_Microwave_Radio_Frequency_Transmissions.pdf

27. http://www.bemri.org/component/docman/doc_download/78-grigoriev-bioeffects07.html?Itemid=4

28. http://www.cellphonetaskforce.org/wp-content/uploads/2012/04/Biol-Effects-EMFs-2012-NZ2.pdf

- Critique of health assessment in the icnirp guidelines for radiofrequency and microwave radiation (100 khz - 300 ghz) - dr neil Cherry http://www.neilcherry.com/documents/90_m4_EMR_ICNIRP_critique_09-02.pdf

- Electromagnetic Hypersensitivity - Norbert Leitgeb 2009 http://diyhpl.us/~nmz787/biological%20radio%20research/Electromagnetic%20Hypersensitivity.pdf [29];

- PUC Docket 2011—- 262 Friedman on Remand Intervenor DW et al Evidence 11 ElectrohyperSensitivity EHS March 5, 2013 - Contains an alphabetical list of peer-reviewed journal articles and their abstracts that have addressed EHS. http://www.mainecoalitiontostopsmartmeters.org/wp-content/uploads/2013/04/EV11-EHS-List-Revised-4-10-13-PUC-470.pdf [30];

- "When health problems are not the responsibility of a health department, how strange!" A personal blog about interacting with the Victorian Chief Health Officer on the EHS 2013 issue: http://stopsmartmeters.com.au/2013/07/02/when-health-issues-are-not-the-responsibility- of-a-health-department-how-bizarre/ [31];

- Electromagnetic hypersensitivity: fact or fiction? Stephen J. Genuis a, Christopher T. Lipp 2011: http://media.withtank.com/c05550c3be/ehs-genuis.pdf [32];

- What are the symptoms of electromagnetic hypersensitivity? http://www.science20.com/florilegium/what_are_symptoms_electromagnetic_hypersensitivity [33]; http://www.electrosensitivity.org.uk/ [34]; http://www.powerwatch.org.uk/health/sensitivity.asp [35];

- Electromagnetic hypersensitivity: a systematic review of challenge studies: http://www.ncbi.nlm.nih.gov/pubmed/15784787 [36];

- Rea et al., 1991, Journal of Bioelectricity, 10 (1 and 2), 241-256. http://www.aehf.com/articles/em_sensitive.html [37];

29. http://diyhpl.us/~nmz787/biological%20radio%20research/Electromagnetic%20Hypersensitivity.pdf

30. http://www.mainecoalitiontostopsmartmeters.org/wp-content/uploads/2013/04/EV11-EHS-List-Revised-4-10-13-PUC-470.pdf

31. http://stopsmartmeters.com.au/2013/07/02/when-health-issues-are-not-the-responsibility-of-a-health-department-how-bizarre/

32. http://media.withtank.com/c05550c3be/ehs-genuis.pdf

33. http://www.science20.com/florilegium/what_are_symptoms_electromagnetic_hypersensitivity

34. http://www.electrosensitivity.org.uk/

35. http://www.powerwatch.org.uk/health/sensitivity.asp

36. http://www.ncbi.nlm.nih.gov/pubmed/15784787

- The Strength - by Lyn Mclean "EMR and Health" - quarterly science and news report - http://www.emraustralia.com.au/EMR_products_EMR_and_health.html [38];

- The myth of contagion – why viruses (including coronavirus) are not the cause of illness. This is a translation of most of the content of the video titled: "Tom Cowan, MD – The Contagion Myth - Why Viruses (including Coronavirus) are Not the Cause of Disease"; "Tom Cowan, MD – The Contagion Myth – Why Viruses (Including Coronavirus) ARE NOT the Cause of Disease": https://www.bitchute.com/video/cI1YJ2GZ984q/ [39].

- Interview with Dr. Juan José Martinez on SER chain about the pandemic and its "sanitary" measures [December 16, 2020]: https://lbry.tv/@ReVelionenlagranja:e/Entrevista-al-Dr.-Juan-Jos%C3%A9-Martinez-in-the-chain-SER:0 [40].

- Weekly Epidemiological Bulletin of Aragon. Public Health Information for health professionals. ISSN 1988-8406. Week 05/2020 (01/27/2020 to 02/02/2020). Available at: https://www.aragon.es/documents/20127/1650151/BEsA_202005.pdf

- Barbara Michiels, Frans Govaerts, Roy Remmen, Etienne Vermeire, Samuel Coenen. A systematic review of the evidence on the effectiveness and risks of inactivated influenza vaccines in different target groups. (2011). Vaccine. 29. 9159-70.10.1016/j.vaccine.2011.08.008. Chiromas® Technical Sheet. Available at: https://cima.aemps.es/cima/pdfs/es/ft/63566/FT_63566.pdf [41].

- Chiroflu® Technical Sheet. Available at: https://cima.aemps.es/cima/pdfs/es/ft/62792/FT_62792.pdf

- Rebecca Helson. Adjuvants: introduction. Translation: Jesús Gil, Würzburg, DE (SEI). Available at: http://inmunologia.eu/vacunas-y-terapias/adyuvantes-introduccion

- Acofarma Technical Information Sheets: TWEEN. Available at: https://www.sefh.es/fichadjuntos/TWEEN80.pdf

- Torisel® Technical Sheet. Available at: https://cima.aemps.es/cima/pdfs/es/ft/07424001/FT_07424001.pdf

- Trangorex® Technical Sheet. Available at: https://cima.aemps.es/cima/pdfs/es/ft/54723/

---

37. http://www.aehf.com/articles/em_sensitive.html

38. http://www.emraustralia.com.au/EMR_products_EMR_and_health.html

39. https://www.bitchute.com/video/cI1YJ2GZ984q/

40. https://lbry.tv/@ReVelionenlagranja:e/Entrevista-al-Dr.-Juan-Jos%C3%A9-Martinez-en-la-cadena-SER:0

41. https://cima.aemps.es/cima/pdfs/es/ft/63566/FT_63566.pdf

54723_ft.pdf

- Technical Data Sheet for Pandemrix® (canceled medication) with its composition, which included Polysorbate 80. Available at: https://www.ema.europa.eu/en/documents/productinformation/pandemrix-epar-product-information_es.pdf

- Gardasil® Technical Sheet. Available at: https://cima.aemps.es/cima/pdfs/es/ft/1151007002/FT_1151007002.pdf

- Prevenar® Technical Sheet. Available at: https://cima.aemps.es/cima/pdfs/ft/09590002/FT_09590002.pdf

- AEMPS Pandemic Vaccine Pharmacovigilance Plan. Available at: https://www.aemps.gob.es/vigilancia/medicamentosUsoHumano/docs/planVacunasPandemicas_gripeA_H1N1.pdf

- Informative Note from the AEMPS on the Pandemrix® flu vaccine and narcolepsy. Available at: https://www.aemps.gob.es/en/informa/notasInformativas/medicamentosUsoHumano/seguro/2011/docs/NI-MUH_05-2011.pdf[42]

- Information about COVID-19. Spanish Society of Immunology. Available at: https://www.inmunologia.org/Upload/Documents/1/5/2/1521.pdf

- Aloysius MM, Thatti A, Gupta A, Sharma N, Bansal P, Goyal H. COVID-19 presenting as acute pancreatitis [published online ahead of print, 2020 May 8]. Pancreatology. 2020; S1424-3903(20)30154-X. doi:10.1016/j.pan.2020.05.003. Available at: https://www.ncbi.nlm.nih.gov/pmc/articles/PMC7207100/pdf/main.pdf

- NASA project, 'Future Strategy for War, 2025': https://www.nogeoingegneria.com/effetti/politicaeconomia/2025-the-future-of-war-guerra-futura-dennis-bushnell-nasa/ [43].

- RTVE. Coronavirus world map. Available at: https://www.rtve.es/noticias/20200614/mapa-mundial-del-coronavirus/1998143.shtml

- Infobae: https://www.infobae.com/america/america-latina/2020/02/28/brasil-adelanto-sucampana-de-vacunacion-contra-la-gripe-por-el-coronavirus/

- Infobae: https://www.infobae.com/america/america-latina/2020/06/10/brasil-reporto-1300-nuevas-muertes-por-coronavirus-y-el-total-roza-las-40000/ 7[44]

Other sources: https://elordenmundial.com/mapas/vacunacion-gripe-en-europa/ [45]; https://www.vaktsineeri.ee/et/taiskasvanutele-vaktsineermine [46]; https://www.heraldo.es/noticias/

---

42. https://www.aemps.gob.es/en/informa/notasInformativas/medicamentosUsoHumano/seguridad/2011/docs/NI-MUH_05-2011.pdf

43. https://www.nogeoingegneria.com/effetti/politicaeconomia/2025-the-future-of-war-guerra-futura-dennis-bushnell-nasa/

44. https://www.infobae.com/america/america-latina/2020/06/10/brasil-reporto-1300-nuevas-muertes-por-coronavirus-y-el-total-roza-las-40000/7

45. https://elordenmundial.com/mapas/vacunacion-gripe-en-europa/

aragon/2020/06/11/aragon-coronavirus-un-total-de-19-residencias-mantienen-casos-de-la-covid-19-en-aragon- 1379967.html[47]

- Weekly Epidemiological Bulletin of Aragon. Public Health Information for health professionals. ISSN 1988-8406. Week 23/2020 (06/01/2020 to 06/07/2020). Available at: https://www.aragon.es/documents/20127/1650151/BOLETIN+ARAGON+232020.pdf/dd19a8fb-e356-036c-9783-086957d6d3bf?t=1591876677118

- Transgenic Covid19 vaccines. Dr Chinda Brandolino explains the risks in 2 minutes. More info at: https://elinvestigador.org/vacunas-covid19-transgenicas-transhumanismo/ [48]or https://lbry.tv/@elinvestigador:0/dra-chinda-brandolino-vacuna-covic19:9?r=3ycuYZfwSuFCGAUCahXKcuZ1zj32oAgT

- Back side N°96 - The vaccine seeks to sterilize the population. Pentagon/DOD leak for a FUNVAX vaccine against "religious fundamentalism".[April 13, 2005]: https://youtu.be/Q0hnIdymFjw [49].

- If first the nanochip and then 5G are established on a global scale, the result is the same, both things work together: nanotechnology and biosensors in vaccines: https://cienciaysaludnatural.com/nanotecnologia-y-biosensores-en-vacunas/

- Nanotechnology and biosensors in Vaccines. Transgenic vaccine, dr. Luis marcelo martínez [former president of the argentine society of medical genetics], chilean/argentine symposium. United for Truth... Chilean/Argentine Medical Symposium. Not to be missed: https://www.bitchute.com/video/9Y0o3SvznJ2J/

- Ginés González García [Minister of Health of Argentina]: "It is very likely that the COVID-19 vaccine will be incorporated into the mandatory schedule in 2022" [December 3, 2020]. In an exclusive interview, the Minister of Health assured that Anmat [National Administration of Medicines, Food and Medical Technology] "is willing to approve the emergency use of any of the candidates who are currently in the final stretch of the race": https://www.infobae.com/salud/2020/...id-19-se-incorpore-al-calendario-obligatorio/

- International control network over the internet, created by Bill Gates to attack information leaks: https://www.libremercado.com/2021-03-02/bill-gates-ministerio- Verdad-microsoft-

46. https://www.vaktsineeri.ee/et/taiskasvanutele-vaktsineermine

47. https://www.heraldo.es/noticias/aragon/2020/06/11/aragon-coronavirus-un-total-de-19-residencias-mantienen-casos-de-la-covid-19-en-aragon-1379967.html

48. https://elinvestigador.org/vacunas-covid19-transgenicas-transhumanismo/

49. https://youtu.be/Q0hnIdymFjw

internet-verificadores-fake-[50]news-6714523/[51].

- In another journalistic report, in this case from the program 60 Minutes, on the North American Television Network CBS, in 1979: https://www.bitchute.com/video/MdHDrrJdpbrd/

- Serious irregularities in the results of the Pfizer vaccine. Video: PCR tests fail seriously: https://cienciaysaludnatural.com/estudios-demuestran- Porque-fallan-los-test-pcr/[52]

- See more: https://cienciaysaludnatural.com/estudios-demuestran- Porque-fallan-los-test-pcr/[53]

- Vaccine side effects: https://cienciaysaludnatural.com/las-vacunas-contra-covid19-Vamos-Emporar-la-enfermedad-tras-la-exposition-al-coronavirus/[54]

- Dangers of the vaccine against covid-19: https://cienciaysaludnatural.com/ley-de-vacuna-contra-el-covid-19-obligatoria-articulos-y-peligros/ [55]and https://cienciaysaludnatural.com/vacuna -against-coronavirus-and-fertility-problems/[56]

- Dr. Luis Marcelo Martinez private meeting with some Argentine senators - Dangers of the COVID-19 Vaccine: https://www.bitchute.com/video/rJDqThtSRJtR/

- Presentation by María José Martínez Albarracín. Physician and surgeon, specialist in diagnostic processes. On the occasion of last weekend's debate in the Basque Country, Dr. Albarracín will talk to us about issues related to vaccines and PCR: https://scabelum.tv/videos/entrevista-con-maria-jose-albarracin/

- Pfizer, the effects will be seen after vaccination. Biologist Fernando López Mirones talks about a Pfizer document: https://superocho.org/watch/tIWzJavrAxGxcLw

- Dr. León is head of the ICU at the Papa Francisco hospital. [from the capital city of the province of Salta, Argentina]. He commented on Via La Mañana TV that hospital professionals were consulted about receiving the COVID 19 vaccine, and many refused. In the therapy area, only 10% agreed to receive the vaccine. What León suggests is that there is a lack of scientific

---

50. https://www.libremercado.com/2021-03-02/bill-gates-ministerio-verdad-microsoft-internet-verificadores-fake-news-6714523/

51. https://www.libremercado.com/2021-03-02/bill-gates-ministerio-verdad-microsoft-internet-verificadores-fake-news-6714523/

52. https://cienciaysaludnatural.com/estudios-demuestran-porque-fallan-los-test-pcr/

53. https://cienciaysaludnatural.com/estudios-demuestran-porque-fallan-los-test-pcr/

54. https://cienciaysaludnatural.com/las-vacunas-contra-covid19-pueden-empeorar-la-enfermedad-tras-la-exposicion-al-coronavirus/

55. https://cienciaysaludnatural.com/ley-de-vacuna-contra-el-covid-19-obligatoria-articulos-y-peligros/

56. https://cienciaysaludnatural.com/vacuna-contra-el-coronavirus-y-problemas-de-fertilidad/

information , "there is a lot of journalistic information." In the coming weeks, more data will be known about phase 3 and it is likely that after that health professionals will agree to be vaccinated. Source: Journalist Cecilia Batista: https://canal7salta.com/2020/12/31/salta-el-jefe-del-uti-del-hospital-papa-francisco-asegura-que-muchos-profesionales-del-hospital- they-refuse-to-receive-the-vaccine/[57]

- High quality documentary, subtitled in Spanish by CounterPropaganda and edited by https://elinvestigador.org

- More info at: https://elinvestigador.org/beneficiarios-del-miedo/ [58]and https://lbry.tv/@elinvestigador:0/Beneficiarios-del-Miedo-Subtitulado-espanol:3

- current concentration camps: https://loveotv.com/watch/los-campos-de-concentraci%C3%B3n-se-extienden-por-todo-el-mundo-reacciona-ya_Tcq64SkIP8N953s.html

- Paraguay Alert - Interview with Geneticist Dr Luis Marcelo Martinez: https://lbry.tv/2020-12-22_Alerta-P...ética-(Fundación-Favaloro)_2473537576282440:c

- Covid fatality rate according to the who: https://www.who.int/bulletin/volumes/99/1/20-265892-ab/es/

- Electromagnetic hypersensitivity syndrome, preliminary study from Spain: https://www.emf-portal.org/en/article/13498

- darpa implants chips in soldiers' brains: https://www.prisonplanet.com/darpa-is-implanting-chips-in-soldiers-brains-according-to-this-new-book.html

- Banker Ronald Bertand exposes the Illuminati: https://newspunch.com/dutch-banker-illuminati-dead/

- 1170 deaths after covid vaccine: https://ejercitoremanente.com/2021/02/14/cdc-1170-muertos-despues-de-inyecciones-de-covid-casi-el-doble-de-muertes-que-las- found-in-vaers/[59]

- Manipulation of climate and people: https://grain.org/es/article/1252

- Jail sentences for deniers: https://www.larazon.es/salud/20210208/35px5bavurgcflq4a7zndw7u44.html

---

57. https://canal7salta.com/2020/12/31/salta-el-jefe-del-uti-del-hospital-papa-francisco-asegura-que-muchos-profesionales-del-hospital-se-niegan-a-recibir-la-vacuna/

58. https://elinvestigador.org/beneficiarios-del-miedo/

59. https://ejercitoremanente.com/2021/02/14/cdc-1170-muertos-despues-de-inyecciones-de-covid-casi-el-doble-de-muertes-que-las-encontradas-en-vaers/

- Bill Gates' vaccine against "religious fanatics": https://www.youtube.com/watch?v=xptxL6xzhRc&feature=youtu.be

- Agenda 21 explained: https://rumble.com/vc1i5s-agenda-21-explained-un-plan-since-1992.html

- There is not even a microphotograph of HIV: https://www.dsalud.com/reportaje/nadie-ha-fotografiado-el-vih-supuesto-virus-del-sida/

- CDC gave cancer via polio vaccine: https://breaking-news.ca/cdc-admits-98-million-americans-were-given-cancer-virus-via-the-polio-shot/

- CIA facilities for mind control studies: https://www.politico.eu/article/the-secret-history-of-fort-detrick-the-cias-base-for-mind-control-experiments/

- Bill Gates against the Kennedy family (anti-vaccine): http://rumormillnews.com/cgi-bin/forum.cgi?read=143670

- Bill Gates appears to have bought the CDC: https://www.armstrongeconomics.com/world-news/corruption/did-bill-gates-buy-the-cdc/?__cf_chl_jschl_tk__=80afe5929e351147bf86da7298e6e59c451a34ce-1614817354-0-Af-aFxkRDA0jH JMb46wO_Yxe5Z4iz7Rta4tST -jHtZJG_0WbLRcdg_OJAFWChY7bDSuOoCnPr2O8 [60]-R-_pxDHxBeKI6Ey8MUHeYJBJUhux8fjMVv4bQzne_rHf_jmmBR64bw7Ii8dmimiBRCWiqnJ_YvhyszS0V4gb21NIkl8rtG9bGYi84gnj4LLyMO BhgvkWTClTWUbcWax_dw408KTl7YAzOjCI0JkSVAic74xJ2Mhn8TfQTsAMoyANbC8XyGMUdq6vs79OgvY6-3M96rfa5XLgbBPyWLxO3PX55AlGOf6PS1r17v8lSsOGU7gIFKcGNqRDDBw9C6rnw5kvHEtpj-w[61]

---

60. https://www.armstrongeconomics.com/world-news/corruption/did-bill-gates-buy-the-cdc/?__cf_chl_jschl_tk__=80afe5929e351147bf86da7298e6e59c451a34ce-1614817354-0-Af-aFxkRDA0jHJMb46wO_Yxe5Z4iz7Rta4tST-jHtZJG_0WbLRcdg_OJAFWChY7bDSuOoCnPr2O8-R-_pxDHxBeKI6Ey8MUHeYJBJUhux8fjMVv4bQzne_rHf_jmmBR64bw7Ii8dmimiBRCWiqnJ_YvhyszS0V24YnoapS036q1PIg9_6lXM6DB1IpVC0hTQsd-4gb21NIkl8rtG9bGYi84gnj4LLyMOBhgvkWTClTWUbcWax_dw408KTl7YAzOjCI0JkSVAic74xJ2Mhn8TfQTsAMoyANbC8XyGMUdq6vs3plRwoYU6ngyaaVPuh7mryNJFkiWxkkhFGyNqiR1P1XU62L5xYb4xGWwcJYdYAGWpp72L79OgvY6-3M96rfa5XLgbBPyWLxO3PX55AlGOf6PS1r17v8lSsOGU7gIFKcGNqRDDBw9C6rnw5kvHEtpj-w

61. https://www.armstrongeconomics.com/world-news/corruption/did-bill-gates-buy-the-

- The CDC would have inflated the figures by up to 1700%: https://tierrapura.org/2021/02/01/el-cdc-habria-inflado-las-cifras-de-covid-hasta-en-un-1600- and-he-is-accused-of-violating-federal-law/[62]

- Former MI6 chief says coronavirus came from Wuhan lab: https://www.youtube.com/watch?v=TGb5inkSkok

- Bill Gates Mass Vaccination Agenda: https://childrenshealthdefense.org/news/government-corruption/gates-globalist-vaccine-agenda-a-win-win-for-pharma-and-mandatory-vaccination/

- Independent review of data from the Israeli Ministry of Health indicates that the Pfizer vaccine killed 40 times more elderly people than Covid: https://www.mentealternativa.com/revision-independiente-de-datos-del-ministerio-de-sanidad-israeli   -indicates-that-the-pfizer-vaccine-killed-40-times-more-elders-than-covid/[63]

- The international medical council of vaccination speaks out harshly against vaccines: https://www.dsalud.com/noticias/el-international-medical-council-on-vaccination-se-pronuncia-muy-duramente-contra-las-vacunas

- Matthew Ehret: Big Pharma Beware: Dr. Montagnier Shines New Light on COVID-19 and The Future of Medicine: https://canadianpatriot.org/2021/02/22/big-pharma-beware-dr-montagnier-shines-new   -light-on-covid-19-and-the-future-of-medicine-2/ [64]. Version translated into Spanish by Mente Alternativa: https://www.mentealternativa.com/covid-19-por-que-el-consejo-atlantico-tilda-de-difusor-de-teorias-conspirativas-al-virologo-y-   nobel-prize-dr-luc-montagnier/ [65].

---

cdc/?__cf_chl_jschl_tk__=80afe5929e351147bf86da7298e6e59c451a34ce-1614817354-0-Af-aFxkRDA0jHJMb46wO_Yxe5Z4iz7Rta4tST-

jHtZJG_0WbLRcdg_OJAFWChY7bDSuOoCnPr2O8-R-

_pxDHxBeKI6Ey8MUHeYJBJUhux8fjMVv4bQzne_rHf_jmmBR64bw7Ii8dmimiBRCWiqnJ_YvhyszS0V24YnoapS036q1PIg9_6lXM6DB1IpVC

0hTQsd-

4gb21NIkl8rtG9bGYi84gnj4LLyMOBhgvkWTClTWUbcWax_dw408KTl7YAzOjCI0JkSVAic74xJ2Mhn8TfQTsAMoyANbC8XyGMUdq6vs3p

lRwoYU6ngyaaVPuh7mryNJFkiWxkkhFGyNqiR1P1XU62L5xYb4xGWwcJYdYAGWpp72L79OgvY6-

3M96rfa5XLgbBPyWLxO3PX55AlGOf6PS1r17v8lSsOGU7gIFKcGNqRDDBw9C6rnw5kvHEtpj-w

62. https://tierrapura.org/2021/02/01/el-cdc-habria-inflado-las-cifras-de-covid-hasta-en-un-1600-y-esta-acusado-de-violar-la-ley-federal/

63. https://www.mentealternativa.com/revision-independiente-de-datos-del-ministerio-de-sanidad-israeli-indica-que-la-vacuna-pfizer-mato-40-veces-mas-ancianos-que-el-covid/

64. https://canadianpatriot.org/2021/02/22/big-pharma-beware-dr-montagnier-shines-new-light-on-covid-19-and-the-future-of-medicine-2/

- La Contra / La Vanguardia: Interview with Richard John Roberts; December 31, 2007; in Pajama Surf: https://pijamasurf.com/2011/02/premio-nobel-de-medicina-farmaceuticas-blockan-farmacos-que-curan- Porque-no-son-rentables [66]/ .

- Alternate Mind: Creator of Quantum Genetics Says What Covid Really Is and Dies Nominated for Nobel in 'The Most Crucial and Precarious Moment in the History of Medicine': https://www.mentealternativa.com/creador-de- quantum-genetics-says-what-covid-really-is-and-nobel-nominee-dies-at-the-most-crucial-and-precarious-moment-in-history- Of medicine/[67]

- Peter P. Garyaev. / Institute of Linguistics of Wave Genetics: LET'S TRY SOMETHING TO DO WITH CORONAVIRUS IN ANOTHER. Until it's not too late: https://wavegenetics.org/en/chto-delat-s-koronavirusom [68]; Version translated into Spanish, in Mente Alternativa: https://www.mentealternativa.com/el-covid-19-como-arma-bioenergetica-y-la-vacuna-cuantica-del-dr-gariaev/

- Israel's Parliament is sued for violating the Numerberg Codes by pressuring the population to accept a vaccine that has not been proven safe: https://israel-news.co.il/archives/24845 [69].

- British study confirms dangers of the covid vaccine: https://www.thegatewaypundit.com/2021/03/british-government-study-confirms-covid-19-vaccine-risk-infections-increase-fortnight-jab/?ff_source= Twitter&ff_campaign=websitesharingbuttons[70]

- Australia abandons vaccine project: https://www.mentealternativa.com/si-la-vacuna-contiene-fragmentos-de-vih-y-mas-australia-abandona-su-proyecto/

- Studies show how and why PCR tests fail and many cases are false positives, the media scares with the number of cases but the deaths are equivalent to previous years. References:

---

65. https://www.mentealternativa.com/covid-19-por-que-el-consejo-atlantico-tilda-de-difusor-de-teorias-conspirativas-al-virologo-y-premio-nobel-dr-luc-montagnier/

66. https://pijamasurf.com/2011/02/premio-nobel-de-medicina-farmaceuticas-bloquean-farmacos-que-curan-porque-no-son-rentables/

67. https://www.mentealternativa.com/creador-de-la-genetica-cuantica-dice-lo-que-realmente-es-el-covid-y-muere-nominado-al-nobel-en-el-momento-mas-crucial-y-precario-de-la-historia-de-la-medicina/

68. https://wavegenetics.org/en/chto-delat-s-koronavirusom

69. https://israel-news.co.il/archives/24845

70. https://www.thegatewaypundit.com/2021/03/british-government-study-confirms-covid-19-vaccine-risk-infections-increase-fortnight-jab/?ff_source=Twitter&ff_campaign=websitesharingbuttons

- 1. Huisman W, Martina BE, Rimmelzwaan GF, Gruters RA, Osterhaus AD. Vaccine-induced enhancement of viral infections. Vaccine. 2009; 27: 505- 512.Crossref CAS PubMed Web of Science°Google Scholar

- 2. Boyoglu-Barnum S, Chirkova T, Anderson LJ. Biology of infection and disease pathogenesis to guide RSV vaccine development. Front Immunol. 2019; 10: 1675.Crossref CAS PubMed Web of Science°Google Scholar

- 3. Chen WH, Hotez PJ, Bottazzi ME. Potential for developing a SARS-CoV receptor-binding domain (RBD) recombinant protein as a heterologous human vaccine against coronavirus infectious disease (COVID)-19. Human Vacc Immunother. 2020; 16: 1239- 1242.Crossref CAS PubMed Web of Science°Google Scholar

- 4. Jiang S, He Y, Liu S. SARS vaccine development. Emerg Infect Dis. 2005; 11: 1016- 1020.Crossref CAS PubMed Web of Science°Google Scholar

- 5. Tseng CT, Sbrana E, Iwata-Yoshikawa N, et al. Immunization with SARS coronavirus vaccines leads to pulmonary immunopathology on challenge with the SARS virus. PLoS One. 2012; 7:e35421.Crossref CAS PubMed Web of Science°Google Scholar

- 6. Wang Q, Zhang L, Kuwahara K, et al. Immunodominant SARS coronavirus epitopes in humans elicited both enhancing and neutralizing effects on infection in non-human primates. ACS Infect Dis. 2016; 2: 361- 376.Crossref CAS PubMed Web of Science°Google Scholar

- 7. Yang JK, Lin SS, Ji XJ, Guo LM. Binding of SARS coronavirus to its receptor damages islets and causes acute diabetes. Diabetol Act. 2010; 47: 193- 199.Crossref CAS PubMed Web of Science°Google Scholar

- 8 . Liu L, Wei Q, Lin Q, et al. Anti-spike IgG causes severe acute lung injury by skewing macrophage responses during acute SARS-CoV infection. JCI insight. 2019; 4:e123158.Crossref PubMed Web of Science°Google Scholar

- 9. Liu ZL, Liu Y, Wan LG, et al. Antibody profiles in mild and severe cases of COVID-19. Clin Chem. 2020; 66: 1102– 1104.Crossref PubMed Web of Science°Google Scholar

- 10. Piccoli L, Park YJ, Tortorici MA, et al. Mapping neutralizing and immunodominant sites on the SARS-CoV-2 spike receptor-binding domain by structure-guided high-resolution serology. Cell. 2020; S0092-8674: 31234-4Google Scholar

- 11. Robbiani DF, Gaebler C, Muecksch F, et al. Convergent antibody responses to SARS-CoV-2 infection in convalescent individuals. bioRxiv. 2020.Google Scholar

- 12. Yong CY, Ong HK, Yeap SK, Ho KL, Tan WS. Recent advances in the vaccine development against middle east respiratory syndrome-coronavirus. Front Microbiol. 2019; 10: 1781.Crossref PubMed Web of Science°Google Scholar

- 13. Corbett KS, Flynn B, Foulds KE, et al. Evaluation of the mRNA-1273 Vaccine against SARS-CoV-2 in Nonhuman Primates. N Engl J Med. 2020; 383: 1544– 1555.Crossref CAS PubMed Web of Science°Google Scholar

- 14. Mulligan MJ, Lyke KE, Kitchin N, et al. Phase 1/2 study of COVID-19 RNA vaccine BNT162b1 in adults. Nature. 2020; 586: 589– 593.Crossref CAS PubMed Web of Science°Google Scholar

- 15. Becerra-Flores M, Cardozo T. SARS-CoV-2 viral spike G614 mutation exhibits higher case fatality rate. Int J Clin Pract. 2020; 74:e13525.Wiley Online Library CAS PubMed Web of Science°Google Scholar

• 16. Korber B, Fischer WM, Gnanakaran S, et al. Tracking changes in SARS-CoV-2 spike: evidence that D614G increases infectivity of the COVID-19 virus. Cell. 2020; 182: 812- 827.e819.Crossref CAS PubMed Web of Science°Google Scholar

• 17. Mansbach RA, Chakraborty S, Nguyen K, Montefiori D, Korber B, Gnanakaran S. The SARS-CoV-2 spike variant D614G favors an open conformational state. bioRxiv. 2020.PubMed Google Scholar

• 18. Zhang L, Jackson C, Mou H, et al. The D614G mutation in the SARS-CoV-2 spike protein reduces S1 shedding and increases infectivity. bioRxiv. 2020.Google Scholar

• 19. Wendler D. What should be disclosed to research participants? Am J Bioeth. 2013; 13: 3- 8.Crossref PubMed Web of Science°Google Scholar

• 20. McNamara D. Three Major COVID Vaccine Developers Release Detailed Trial Protocols. https://wwwmedscapecom/viewarticle/937845 ; 2020.Google Scholar.

<< Let no one deceive you in any way; because it will not come unless the apostasy first comes, and the man of sin is revealed, the son of perdition, who opposes and exalts himself against everything that is called God or is an object of worship; so much so that he sits in the temple of God as God, showing himself to be God... And now you know what holds him back, so that he may be revealed in due time. Because the mystery of iniquity is already at work; Only there is someone who currently stops him, until he in turn is taken out of the way. And then that wicked one will be revealed, whom the Lord will kill with the spirit of his mouth, and destroy with the brightness of his coming; wicked one whose coming is by the work of Satan, with great power and signs and lying wonders, and with all deception of wickedness for those who are perishing, because they did not receive the love of the truth to be saved. For this reason God sends them a deceptive power, so that they believe the lie, so that all those who did not believe the truth, but took pleasure in unrighteousness, may be condemned. >>

(2nd Letter of the Apostle Paul to the Thessalonians, chapter 2:1-12,

New Testament, The Bible)

[]

Don't miss out!

Visit the website below and you can sign up to receive emails whenever Frederick Guttmann publishes a new book. There's no charge and no obligation.

https://books2read.com/r/B-A-DKUGB-RJCBD

BOOKS 2 READ

Connecting independent readers to independent writers.

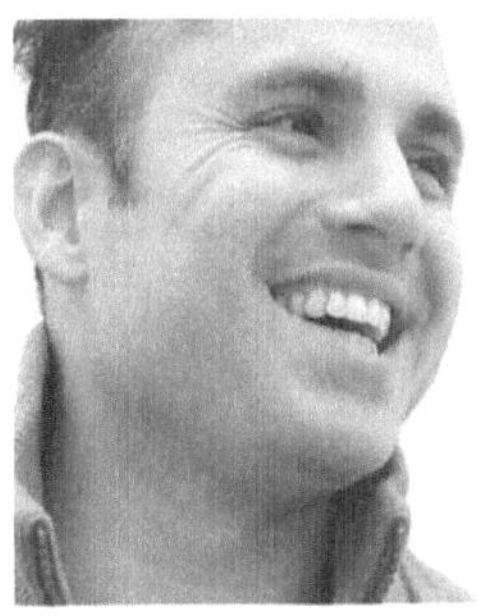

About the Author

Israeli writer, researcher, disseminator, documentary filmmaker and influencer. He is the writer of more than 35 books, mostly research and dissemination theses.

Read more at https://www.frederickguttmann.com.